George A. Howell III

Breastfeeding Updates for the Pediatrician

Editors

ARDYTHE L. MORROW
CAROLINE J. CHANTRY

PEDIATRIC CLINICS OF NORTH AMERICA

www.pediatric.theclinics.com

February 2013 • Volume 60 • Number 1

ELSEVIER

1600 John F. Kennedy Boulevard • Suite 1800 • Philadelphia, Pennsylvania 19103-2899

http://www.theclinics.com

THE PEDIATRIC CLINICS OF NORTH AMERICA Volume 60, Number 1
February 2013 ISSN 0031-3955, ISBN-13: 978-1-4557-7133-2

Editor: Kerry Holland
Developmental Editor: Donald Mumford

The Pediatric Clinics of North America (ISSN 0031-3955) is published bimonthly by Elsevier Inc., 360 Park Avenue South, New York, NY 10010-1710. Months of issue are February, April, June, August, October, and December. Periodicals postage paid at New York, NY and additional mailing offices. Subscription prices are $191.00 per year (US individuals), $444.00 per year (US institutions), $259.00 per year (Canadian individuals), $591.00 per year (Canadian institutions), $308.00 per year (international individuals), $591.00 per year (international institutions), $93.00 per year (US students and residents), and $159.00 per year (international and Canadian residents and students). To receive students/resident rare, orders must be accompanied by name of affiliated institution, date of term, and the signature of program/residency coordinator on institution letterhead. Orders will be billed at individual rate until proof of status is received. Foreign air speed delivery is included in all *Clinics* subscription prices. All prices are subject to change without notice. **POSTMASTER:** Send address changes to *The Pediatric Clinics of North America*, Elsevier Health Sciences Division, Subscription Customer Service, 3251 Riverport Lane, Maryland Heights, MO 63043. **Customer Service: 1-800-654-2452 (US and Canada). From outside of the US and Canada: 1-314-447-8871. Fax: 1-314-447-8029. For print support, E-mail: JournalsCustomerService-usa@elsevier.com. For online support, E-mail: JournalsOnlineSupport-usa@elsevier.com.**

Reprints. For copies of 100 or more, of articles in this publication, please contact the Commercial Reprints Department, Elsevier Inc., 360 Park Avenue South, New York, NY 10010-1710. Tel.: 212-633-3812; Fax: 212-462-1935; E-mail: reprints@elsevier.com.

The Pediatric Clinics of North America is also published in Spanish by McGraw-Hill Inter-americana Editores S.A., Mexico City, Mexico; in Portuguese by Riechmann and Affonso Editores, Rua Comandante Coelho 1085, CEP 21250, Rio de Janeiro, Brazil; and in Greek by Althayia SA, Athens, Greece.

The Pediatric Clinics of North America is covered in *MEDLINE/PubMed (Index Medicus), Excerpta Medica, Current Contents, Current Contents/Clinical Medicine, Science Citation Index, ASCA, ISI/BIOMED,* and *BIOSIS.*

Printed in the United States of America.

PROGRAM OBJECTIVE:

The goal of the *Pediatric Clinics of North America* is to keep practicing physicians and residents up to date with current clinical practice in pediatrics by providing timely articles reviewing the state-of-the-art in patient care.

TARGET AUDIENCE

All practicing pediatricians, physicians and healthcare professionals who provide patient care to pediatric patients.

ACCREDITATION

The Elsevier Office of Continuing Medical Education (EOCME) is accredited by the Accreditation Council for Continuing Medical Education (ACCME) to provide continuing medical education for physicians.

The EOCME designates this journal-based CME activity for a maximum of 15 *AMA PRA Category 1 Credit*(s)™. Physicians should claim only the credit commensurate with the extent of their participation in the activity.

All other health care professionals completing continuing education credit for this activity will be issued a certificate of participation.

DISCLOSURE OF CONFLICTS OF INTEREST

The EOCME assesses conflict of interest with its instructors, faculty, planners, and other individuals who are in a position to control the content of CME activities. All relevant conflicts of interest that are identified are thoroughly vetted by EOCME for fair balance, scientific objectivity, and patient care recommendations. EOCME is committed to providing its learners with CME activities that promote improvements or quality in healthcare and not a specific proprietary business or a commercial interest.

The planning committee, staff, authors and editors listed below have identified no financial relationships or relationships to products or devices they or their spouse/life partner have with commercial interest related to the content of this CME activity:

Teresa Baker, MD; Olivia Ballard, JD; Harold R. Bigger, MD; Maya Bunik, MD, MSPH; Caroline J. Chantry, MD; Nicole Congleton; Christine M. Dieterich, MS, MD; Janet L. Engstrom, PhD, RN, CNM, WHNP-BC; Lori Feldman-Winter, MD, MPH; Julia P. Felice, BS; Valerie J. Flaherman, MD, MPH; Thomas W. Hale, PhD; Deepali Handa, MBBS; Alison V. Holmes, MD, MPH; Cynthia R. Howard, MD, MPH; Indu Kumari; Miriam H. Labbok, MD, MPH, IBCLC; Robert M. Lawrence, MD; Henry C. Lee, MD, MS; Jill McNair; Marianne Neifert, MD, MTS; Elizabeth O'Sullivan, BA, BS; Aloka L. Patel, MD; Kathleen M. Rasmussen, AB, ScM, ScD, RD; Beverly Rossman, PhD, RN; Hilary Rowe, BSc(Pharm), PharmD, ACPR; Richard J. Schanler, MD; Katelynn Steck; Mark A. Underwood, MD, MAS; Christina J. Valentine, MD, MS, RD; Carol L. Wagner, MD.

The planning committee, staff, authors and editors listed below have identified financial relationships or relationships to products or devices they or their spouse/life partner have with commercial interest related to the content of this CME activity:

Ben T. Hartmann, PhD received travel reimbursement from Medela to be a conference speaker.
Susan Landers, MD is a consultant/advisor for Medela Breastfeeding USA.
Paula P. Meier, PhD, RN is a consultant/advisor for Medela.
Ardythe L. Morrow, PhD, MSc received a research grant from Mead Johnson Nutrition, Inc.

UNAPPROVED / OFF-LABEL USE DISCLOSURE

The EOCME requires CME faculty to disclose to the participants:

1. When products or procedures being discussed are off-label, unlabelled, experimental, and/or investigational (not US Food and Drug Administration (FDA) approved; and
2. Any limitations on the information presented, such as data that are preliminary or that represent ongoing research, interim analyses, and/or unsupported opinions. Faculty may discuss information about pharmaceutical agents that is outside of DA-approved labelling. This information is intended solely for CME and is not intended to promote off-label use of these medications. If you have any questions, contact the medical affairs department of the manufacturer for the most recent prescribing information.

TO ENROLL

To enroll in the *Pediatric Clinics of North America* Continuing Medical Education program, call customer service at 1-800-654-2452 or sign up online at http://www.theclinics.com/home/cme. The CME program is available to subscribers for an additional annual fee of $261 USD.

METHOD OF PARTICIPATION

In order to claim credit, participants must complete the following:

1. Complete enrolment as indicated above.
2. Read the activity.
3. Complete the CME Test and Evaluation. Participants must achieve a score of 70% on the test. All CME Tests and Evaluations must be completed online.

CME INQUIRIES/SPECIAL NEEDS

For all CME inquiries or special needs, please contact elsevierCME@elsevier.com.

Contributors

GUEST EDITORS

ARDYTHE L. MORROW, PhD, MSc
Professor of Pediatrics and Nutrition, Director, Center for Interdisciplinary Research of Human Milk and Lactation, Perinatal Institute, Cincinnati Children's Hospital Medical Center, University of Cincinnati College of Medicine and College of Allied Health Sciences, Cincinnati, Ohio

CAROLINE J. CHANTRY, MD
Professor of Clinical Pediatrics, University of California Davis Medical Center, Sacramento, California

AUTHORS

TERESA BAKER, MD
Associate Professor of Obstetrics and Gynecology, Texas Tech University School of Medicine, Amarillo, Texas

OLIVIA BALLARD, JD, PhD (candidate)
Division of Immunobiology, Center for Interdisciplinary Research in Human Milk and Lactation, Cincinnati Children's Hospital Medical Center, Cincinnati, Ohio

HAROLD R. BIGGER, MD
Assistant Professor, Department of Pediatrics, Section of Neonatology, Rush University Medical Center, Chicago, Illinois

MAYA BUNIK, MD, MSPH
Associate Professor, Children's Outcomes Research, Department of Pediatrics, Children's Hospital Colorado, University of Colorado Denver, Aurora, Colorado

CAROLINE J. CHANTRY, MD
Professor of Clinical Pediatrics, University of California Davis Medical Center, Sacramento, California

CHRISTINE M. DIETERICH, MS, RD
Division of Nutritional Sciences, Cornell University, Ithaca, New York

JANET L. ENGSTROM, PhD, RN, CNM, WHNP-BC
Associate Dean for Research, Frontier Nursing University, Hyden, Kentucky; Professor and Researcher, Department of Women, Children and Family Nursing, Rush University Medical Center, Chicago, Illinois

LORI FELDMAN-WINTER, MD, MPH
Professor of Pediatrics, Cooper Medical School of Rowan University; Division Head, Adolescent Medicine, Children's Regional Hospital at Cooper University Hospital, Camden, New Jersey

JULIA P. FELICE, BS
Division of Nutritional Sciences, Cornell University, Ithaca, New York

VALERIE J. FLAHERMAN, MD, MPH
Assistant Professor of Pediatrics, Department of Pediatrics, University of California San Francisco, San Francisco, California

THOMAS W. HALE, PhD
Professor, Department of Pediatrics, Texas Tech University School of Medicine, Amarillo, Texas

DEEPALI HANDA, MBBS
Fellow, Division of Neonatal-Perinatal Medicine, Cohen Children's Medical Center of New York, New Hyde Park, New York

BEN T. HARTMANN, PhD
Neonatology Clinical Care Unit, Perron Rotary Express Milk Bank, King Edward Memorial Hospital, Subiaco, Western Australia; Centre for Neonatal Research and Education, The University of Western Australia, Perth, Western Australia

ALISON V. HOLMES, MD, MPH, FABM
Assistant Professor of Pediatrics and Community and Family Medicine, Division of Pediatric Hospital Medicine; Associate Director of Pediatric Medical Education, The Geisel School of Medicine at Dartmouth, Hanover, New Hampshire

CYNTHIA R. HOWARD, MD, MPH
Associate Professor of Pediatrics and Community and Preventive Medicine, University of Rochester, Rochester, New York

MIRIAM H. LABBOK, MD, MPH, IBCLC, FACPM, FABM, FILCA
Professor, and Director, Carolina Global Breastfeeding Institute (CGBI); Department of Maternal and Child Health, Gillings School of Global Public Health, University of North Carolina, Chapel Hill, North Carolina

SUSAN LANDERS, MD, FABM
Pediatrix Medical Group, Sunrise, Florida; Neonatologist, Seton Family of Hospitals, Department of Neonatology, Austin, Texas

ROBERT M. LAWRENCE, MD
Clinical Professor, Pediatric Infectious Diseases, Department of Pediatrics, Health Science Center, University of Florida, Gainesville, Florida

HENRY C. LEE, MD, MS
Assistant Professor of Pediatrics, Division of Neonatal and Developmental Medicine, Stanford University School of Medicine, Stanford, California

PAULA P. MEIER, PhD, RN
Director for Clinical Research and Lactation, Neonatal Intensive Care Unit; Professor, Departments of Pediatrics and Women, Children and Family Nursing, Rush University Medical Center, Chicago, Illinois

ARDYTHE L. MORROW, PhD, MSc
Professor of Pediatrics and Nutrition, Director, Center for Interdisciplinary Research of Human Milk and Lactation, Perinatal Institute, Cincinnati Children's Hospital Medical Center, University of Cincinnati College of Medicine and College of Allied Health Sciences, Cincinnati, Ohio

MARIANNE NEIFERT, MD, MTS
Department of Pediatrics, University of Colorado Denver, Aurora, Colorado; Dr. Mom®
Presentations LLC, Parker, Colorado

ELIZABETH O'SULLIVAN, BA, BS
Division of Nutritional Sciences, Cornell University, Ithaca, New York

ALOKA L. PATEL, MD
Associate Professor, Department of Pediatrics, Section of Neonatology, Rush University
Medical Center, Chicago, Illinois

KATHLEEN M. RASMUSSEN, AB, ScM, ScD, RD
Professor, Division of Nutritional Sciences, Cornell University, Ithaca, New York

BEVERLY ROSSMAN, PhD, RN
Research Specialist, Department of Women, Children and Family Nursing, Rush
University Medical Center, Chicago, Illinois

HILARY ROWE, BSc(Pharm), PharmD, ACPR
Clinical Pharmacy Specialist, Maternal Fetal Medicine, Fraser Health, Surrey, British
Columbia, Canada

RICHARD J. SCHANLER, MD
Professor of Pediatrics, Division of Neonatal-Perinatal Medicine, Cohen Children's
Medical Center of New York, New Hyde Park, New York; Hofstra North Shore-LIJ School
of Medicine, Hempstead, New York

MARK A. UNDERWOOD, MD, MAS, FAAP
Associate Professor of Clinical Pediatrics, Department of Pediatrics, University of
California Davis, Sacramento, California

CHRISTINA J. VALENTINE, MD, MS, RD
Assistant Professor, Perinatal Institute, Division of Neonatology, Cincinnati Children's
Hospital Medical Center, Cincinnati, Ohio

CAROL L. WAGNER, MD
Professor, Department of Neonatology, Medical University of South Carolina, Charleston,
South Carolina

Contents

biological norm for infant nutrition. Human milk also contains many hundreds to thousands of distinct bioactive molecules that protect against infection and inflammation and contribute to immune maturation, organ development, and healthy microbial colonization. Some of these molecules (eg, lactoferrin) are being investigated as novel therapeutic agents. Human milk changes in composition from colostrum to late lactation, within feeds, by gestational age, diurnally, and between mothers. Feeding infants with expressed human milk is increasing.

Clinical guidelines are developed to provide clinicians with guidance that enables quality and consistency of practice based on the systematic review of available evidence. An important development over the past 13 years in the clinical management of breastfeeding has been the development of clinical protocols by the Academy of Breastfeeding Medicine (ABM). Here we review the clinical guidelines developed by ABM, the process of protocol development, and their current Internet usage rates. Protocol summaries include the purpose, content, evidence level, and associated research gaps.

Although a large majority of US mothers now begin breastfeeding, exclusive breastfeeding rates fall far below national health objectives, with vulnerable populations being least likely to breastfeed exclusively. This article explores common personal and societal barriers to exclusive breastfeeding and offers evidence-based strategies to support mothers to breastfeed exclusively, such as ensuring prenatal education, supportive maternity practices, timely follow-up, and management of lactation challenges. The article also addresses common reasons nursing mothers discontinue exclusive breastfeeding, including the perception of insufficient milk, misinterpretation of infant crying, returning to work or school, early introduction of solid foods, and lack of support.

The first days after delivery of a newborn infant are critical for breastfeeding establishment. Successful initiation and continuation—especially of exclusive breastfeeding—have become public health priorities, but it is fraught with many individual- and systems-level barriers. In this article, we review how hospital newborn services can be constructed or restructured to support the breastfeeding mother–infant dyad so that they can achieve high levels of breastfeeding success. Important positive and negative factors from the prenatal period, and the preparation for hospital discharge are also discussed.

Considerable progress has been made in the past decade in developing comprehensive support systems to enable more women to reach their

breastfeeding goals. Given that most women in the United States participate in some breastfeeding, it is essential that each of these support systems be rigorously tested and if effective replicated. Additional research is
needed to determine the best methods of support during the preconception period to prepare women to exclusively breastfeed as a cultural norm.

Premature infants are at risk for growth failure, developmental delays, necrotizing enterocolitis, and late-onset sepsis. Human milk from women
delivering prematurely has more protein and higher levels of bioactive molecules. Human milk must be fortified for premature infants to achieve
adequate growth. Mother's own milk improves growth and neurodevelopment, decreases the risk of necrotizing enterocolitis and late-onset sepsis,
and should be the primary enteral diet for premature infants. Donor milk is
a resource for premature infants whose mothers are unable to provide an
adequate supply of milk. Challenges include the need for pasteurization,
nutritional and biochemical deficiencies, and limited supply.

The translation of the evidence for the use of human milk (HM) in the neonatal intensive care unit (NICU) into best practices, toolkits, policies and
procedures, talking points, and parent information packets is limited,
and requires use of evidence-based quality indicators to benchmark the
use of HM, consistent messaging by the entire NICU team about the importance of HM for infants in the NICU, establishing procedures that protect maternal milk supply, and incorporating lactation technologies that
take the guesswork out of HM feedings and facilitate milk transfer during
breastfeeding.

This article provides the pediatric community with a practical overview of
milk expression and an update on the recent literature. Approaches for
working mothers, preterm infants, critically ill infants, and mothers before
lactogenesis II are presented separately, as these groups may benefit from
practices tailored to individual needs.

Donor human milk has emerged as the preferred substrate to feed
extremely preterm infants, when mother's own milk is unavailable. This
article summarizes the clinical data demonstrating the safety, efficacy,
and cost-effectiveness of feeding donor human milk to premature babies.
It describes the current state of milk banking in North America, as well as

other parts of the world, and the differing criteria for donor selection, current pasteurization techniques, and quality control measures. A risk assessment methodology is proposed, which would allow milk banks globally to assess the safety of their process and respond appropriately to differing risk environments.

Milk is successfully produced by mothers regardless of their nutritional status. Nevertheless, the concentrations of some nutrients, specifically vitamins A, D, B1, B2, B3, B6, and B12, fatty acids, and iodine, in human milk depend on or are influenced by maternal diet. A healthy and varied diet during lactation ensures adequate maternal nutrition and optimal concentration of some nutrients in human milk. Exclusive breastfeeding meets the nutritional needs of infants for 6 months of life with the exception of vitamins D and K, which should be given to breastfed infants as supplements.

This article reviews the necessary skills required for clinicians to make informed decisions about the use of medications in women who are breastfeeding. Even without specific data on certain medications, this review of kinetic principles, mechanisms of medication entry into breast milk, and important infant factors can aid in clinical decision making. In addition, common medical conditions and suitable treatments of depression, hypertension, infections and so forth for women who are breastfeeding are also reviewed.

This article reviews risks of illness or exposures to breastfed infants. Galactosemia in an infant is a contraindication to breastfeeding. There are no medical conditions in the mother that are contraindications, although diagnostic procedures, treatment, or illness can interfere. Restrictive diets or malnutrition are not contraindications but are opportunities to provide nutritional counseling. Environmental toxic exposures within the United States are uncommon; breastfeeding is not usually contraindicated. In any concerning situation, an assessment and discussion of risks and benefits for the mother-infant dyad (breastfed or formula fed) is indicated. Coordinated medical care and lactation assistance can facilitate successful breastfeeding.

PEDIATRIC CLINICS OF NORTH AMERICA

RELATED INTEREST

Gastroenterology Clinics of North America December 2012 (Volume 41:4)
Clinical Applications of Probiotics in Gastroenterology: Questions and Answers
Gerald Friedman, MD, PhD, MS, FACP, MACG, AGAF, *Guest Editor*
http://www.gastro.theclinics.com/issues?issue_key=S0889-8553(11)X0009-2

NOW AVAILABLE FOR YOUR iPhone and iPad

Preface

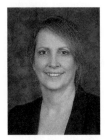 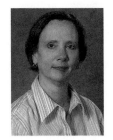

Ardythe L. Morrow, PhD, MSc   Caroline J. Chantry, MD
Guest Editors

In the 12 years since *Pediatric Clinics of North America* last addressed the topic of breastfeeding, the percentage of women who initiated breastfeeding climbed nearly 1% per year and is now approaching 80% of the U.S. population. This is a historic high and something to celebrate! The evidence is clear that not breastfeeding increases the risk of infant and maternal diseases, and research on the biology of human milk demonstrates its unique match to the developmental needs of the infant. Public health programs and data systems have been greatly strengthened to support optimal infant feeding. Hospitals are shifting toward breastfeeding and away from unnecessary formula feeding, encouraged by changing norms and accreditation standards. Human milk banks have been increasing in North America to provide pasteurized, donor human milk for high-risk infants. North American culture appears to be incrementally shifting toward breastfeeding as the norm for infant feeding.

Tempering this enthusiasm for our progress over the past 10 to 12 years is recognition that breastfeeding rates remain suboptimal. Exclusive breastfeeding rates are low; only about one-third of mothers breastfeed to 1 year, and <60% of African American mothers initiate breastfeeding. The toll on health and society is real. Suboptimal breastfeeding in the United States results in more than 900 deaths per year and costs the economy about $13 billion per year.[1] Most women are convinced to begin breastfeeding, but too many women struggle and fail to meet their own goals for breastfeeding. There remain real threats and continuing barriers to breastfeeding, including lack of maternity leave, inconsistent messages, and lack of knowledgeable, accessible support for breastfeeding by trained health care professionals. And, while breastfeeding has been increasing, so has the expression and storage of breast milk, so that "breastfeeding" is often sustained by feeding the infant mother's milk by bottle. The evidence base has not caught up to practice: What are the consequences to the infant of routinely feeding human milk by bottle versus feeding at the breast of his own mother? What are the consequences of Internet-based milk sharing that has arisen in this era?

Thus, the pediatrician's role in support of breastfeeding is more important than ever. The lead article of this issue cogently argues that pediatricians should provide effective support and management of breastfeeding and should be knowledgeable advocates

Pediatr Clin N Am 60 (2013) xv–xvii
http://dx.doi.org/10.1016/j.pcl.2012.10.011
0031-3955/13/$ – see front matter © 2013 Published by Elsevier Inc.

pediatric.theclinics.com

for breastfeeding, the position of the American Academy of Pediatrics.[2] In this issue, 14 articles from experts across North America address topics that may help pediatricians and other child health professionals in their critical role. Articles address the evidence regarding the risk of not breastfeeding and benefits of breastfeeding, evidence-based approaches to clinical management of breastfeeding, the impact of public health policy, and the promotion and support of breastfeeding from a health system and community-wide view. A major advance has been the development of evidence-based protocols by the Academy of Breastfeeding Medicine, addressing many specific circumstances, which we are pleased to introduce in this issue. Other clinically relevant topics include how to establish successful breastfeeding in the newborn period, and how to remove clinical barriers to exclusive breastfeeding. Guidance is provided regarding nutrition for the breastfeeding dyad and breastfeeding when the mother is taking medications or recreational drugs. Also addressed are methods of expressing human milk, which is of interest to mothers in general but is especially important for maximizing early milk supply in mothers of high-risk infants who are not suckling at the breast. Human milk feeding is so critical to the health and survival of high-risk infants that several excellent articles address elements of that topic: Provision of human milk to premature infants, how to optimize breastfeeding in the setting of the neonatal intensive care unit, and developments regarding donor human milk banks. And while breastfeeding is the goal, an expert clarifies the few circumstances when breastfeeding is contraindicated.

We wish to thank Kerry Holland and Elsevier for publishing this much-needed update on breastfeeding, as so much has happened since the last issue. We are especially grateful to our colleagues for contributing their time and expertise. Each article provides a depth of information, and this issue provides a wonderful reference for pediatricians and other child health professionals concerned with mothers and infants. We began this preface with a view to developments over the past 10 to 12 years. But we close with data and perspective from a century ago, which provides a very different perspective on our "progress."

From the article by Dr Davis in 1912 (**Box 1**), we learn that the "high" breastfeeding rates of North America today do not yet represent a return to the higher breastfeeding rates that he reported a century ago, when more than twice as many mothers continued breastfeeding to 1 year of age. In the commentary by Dr Chapin, we see that the breastfeeding issues of that time remain relevant today: "How to secure more breastfeeding" remains our "great problem," and how to best assist mothers in "securing a good secretion of breast milk and maintaining it" remains the heart of the matter. In order to provide effective advocacy and ensure evidence-based clinical support, it is still "a great help to us to have home figures"; indeed, our clinical

---

Box 1

Breastfeeding in North America, 100 years ago

In 1912, William Davis, MD of the Boston Board of Health, published a careful population-based study that documented a 6-fold higher mortality rate in bottle-fed compared to breastfed infants.[3] At that time, breastfeeding was practiced by more than 60% of mothers to 1 year of age. In a commentary following that article, Dr Chapin noted: "We all realize, I think, from these figures, as we have to some extent before, the great advantage of breast feeding. How to secure more breast feeding has been the great problem... We have, in order to assist mothers in this respect, prepared a circular explaining the best way of securing a good secretion of breast milk and maintaining it, and that circular has been used very largely by the nurses in instructing the mothers. But it is certainly a great help to us to have home figures with which to back up our arguments."

evidence base remains lacking, and more quality improvement studies are needed to advance the field. We take as a lesson that the promotion, protection, and support of breastfeeding remains the job of every generation as social and medical circumstances change. The changes of our own era provide us with new opportunities and new challenges. Let us continue the progress made in the past decade that has enabled more mothers to breastfeed. Let us promote an evidence-based culture of breastfeeding. We can be assured that the children and mothers whom we serve will benefit, now and in the future.

Ardythe L. Morrow, PhD, MSc
Center for Interdisciplinary Research of Human Milk and Lactation
Perinatal Institute
Cincinnati Children's Hospital Medical Center
University of Cincinnati College of Medicine and
College of Allied Health Sciences
Cincinnati, OH 45229, USA

Caroline J. Chantry, MD
Ticon II, Suite 334
University of California Davis Medical Center
2516 Stockton Blvd.
Sacramento, CA 95817, USA

E-mail addresses:
Ardythe.Morrow@cchmc.org (A.L. Morrow)
Caroline.Chantry@ucdmc.ucdavis.edu (C.J. Chantry)

REFERENCES

1. Bartick M, Reinhold A. The burden of suboptimal breastfeeding in the United States: A pediatric cost analysis. Pediatrics 2010;125(5):e1048–56.
2. American Academy of Pediatrics, Section on breastfeeding. Breastfeeding and the use of human milk. Pediatrics 2012;129:e827–41.
3. Davis W. Prevention of infant mortality by breast feeding. Am J Public Health 1912; 2:67–71.

Role of the Pediatrician in Breastfeeding Management

Deepali Handa, MBBS[a], Richard J. Schanler, MD[a,b],*

KEYWORDS

- Breastfeeding - Pediatrician - Role - Lactation

KEY POINTS

- The pediatrician champions children's health.
- The encouragement of breastfeeding to families and to the community at large is an important aspect of the pediatrician's profession.
- The pediatrician must be equipped with optimal resources to achieve this goal.

INTRODUCTION

Breastfeeding is beneficial to the health of the maternal–infant dyad; it improves psychosocial interactions, reduces economic burdens, and is valuable to society. The American Academy of Pediatrics (AAP) and the World Health Organization (WHO) strongly endorse breastfeeding. How is breastfeeding supported in the hospital, in the home, and in the community? It is the responsibility of the leader of the health care team, the pediatrician, to understand the importance of breastfeeding, advocate for breastfeeding, and be comfortable in directing its assessment and management, to enable mothers to achieve their breastfeeding goals.

In the 2012 policy statement, "Breastfeeding and the Use of Human Milk" the AAP supports the recommendation of exclusive breastfeeding for about 6 months, followed by continued breastfeeding as complementary foods are introduced, with continuation of breastfeeding for 1 year or longer as mutually desired by mother and infant.[1] The policy statement emphasizes the critical role that pediatricians play in their practices and communities:

To advocate for breastfeeding
To optimize their knowledge about the health risks of not breastfeeding

The authors have nothing to disclose.
[a] Division of Neonatal-Perinatal Medicine, Cohen Children's Medical Center of New York, 269-01 76th Avenue, New Hyde Park, NY 11040, USA; [b] Hofstra North Shore-LIJ School of Medicine, 900 Fulton Avenue, Hempstead, NY 11550, USA
* Corresponding author. Division of Neonatal-Perinatal Medicine, Cohen Children's Medical Center of New York, 269-01 76th Avenue, New Hyde Park, NY 11040.
E-mail address: schanler@nshs.edu

Pediatr Clin N Am 60 (2013) 1–10
http://dx.doi.org/10.1016/j.pcl.2012.10.004
0031-3955/13/$ – see front matter © 2013 Elsevier Inc. All rights reserved.

To promote the economic benefits to society of breastfeeding

To train mothers and health care providers in the management of the breastfeeding dyad

To train health care providers in the support of the breastfeeding dyad

The AAP recommendations for breastfeeding stress that all breastfed newborns be seen by a knowledgeable health care provider at 3 to 5 days of age, which is within 48 to 72 hours after discharge from the hospital. This visit should stress hydration, body weight changes, and elimination patterns; additionally the pediatrician should discuss maternal and/or infant issues and observe a breastfeeding. The pediatrician is the optimal person to promote breastfeeding as the norm for infant feeding. To do so, the physician must be knowledgeable in the principles and management of lactation and breastfeeding, and have developed the skills necessary for assessing the adequacy of breastfeeding. Pediatricians are in the prime position to support lactation education and training for medical students, residents, and postgraduate physicians. As members of their medical staffs, they are in positions to promote hospital policies that are compatible with the AAP and Academy of Breastfeeding Medicine Model Hospital Policy and the WHO/United Nations Children's Fund (UNICEF) "Ten Steps to Successful Breastfeeding."[2,3] In the community, the pediatrician should collaborate with the obstetricians to develop optimal breastfeeding programs and encourage community-based uniform and comprehensive breastfeeding.[1]

NORM

On January 20, 2011, Surgeon General Regina M. Benjamin released "The Surgeon General's Call to Action to Support Breastfeeding," which outlined steps that should be taken to remove obstacles faced by women who want to breastfeed their infants.[4] The call to action states that families, communities, employers, and health care professionals (pediatricians) can improve breastfeeding rates and increase support for breastfeeding by the following actions:

Educate mothers and their families on the importance of breastfeeding

Provide ongoing support to the mothers and their families

Encourage communities to support breastfeeding

Provide and train peer counseling support

Promote breastfeeding in the community organizations and media

Remove commercial barriers to breastfeeding

Adopt evidence-based practices (baby-friendly hospital initiative)

Provide health professional education

Assure access to lactation services

Support the increased availability of banked donor milk

Encourage paid maternity leave

Encourage worksite accommodations for breastfeeding

Allocate more resources for research

Address disparities in breastfeeding

Support the use of surveillance methods to highlight the economic impact of breastfeeding

Support national campaigns to promote breastfeeding

Advocate for enhanced national leadership of breastfeeding

It should be emphasized that national leadership for promotion of breastfeeding is emerging. First Lady Michelle Obama's "Let's Move" campaign begins the obesity prevention initiative by noting that the odds of being overweight are reduced by 30% with breastfeeding for 9 months.

The rates of breastfeeding initiation continue to increase in the United States. This shift is based on the knowledge of breastfeeding as the optimal nutrition for infants. The choice to breastfeed is not merely a lifestyle choice but rather a key health issue and should receive strong endorsement and support. The risks of not breastfeeding should be discussed:

There should be no encouragement of formula feeding as an acceptable alternative to breastfeeding.
Formula feeding interferes with the establishment of maternal milk supply
Formula feeding delays lactogenesis
Formula feeding increases the risk of engorgement
Formula feeding undermines maternal confidence
Formula feeding shortens the duration of exclusive or any breastfeeding
Formula feeding alters infant intestinal flora
Formula feeding affects bioactive factor interactions within the intestine
Formula feeding is associated with increased childhood acute and chronic illnesses

In brief, breastfeeding should be advocated as the norm and not the exception. "The Surgeon General's Call to Action to Support Breastfeeding" outlines steps to promote breastfeeding. Pediatricians can ensure increments in breastfeeding rates by following these guidelines.

SCOPE OF PROBLEM

Breastfeeding statistics are collected via the Centers for Disease Control and Prevention (CDC) National Immunization Survey (http://www.cdc.gov/breastfeeding/). From these data, the CDC produces a yearly Breastfeeding Report Card for the United States that provides national statistics for breastfeeding.[5] In 2011, 74.6% of infants were ever breastfed, and 14.6% of infants were breastfeeding exclusively at 6 months. It should be noted that average rates do not reflect wide disparities in breastfeeding among racial/ethnic groups and by socioeconomic status. The United States may be approaching the targets for The Healthy People 2020 goals for breastfeeding initiation rates, but remains far behind the other targets (http://www.cdc.gov/breastfeeding/policy/hp2010.htm). The Healthy People 2020 target for breastfeeding initiation is approximately 82%, and for exclusive breastfeeding at 6 months, the goal is 26%. By 2020, the goal is to increase births in a baby-friendly center from 2.9% (2007) to 8%, increase worksite lactation support facilities from 25% (2009) to 38%, and reduce formula use in breastfed newborns in the first 48 hours from 24% (2006) to 14%.

The biannual CDC National Survey of Maternity Practices in Infant Nutrition and Care (mPINC) identifies major practices in hospitals and birth centers that warrant changes to more fully support breastfeeding. For example, the 2009 survey reported that[6]

25% of the birth facilities routinely provide formula supplementation to breastfeeding infants
Few/some mothers have more than 30 minutes of skin-to-skin contact with their infant
Fewer than 50% mothers begin feeding within 1 hour after a vaginal delivery
Fewer than 50% mothers begin feeding 2 hours after a Cesarean delivery
Most hospitals separate mothers and babies in the first 30 minutes for routine procedures

Healthy newborns room-in with mother 24/7 in less than 50% of facilities
Only 44% of facilities have policies about pacifiers
Formula is provided to breastfeeding infants in 74% of facilities
More than 50% of the facilities give discharge packs containing formula samples
Almost all facilities receive formula at no cost
Breastfeeding training of new and existing staff is inadequate
Few hospitals have a written breastfeeding policy
Few US births occur in a baby-friendly hospital

The mPINC report serves as a background for pediatricians to use to develop and advocate for a specific breastfeeding policy in their hospital. The joint commission also has added the measurement of exclusive breastfeeding in their perinatal care core measures. They have initiated a "Speak-Up Campaign" to encourage mothers to let their plan for exclusive breastfeeding be known to hospital staff and to speak up if they find obstacles.

In brief, the CDC breastfeeding report card and mPINC study indicate areas that need improvement to achieve the Healthy People 2020 goals.

KNOWLEDGE

Pediatricians should have the knowledge base to support their staff in breastfeeding management. Periodic surveys from the AAP pertaining to breastfeeding issues, however, identified a diverse knowledge base among pediatrician respondents. In 1995, the survey identified that 45% of pediatrician respondents said that breastfeeding and formula feeding were equally acceptable methods for feeding infants.[7] After a best practices campaign for breastfeeding in the pediatric office, the survey was repeated in 2005. Ten years later, the survey again identified that 45% of pediatrician respondents claimed that breastfeeding and formula feeding were equally acceptable methods for feeding infants.[8] Thus, education of the leader of the health care team is imperative.

Not breastfeeding is associated with multiple health risks for both the infant and the mother. Systematic reviews and meta-analyses have documented the evidence to support the risks of not breastfeeding, both in the short term and in the long term. The Agency for Health care Research and Quality (AHRQ) published the "Evidence Report on Breastfeeding and Maternal and Infant Health Outcomes in Developed Countries," which provides sufficient data to conclude that the beneficial aspects of breastfeeding are substantial.[9] The report summarizes the link between breastfeeding and reductions in acute morbidity and long-term morbidity. The data specifically suggest a dose–response relationship between breastfeeding and reductions in otitis media, respiratory tract infections, asthma, bronchiolitis, atopic dermatitis, gastroenteritis, inflammatory bowel disease, celiac disease, diabetes, leukemia, and mortality (sudden infant death syndrome).[1] Evidence for infant protection following exclusive breastfeeding is seen in otitis, respiratory disease, gastroenteritis, atopic disease, sudden infant death syndrome, and cognitive development.[10,11] For maternal outcomes, a history of lactation was associated with a reduced risk of type 2 diabetes and breast and ovarian cancers. Additional data support reductions in maternal cardiovascular disease with breastfeeding.[12] Early cessation of breastfeeding is associated with increased risk of postpartum depression. Mothers also benefit from exclusive breastfeeding by delays in menses and favorable postpartum weight loss.[10,11]

In brief, breastfeeding reduces short- and long-term morbidities in children, and benefits mothers. The pediatrician should be well equipped with the appropriate knowledge base to enable and support the optimal management of breastfeeding.

SKILLS

In 2009, the AAP endorsed the WHO/UNICEF "Ten Steps to Successful Breastfeeding."[3] A key aspect of this program is the training all health care staff in the skills necessary to implement the 10 steps. Mothers comment that the support received from health care providers is the single most important intervention the health care system could have offered to have them breastfeed.[11] Since the pediatrician is the leader of the health care team, management skills and advocacy should be enhanced in their education, as they are responsible for delegating these to others in their office or community. Clinician education through reputable breastfeeding courses, conferences, books, and on the Internet can introduce the basics of breastfeeding and expand knowledge of management and diagnosis for the more sophisticated physician. It is important that physicians provide age-appropriate breastfeeding intervention and anticipatory guidance as part of every routine health supervision visit for mother and baby. Breastfeeding counseling can be discussed and reinforced antenatally, but few pediatricians see expectant families. Nevertheless, these visits serve an important role in recruitment of patients, since families may be searching for a health care provider who is knowledgeable about breastfeeding and has an office that is deemed breastfeeding friendly.

Each visit is a valuable opportunity to provide initial and ongoing support. Most women make their feeding choice early. In fact, 1 study reported that 78% of women made their feeding decision before the pregnancy or during the first trimester.[13] Transforming the physician's office, including the décor and advertising literature and designating areas for breastfeeding mothers sends a strong message in support of breastfeeding. The AAP indicates that pediatric practice should not dispense formula company literature or promote formula to avoid undue influence of families.

Office medical practices should be directed to support the goal of Healthy People 2020, to increase the percentage of women who initiate feeding and who continue exclusive breastfeeding for 6 months and then with complementary foods for a year or longer. Tracking breastfeeding rates in the practices may be a good way to critically look at the effectiveness of promoting and supporting breastfeeding. It points toward critical time points in well visits when more support for breastfeeding is needed. It also allows the practice to measure up against the national breastfeeding goals and work to improve on their practices.

The hospital is a key education opportunity, but many mothers do not remember all that is taught in such a short time. Therefore, the first pediatric health supervision visit at 3 to 5 days of age is a critical time to review education provided in the hospital. At that visit, the pediatrician observes a breastfeeding, comments on latch and position, and discusses elimination patterns and maternal/infant issues. The pediatrician should ask questions that anticipate return to work or school and help mothers develop a plan to maintain lactation and store breast milk in advance of circumstances that separate the mother and infant. The mother's goals for breastfeeding should be discussed and decisions about exclusive breastfeeding reinforced.

In summary, initiating discussions about breastfeeding from the early prenatal period and continuing it at every well visit during the first year of life is important. Discussions may involve problem solving, reassurance, or complimenting the mother on her success. Clinician education through reputable breastfeeding courses, conferences, books, and on the Internet can introduce the basics of breastfeeding for physicians and expand the skill set and knowledge of management and diagnosis for more sophisticated physicians.

EDUCATION

Clinicians are consistently identified by mothers as the trusted source for information and guidance regarding breastfeeding. Therefore, it is important for clinicians, especially pediatricians, to demonstrate competency in supporting lactation and breastfeeding. Inadequate education and inadequate training of clinicians have been identified as major barriers to breastfeeding, and education on breastfeeding is not a core element of most medical school or residency programs. A few implementation strategies that have been recommended include improving the breastfeeding content in undergraduate and graduate education and training for health professionals; establishing and incorporating minimum requirements for competency in lactation care into health professional credentialing, licensing, and certification processes; and increasing opportunities for continuing education on the management of lactation to ensure the maintenance of minimum competencies and skills.[4]

A survey was conducted by the AAP in 2004 regarding mothers' and clinicians' perspectives on breastfeeding counseling during routine preventative visits.[14] The prospective cohort study of low-risk mothers in a large multispecialty group practice reported that although nearly all obstetric (91%) and pediatric (97%) clinicians said they usually/always discuss plans to continue breastfeeding after returning to work, only 55% of the mothers reported that the topic was actually discussed. Only a few mothers reported discussing specific steps to maintain lactation after returning to work. These results indicate the gaps that the clinicians have in communicating effectively about the importance of breastfeeding and maintaining lactation. Discussions on breastfeeding are a significant part of the office visit, and yet insufficient time (by any of the office personnel) is spent in supporting lactation. Importantly, as leader of the health care team, the pediatrician often delegates lactation counseling to office specialists but remains responsible for their training and the education they provide.

Physicians have requested more education in breastfeeding.[7,8] Education can begin or be enhanced during residency programs. Through collaborations with the American College of Obstetricians and Gynecologists (ACOG), the American Academy of Family Physicians (AAFP), and the Association of Pediatric Program Directors, the AAP developed a curriculum for breastfeeding that has been tested in residency programs. The trial breastfeeding curriculum contained sections on advocacy, community outreach and coordination of care, anatomy and physiology, basic skills, peripartum support, ambulatory management, and cultural competency. Trained residents were more likely to show improvements in knowledge, breastfeeding practice patterns, and confidence than residents at control sites. Implementation of the curriculum also had a significant effect on increasing the rates of exclusive breastfeeding at intervention sites.[15] This curriculum is available online at http://www2.aap.org/breastfeeding/curriculum/.

Wellstart International provides a resource to promote breastfeeding through education of health professionals. The Lactation Management Education Program (LMEP) is available to provide education to leaders in medical, nursing, and nutrition (http://www.wellstart.org/resources.html). "Breastfeeding Basics (http://www.breastfeedingbasics.org)" is an academic noncommercial short course on the fundamentals of breastfeeding, geared to training medical practitioners.

The Academy of Breastfeeding Medicine (ABM) physician education statement (http://www.bfmed.org/Resources/Protocols.aspx) is used to promote physician education on breastfeeding, and to develop and disseminate standard approaches for physicians about breastfeeding issues. Detailed guidelines for undergraduate, graduate and postgraduate training are described in this statement.

In brief, residents who receive training are more likely to show improvements in knowledge, breastfeeding practice patterns, and confidence. Optimizing education and training of pediatricians would improve their competency in supporting lactation and breastfeeding.

HOSPITAL POLICY

Hospital policies must be conducive to breastfeeding. The pediatrician can insist on having a breastfeeding policy for their affiliated hospitals and help to create it. A positive maternity care experience is important to enable mothers to meet their breastfeeding goals. Importantly, nearly two-thirds of mothers who desired to breastfeed exclusively while in the hospital failed to do so because of hospital practices.[16] New York State has advanced a "Model Breastfeeding Policy", as have the AAP and the Academy of Breastfeeding Medicine:

New York: http://www.health.ny.gov/community/pregnancy/breastfeeding/docs/ model_hospital_breastfeeding_policy.pdf

AAP: http://www2.aap.org/breastfeeding/curriculum/documents/pdf/Hospital% 20Breastfeeding%20Policy_FINAL.pdf

Academy of Breastfeeding Medicine: http://www.bfmed.org/Media/Files/ Protocols/Protocol%207%20-%20Model%20Hospital%20Policy%20(2010% 20Revision).pdf

Box 1 highlights 11 steps adapted from the New York State "Model Breastfeeding Policy." These steps can be tailored to specific institutions to help mothers meet their breastfeeding goals.

It is important for practicing pediatricians to recognize that their influence is important; pediatricians can insist upon, and help create, a breastfeeding policy for their affiliated hospitals.

COMMUNITY

Normative health benefits are heavily influenced by one's environment. Changing the perception regarding breastfeeding in the society at large would in turn make it easier for mothers to adopt it as a norm. National initiatives have strengthened support for breastfeeding in the United States. The Healthy People 2020 goals include increases in breastfeeding initiation rates, rates of exclusive breastfeeding, lactation support in the workplace, and increasing the number of baby-friendly hospitals. The "Surgeon General's Call to Action," (http://www.surgeongeneral.gov/library/calls/breastfeeding/ index.html) prompts families, clinicians, hospitals, and communities to support and promote breastfeeding. The CDC mPINC survey enables hospitals to gauge their breastfeeding efforts against similar hospitals in their region and the United States. The joint commission (www.usbreastfeeding.org/Portals/0/.../BTT-29-Handout.pdf) includes in-hospital rates of exclusive breastfeeding in their perinatal care core measures and asks women to speak up (http://www.jointcommission.org/speakup_ breastfeeding/) when desiring to breastfeed in their birthing hospitals.

The media is beginning to notice as well. "Babies Were Born to Be Breastfed" is the campaign tag line of the US National Breastfeeding Awareness Campaign (http:// www.womenshealth.gov/breastfeeding/government-in-action/national-breastfeeding- campaign/) launched by the US Department of Health and Human Services' Office on Women's Health and the Advertising Council. This campaign targets first-time parents through television, radio, out-of-home, Internet, and print advertising to highlight the health consequences of not breastfeeding. Both federal and state laws have been

Box 1
11 steps from the New York State "Model Breastfeeding Policy"

1. Training for staff in hospitals that provide maternity services

   a. At least 1 thoroughly trained person must ensure the implementation of a program

   b. At least 1 maternity staff member should be thoroughly trained in breastfeeding physiology, and management should be available at all times to assist and encourage mothers with breastfeeding

2. Breastfeeding education for mothers in maternal and prenatal settings

   a. Assure the availability of prenatal childbirth education classes, specifically addressing subjects related to breastfeeding: nutritional and physiologic aspects of human milk, dietary requirements for breastfeeding, and diseases and medication or other substances that may have an effect on breastfeeding

   b. Provide mothers with complete commercial-free information about the benefits of breastfeeding, for mother and baby, to inform their feeding decisions, including nutritional, medical, and emotional benefits of BF for mother and baby; breastfeeding preparation; and potential breastfeeding problems

3. Breastfeeding initiation and skin-to-skin contact

   a. Prohibit the application of standing orders for antilactation drugs

   b. Encourage and assist mothers to place infants skin to skin soon after delivery

4. Breastfeeding instruction and assistance—provide instruction and assistance to each maternity patient who has chosen to breastfeed (establishing lactation care of breasts and breast examination common problems associated with breastfeeding; frequency of feeding, mother's nutrition and exercise; infant care, including taking temperature, feeding, bathing and diapering; infant growth and development; parent–infant relationship; and sanitary procedures for milk expression, collection, and storage of human milk)

5. Feeding on demand—provide for infants to be fed on demand

6. Rooming-in—establish and implement rooming-in for each patient unless medically contraindicated; the hospital must allow mothers to breastfeed their babies at any time day or night

7. Separation of mother and baby

   a. The hospital must provide mothers, including those who have infants with special needs, with full information about their breastfeeding progress and how to obtain help to improve their breastfeeding skills from a hospital staff member, trained in breastfeeding support and breast milk expression

   b. Allow mothers to breastfeed their babies in the neonatal intensive care unit (NICU) unless medically contraindicated. If nursing is not possible, the babies receive their mother's pumped milk. If a mother or baby is rehospitalized in a maternal care facility after the initial delivery stay, the hospital must make every effort to continue to support breastfeeding and provide hospital-grade electric pumps and rooming-in facilities

8. Supplementation and formula feeding

   a. Restrict formula feedings to those indicated by medical condition; hospital maternity staff must inform mothers if their doctor or pediatrician is advising against breastfeeding before any feeding decisions are made

   b. The hospital must allow mothers to have their baby not receive any formula and to have a sign on their baby's crib clearly stating that their baby is breastfeeding and that no formula bottles are to be offered; signs without advertisement are available from the CDC Web site

9. Pacifier use- Except for pain management and painful procedures, do not offer pacifiers routinely

10. Discharge support- Provide mothers with information about breastfeeding resources in their community, including information on availability of breast pumps; the hospital must ensure that follow-up medical visits are made for mother and infant within an appropriate timeframe, 3 to 5 days of age

11. Formula discharge packs—mothers should not be given discharge packs containing infant formula or formula coupons

enacted that specifically allow women to breastfeed in any place they are otherwise legally allowed to be. The United States Breastfeeding Committee (USBC) affirms that conditions in the workplace have a substantial effect on breastfeeding duration. In 2010, women compromised 47% of the total labor force in the United States. Seventy-three percent of employed women worked full-time jobs, while 27% worked on a part-time basis (http://www.dol.gov/wb/stats/stats_data.htm). Three out of 4 US mothers initiate breastfeeding, and more than half of mothers participate in the labor force before their children reach their first birthday.[17] Thus, the workplace issues are important. Many employers see less absenteeism and greater worker retention rates when they support a workplace lactation program, leading to a noticeable return on investment. Less illness in breastfed infants accounts for less employee absenteeism, improved employee productivity, and greater company loyalty. Pediatricians can be instrumental in promoting the business model plan for breastfeeding to businesses in their community. They are able to offer guidance to businesses by directing them to available resources like the business case for breastfeeding (http://www.womenshealth.gov/breastfeeding/government-in-action/business-case-for-breastfeeding/). This comprehensive program offers guidance to employers about supporting lactating mothers at the workplace.

Pediatricians have a powerful role in their communities, and their involvement in breastfeeding promotion has the potential to transform the experience of breastfeeding and improve its outcomes. Being a major part of the workforce, lactating mothers should have a workplace conducive to breastfeeding. Pediatricians can be instrumental in promoting the business model plan for breastfeeding in their community.

SUMMARY

The pediatrician champions children's health. The encouragement of breastfeeding to families and to the community at large is an important aspect of their profession. Thus, the pediatrician must be equipped with optimal resources to achieve this goal.

REFERENCES

1. Eidelman AI, Schanler RJ. American Academy of Pediatrics, Section on Breastfeeding Executive Committee. Breastfeeding and the use of human milk. Pediatrics 2012;129:e827–41.
2. Philipp BL, Chantry CJ, Howard CR. Academy of Breastfeeding Medicine Protocol Committee. Model Breastfeeding Policy. In: Lawrence RA, Lawrence RK, editors. Breastfeeding: A guide for the medical profession. 6th edition. Philadelphia: Elsevier; 2005. p. 1081–6.
3. World Health Organization. Evidence for the ten steps to successful breastfeeding. Geneva: World Health Organization; 1998.

4. US Department of Health and Human Services. The Surgeon General's Call to Action to Support Breastfeeding. Available at: http://www.surgeongeneral.gov/library/calls/breastfeeding/index.html. Accessed October 24, 2012.

5. Centers for Disease Control and Prevention, Centers for. Breastfeeding report card—United States. 2010. Available at: http://www.cdc.gov/breastfeeding/data/reportcard/reportcard2011.htm. Accessed October 24, 2012.

6. Available at: http://www.cdc.gov/breastfeeding/data/mpinc/index.htm. Accessed October 24, 2012.

7. Schanler RJ, O'Connor KG, Lawrence RA. Pediatricians' practices and attitudes regarding breastfeeding promotion. Pediatrics 1999;103:e35.

8. Feldman-Winter LB, Schanler RJ, O'Connor K, et al. Pediatrics and the promotion and support of breastfeeding. Arch Pediatr Adolesc Med 2008;162:1142–9.

9. Ip S, Chung M, Raman G, et al. Breastfeeding and maternal and infant health outcomes in developed countries. Agency for Healthcare Research and Quality 2007;153:1–186.

10. Eidelman AI, Schanler RJ. Section on breastfeeding executive committee. Breastfeeding and the use of human milk: executive summary. Pediatrics 2012;129:598–601.

11. Hauck FR, Thompson JM, Tanabe KO, et al. Breastfeeding and reduced risk of sudden infant death syndrome: a meta-analysis. Pediatrics 2011;128:1–8.

12. Schwarz EB, Ray RM, Stuebe AM, et al. Duration of lactation and risk factors for maternal cardiovascular disease. Obstet Gynecol 2009;113:974–82.

13. Arora S, McJunkin C, Wehrer J, et al. Major factors influencing breastfeeding rates: mother's perception of father's attitude and milk supply. Pediatrics 2000;106:e67.

14. Taveras EM, Li R, Grummer-Strawn L, et al. Mothers' and clinicians' perspectives on breastfeeding counseling during routine preventive visits. Pediatrics 2004;113:e405–11.

15. Feldman-Winter L, Barone L, Milcarek B, et al. Residency curriculum improves breastfeeding care. Pediatrics 2010;126:289–97.

16. Perrine CG, Scanlon KS, Li R, et al. Baby-friendly hospital practices and meeting exclusive breastfeeding intention. Pediatrics 2012;130:54–60.

17. Available at: http://www.bls.gov/opub/ted/2009/may/wk4/art04.htm. Accessed October 24, 2012.

Breastfeeding: Population-Based Perspectives

Miriam H. Labbok, MD, MPH, IBCLC, FACPM, FABM, FILCA

KEYWORDS

- Breastfeeding • Innocenti • Public health frameworks • Policy • Programs
- Woman-centered care

KEY POINTS

- Breastfeeding initiation has increased over the last 2 decades in the United States; increases in optimal breastfeeding lag.
- The number of published research studies has increased significantly, despite little dedicated federal funding for breastfeeding translational and programmatic research.
- Sociocultural factors, such as migration, ethnic belief systems, subtle discrimination, and social and other media, as well as political factors, such as laws and regulations, also create barriers to breastfeeding decisions and practices.
- The lack of guaranteed paid maternity leave and governmental provision of free formula immediately after birth in the United States, in contrast to the rest of North America and most countries in the world, creates an artificial short-term economic benefit for the use of human milk substitutes.
- The US Affordable Care Act offers new support for preventive health, including support for breastfeeding and for maintaining lactation after return to work.
- Health care practices and systems must change to cease creating barriers to breastfeeding.
- Clinicians have an essential role to play today in supporting needed changes in medical education and practice modifications based on the new and increasing research on how best to support optimal infant feeding.

INTRODUCTION

Optimal infant feeding is defined as exclusive breastfeeding for 6 months, followed by continued breastfeeding with age-appropriate complementary feeding for at least 1 year[1] or up to 2 years or longer.[2] Immediate postpartum skin-to-skin contact with early initiation is also considered among the optimal practices for breastfeeding success.[3] For infants, lack of optimal breastfeeding is associated with increased infectious

Disclosures: No disclosures.
Carolina Global Breastfeeding Institute (CGBI), Department of Maternal and Child Health, Gillings School of Global Public Health, University of North Carolina, CB#7445, Chapel Hill, NC 27599-7445, USA
E-mail address: labbok@unc.edu

Pediatr Clin N Am 60 (2013) 11–30
http://dx.doi.org/10.1016/j.pcl.2012.09.011
0031-3955/13/$ – see front matter © 2013 Elsevier Inc. All rights reserved.

diseases, gut diseases, diabetes, certain cancers,[4] and heart health risks such as obesity and hypertension.[5] Mothers, too, suffer from lack of breastfeeding in that they have increased risk of breast and ovarian cancers, slower postpartum uterine recovery, diabetes, and other risks.[4] These findings have created an increased interest among pediatricians and other clinicians in supporting breastfeeding.

Interest in breastfeeding increased at the global policy level in the 1990s. Mr James Grant, Executive Director of the United Nations Children's Fund (UNICEF), 1980 to 1995, often noted that "breastfeeding is the only natural safety net against being born into poverty." He considered breastfeeding "the great equalizer," because babies from all social or economic backgrounds who are optimally fed have an equal start on a healthy life. Although less was known in that decade about the specific health impacts of breastfeeding, population-level data were clear that lack of breast-feeding is extremely costly, in terms of excess mortality[6] and excess health care costs for mother and child, resulting in loss of productive life years. Breastfeeding not only reduces risk of disease, it also supports some natural birth spacing by suppressing the hormones that induce ovulation. Breastfeeding plays an important role in slowing population growth, especially in the poorer countries. As Mr Grant also observed, "How many of us are aware that if there were no breastfeeding tomorrow, births would increase by an estimated 20 to 30 per cent?"[7]

This population-based perspective was vital to support global action to protect, promote, and support breastfeeding, and served as the basis for the World Health Organization (WHO)/UNICEF Policymakers Meeting on "Breastfeeding in the 1990s: A Global Initiative," which led to the signing of the Innocenti Declaration on the Protection, Promotion and Support of Breastfeeding on August 1, 1990.[8] At that time, less than optimal breastfeeding was estimated to cause 3000 to 4000 deaths in infants and young children each day. As a result of the progress that has been made in support of exclusive breastfeeding and other child survival interventions in the last 2 decades, the daily death count has been reduced by about 35%,[9] allowing a reduced estimate number of daily deaths from less than optimal breastfeeding of around 2000 each day. Although this figure reflects the real improvement in breastfeeding,[10] it also remains a highly unacceptable toll from a preventable cause.

The observed progress in breastfeeding rates over the last 20 years was spear-headed globally by UNICEF and WHO, working together for change. The 1990 WHO/UNICEF/US Agency for International Development/Sida Innocenti Declaration called for all nations to implement 4 operational goals by 1995: (1) appoint a national breastfeeding coordinator of appropriate authority, and establish a multisectoral national breastfeeding committee composed of representatives from relevant government departments, nongovernmental organizations (NGOs), and health professional associations; (2) ensure that every facility providing maternity services fully practices all 10 of the *Ten Steps to Successful Breastfeeding* set out in the joint WHO/UNICEF statement *Protecting, Promoting and Supporting Breastfeeding: the Special Role of Maternity Services*; (3) take action to give effect to the principles and aim of all articles of the *International Code of Marketing of Breast-Milk Substitutes* and subsequent relevant World Health Assembly resolutions in their entirety; and (4) enact imaginative legislation protecting the breastfeeding rights of working women and establish means for its enforcement.[11]

The United States, although a signatory on the Innocenti Declaration of 1990, has been slower or has taken no action on the 4 Innocenti operational targets: development of a national committee and authority, the baby-friendly hospital initiative, legislation supporting the *International Code of Marketing of Breast-Milk Substitutes*, and paid maternity leave with workplace accommodation. Other countries have been more closely in tune with the global action plan. Infant mortality in the United States is the highest among countries of similar economic status. Although much of this mortality is attributable to a high rate of prematurity and low birth weight, the United States does better than most countries at keeping these newborns alive. In contrast, the mortality among full-term births is higher than other countries,[12] and a substantial part of this is caused by illnesses such as respiratory disease, sudden infant death syndrome, and sepsis, which could be reduced by increased breastfeeding.

This article explores the progress and trends in breastfeeding rates and research over the past decades, highlighting the sociocultural issues, politics, and public health thinking over the last decade that are increasingly supporting an enabling environment in which all women in North America have unbiased information on which to decide their feeding plan and succeed with their plans.

PROGRESS

In the United States, the Healthy People 2010 goals for breastfeeding were to have 75% of mothers breastfeed in the early postpartum, continued breastfeeding by 50% at 6 months and 25% at 1 year, with exclusive breastfeeding by 40% at 3 months and 17% at 6 months.[13] Public health goals for breastfeeding are set to stimulate action both in clinical practices and in public health programming. Because of progress in breastfeeding rates, new US public health goals are now:

- Initiation of any breastfeeding, 81.9%; continued breastfeeding to 6 months, 60.6%; continued breastfeeding to 1 year, 34.1%; exclusive breastfeeding to 3 months, 46.2%; and exclusive breastfeeding to 6 months, 25.5%.[13]

Additional goals set include:

- Increase the proportion of employers who have worksite lactation support programs to 38%;
- Reduce the proportion of breastfed newborns who receive formula supplementation within the first 2 days of life to 14.2%; and
- Increase the proportion of live births that occur in facilities that provide recommended care for lactating mothers and their babies to 8.1%.

How did the need to set new goals arise? Breastfeeding, over the last 2 decades, has increasingly been recognized as a major component of reducing infant and child mortality globally[6,14,15] and increasingly recognized in national public health programs in North America. The trends in breastfeeding initiation and exclusive breastfeeding from 1999 to 2009 are shown in **Fig. 1** and **Table 1**. These data are not fully comparable, because the definition used internationally is generally the rate of exclusive breastfeeding among all infants aged 0 to 5 months, and the definition used in the Canadian and US data is exclusive breastfeeding until the sixth month of life.

Rates of breastfeeding initiation are on the increase in North America. Specifically in the United States, breastfeeding initiation has increased above the 2010 goal, although increases in optimal breastfeeding exclusivity and duration are lagging. Historically, the United States experienced a setback in the 1980s, such that the rate achieved by 1982 was not seen again until the latter half of the 1990s. The full explanation of this setback has not been adequately studied, but may have been a combination of 3 factors: increasing special supplemental nutrition program for women, infants, and children (WIC) enrollment, with concomitant free supplies of commercial formula; increased advertising to the public and to hospitals by formula

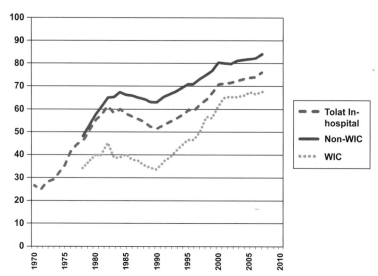

Fig. 1. Trends in breastfeeding initiation in the United States: national/total, women, infants, and children (WIC) population, and non-WIC populations: Ross survey data to 1999. (*Courtesy of* CDC National Immunization Survey 2000–2007; with permission.)

companies; and, possibly, attempts by many women to breastfeed in the 1970s with little support, resulting in lack of attempts with subsequent children.

In 1990, 2 important contributions to breastfeeding support occurred. The Innocenti Declaration was signed by the United States, and Dr Audrey Nora, at the time Associate Administrator, Maternal and Child Health, Health Services and Research Administration, attempted to jumpstart activities. However, the inclusion of formula companies in the US effort may have contributed to its short duration. The second important contribution was that of Catherine Bertini, then Assistant Secretary of

Table 1
Reported breastfeeding rates (%) in selected countries: rates of initiation, or any, breastfeeding and rates of exclusive breastfeeding in the first 6 months of life

| Year | Breastfeeding Initiation Rates | | | Exclusive Breastfeeding in the First 6 mo | | |
	Canada[a]	Mexico[b]	United States[c]	Canada	Mexico	United States
1999	—	92.3	67.2	—	20.3	—
2001	81.5	—	71.6	—	—	—
2003	84.9	—	72.6	17.3	—	10.3
2005	86.9	—	74.1	20.3	—	12.3
2007	87.9	—	76.0	23.1	—	13.8
2009	87.3	—	76.9	25.9	—	16.3

[a] Health Canada: data source: Statistics Canada, Canadian Community Health Survey, 2001, 2003, 2005, 2007–2008, 2009–2010. Available at: http://www.hc-sc.gc.ca/fn-an/surveill/nutrition/commun/prenatal/trends-tendances-eng.php. Accessed September 5, 2012.
[b] Child-info: nutritional status statistical tables. Available at: http://www.childinfo.org/undernutrition_nutritional_status.php. Accessed September 5, 2012.
[c] CDC National Immunization Surveys Breastfeeding among US children. Available at: http://www.cdc.gov/breastfeeding/data/nis_data/. Accessed September 5, 2012.

Agriculture for Food and Consumer Services at the US Department of Agriculture. In private conversations, she noted that when she first went to see a WIC program, she was shown storehouses full of formula and asked what was given to the breastfeeding mothers, with no response. Motivated in part by this experience, she oversaw the creation of the first food packages for low-income breastfeeding mothers.[15] As is shown in **Fig. 1**, the initiation of this package correlated with subsequent increases in the percentage of low-income American mothers who initially breastfed their infants.

The founding of the Academy of Breastfeeding Medicine, the increase in the number of International Board Certified Lactation Consultants and other forms of breastfeeding support training, and the growth of breastfeeding interest groups in pediatric professional organizations also have had an impact by greatly strengthening clinical support for breastfeeding. Clinicians have a vital role to play in creating the confidence among new mothers and in supporting behaviors associated with breastfeeding success. It will be necessary for clinical curricula to catch up with the increasing knowledge base and for all health care providers to consider the importance of breastfeeding in working with the mother/child dyad.

The US Breastfeeding Committee has been growing steadily and responds in part to the Innocenti call for a national committee and authority. With the increasing role of federal agencies in this committee, the impact is being multiplied. The US Centers for Disease Control and Prevention (CDC), along with the Surgeon General, the Office of Women's Health, the Food and Drug Administration, the Agency for Healthcare Research and Quality (AHRQ), and Maternal and Child Health Bureau, now participate in the US Breastfeeding Committee and have taken major steps to support breastfeeding in the new millennium. Since 2000, the CDC collects breastfeeding trend data, supports study of the issue, and actively supports hospitals to initiate the 10 steps called for in the Innocenti Declaration and codified in the Breastfeeding-Friendly Hospital Initiative. The CDC report card,[16] which includes several breastfeeding-related process indicators, also highlights the Maternity Practices in Infant Nutrition and Care survey of hospital practices.[17]

The numbers of studies and journals that report on breastfeeding have also taken a rapid upward turn in recent years. **Fig. 2** shows the number of articles published

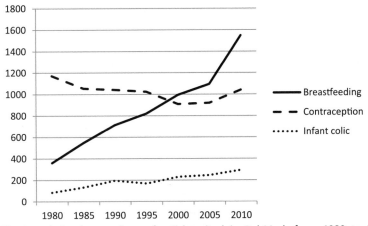

Fig. 2. The trends in the numbers of articles cited in PubMed, from 1980 to 2010 in 5-year intervals, using the indicated search term. (*From* PubMed, US National Library of Medicine. Available at: http://www.ncbi.nlm.nih.gov.libproxy.lib.unc.edu/sites/entrez?dr=abstract&otool=uncchlib&holding=_fft; with permission.)

and reported by the US National Library of Medicine at 5-year intervals over 3 decades for 3 common terms associated with maternal or child health: breastfeeding, contraception, and infant colic. Although there has been some uptick in the number for colic, possibly because of emerging pharmaceutical research, the number for contraception has been steady or declining. In contrast, the rate of publication on breastfeeding has shown a steady increase, with a possible impetus in the last decade from the emergence of 2 new journals: *Breastfeeding Medicine* (the journal of the Academy of Breastfeeding Medicine) and the *International Breastfeeding Journal*.

Another major trend in the United States has been in the use of electronic pumps to express milk, rather than continued feeding at the breast.[18] By the year 2000, 85% of breastfeeding mothers of infants aged 1.5 to 4.5 months had expressed milk at some time since their infant was born, and a high proportion used the pump regularly and over a long period.[19] Nearly 5% of mothers fed their infants human milk exclusively by expression. In this same study, women most often stated that they expressed their milk so that some other person might feed the infant. Although shared caretaking is an important strategy, especially when mothers must return to work soon after the birth, little is known about the relative impact on the health parameters attributed to breastfeeding. The composition of milk changes during the course of a feeding and over time. Human milk components may influence sleep and growth patterns, and feeding by bottle does not foster so much control by the infant, allowing more ready overfeeding.[20,21] Further, the risks of pump usage should be monitored, because trauma and infection may result from improper usage. Public health planning and pediatric counseling would benefit from more research on such trends, as well as the impact of such trends on mother and child health.

PERCEPTIONS

The pediatrician's role in support of breastfeeding is more important than ever. Increasingly, women are initiating breastfeeding; however, rates are far from optimal and barriers to successful breastfeeding persist. These barriers fall in 3 categories: (1) health system, (2) sociocultural and (3) economic/political barriers. The following sections consider how these barriers affect breastfeeding.

Health Systems

Passive and active barriers to breastfeeding occur throughout our health care systems. The passive barriers result from lack of recognition and support for breastfeeding among all of our patients, the lack of clinician energy exerted to stay up to date in breastfeeding support skills, and the quiet acceptance of formula company advertising into our practices and hospitals. The active barriers include lack of clarity in reimbursement for breastfeeding support, prenatally, in maternity care, and throughout the continuum of health care for as long as the mother and child continue breastfeeding; the inattention to the importance of breastfeeding by other health providers, including the too-easy recommendation to stop breastfeeding for procedures when this is not warranted; and inappropriate contraceptive use during breastfeeding.

These barriers create an unnecessary tension for the mother who intends to breastfeed, contributing to lower achieved breastfeeding compared with maternal intentions. Recent studies confirm that quality-of-care practices, known as the *Ten Steps for Successful Breastfeeding* (see articles elsewhere in this issue by Chantry and Howard, Holmes, and Bunik), can reduce this tension and create an enabling environment in which the mother who intends to breastfeed can achieve her intention.[22,23]

Biologically and physiologically, all newborns and their mothers intend to breastfeed; infant and maternal reflexes bring the baby to the breast, and the urge to latch on is strong in the infant in the time immediately after birth. When these practices are disallowed by hospital procedures, it leads to breastfeeding failure, and maternal discontent with her treatment. The call for patient satisfaction alone should encourage these practice changes. There are many compelling reasons for immediate action to implement these steps, outlined in **Box 1**. In addition, new data are allowing us to see which of the steps might have the greatest impact on breastfeeding initiation and duration.[24,25] Specifically, step 1 (calling for consistent policy), step 2 (calling for training of all hospital staff), step 4 (calling for immediate postpartum skin-to-skin contact), step 6 (calling for limiting use of human milk substitutes), and step 9 (calling for restriction of the use of artificial nipples and pacifiers) seem to be most associated with achieving breastfeeding intentions in the hospital, in terms of exclusivity, and beyond, in terms of duration. These insights may help inform clinical practice change during the perinatal period.

All of the barriers merit active intervention. First, there is a critical need for including breastfeeding support skills in all undergraduate clinical training curricula, as well as in residencies for any specialty that may come into contact with a breastfeeding dyad. Next, clinicians should consider eliminating the ambiguous message given when they tell their patients that they support breastfeeding and yet offer formula marketing materials in their practice area and hospital. Pediatricians might consider instituting the 10 steps in every maternity setting, and adopting protocols that may enhance your practice, such as *The Breastfeeding-Friendly Physicians' Office: Optimizing Care for Infants and Children*, which may be located along with many other useful protocols at the Academy of Breastfeeding Medicine Web site.[26]

Sociocultural

The general public and clinicians, alike, remain conflicted about breastfeeding and its importance in North America. This conflict is perhaps shown by a recent *Today Show* survey that asked, "Should mothers breastfeed their children" with an impossible choice of responses: 'It's the mother's choice. If she chooses not to breastfeed that's fine.' versus 'Yes, the health benefits are proved.' The options provided are neither comprehensive nor complementary; it is feasible that a person would agree with both. And yet more than 7500 responses came in choosing one or the other answer. By a slim margin of 56% to 43 %, the "yeses" won (**Fig. 3**). What does it mean that our society would accept this question, or that a thinking person would consider that these answers are mutually exclusive?

Perhaps our confusion stems in part from our sociocultural mix, acceptance of media and advertising, and love of technologies, sprinkled with a touch of gender discrimination and unrealistic expectations of women to perform as high-achieving nurturers and successful income generators, simultaneously. In North America, we have regional and community cultures and a high level of in-migration. Media, including television, advertisements, print media, and even cartoons, influence normative behavior in many areas of human behavior in North America. Research on how the media portray breastfeeding has shown that negative cultural attitudes toward breastfeeding have been reinforced by media messages. A textual analysis was conducted on 53 fictional television breastfeeding representations, ranging in genre and audience, from *Beavis and Butthead* to *Criminal Minds*.[27] Findings indicate that breastfeeding depictions are increasing in number and are generally positive, but limited in scope to educated, older, White women breastfeeding newborns, with little discussion about how to overcome problems. Extended breastfeeding and nursing in public

Box 1
Reasons for implementation of the *Ten Steps for Successful Breastfeeding*

- Increasing interest and measurement of quality of care in all facilities: the 10 steps are a quality-of-care standard
- Reputation and public relations: implementation of the steps are now recognized by many states and provinces with either baby-friendly hospital status or other recognition
- Patient satisfaction[a]: women who wish to breastfeed express increased satisfaction with their hospital stay if they perceive that they are receiving support for their intentions
- Return hospitalizations among breastfed infants tend to be for less severe and costly reasons; formula-fed newborns had a higher incidence of positive diagnostic results and a longer hospital stay[b]
- Pharmacologic/ethical considerations: research shows that detail men successfully influence physician prescribing, and the same applies to formula sales personnel[c]
- Minimal cost with significant positive health outcomes
- New growth standards in use are based on breastfed infants' growth rates
- In the United States:
  - AHRQ Prevention Guidelines[d]
  - American Academy of Pediatrics, American Academy of Family Physicians, and American College of Obstetricians and Gynecologists statements and updates
  - Magnet status for nurses
  - *Clinical Preventive Services for Women: Closing the Gaps*[e]
  - Existence of Diagnostic and Statistical Manual (DSM) codes for prenatal nutrition counseling reimbursement
  - The *Surgeon General's Call to Action to Support Breastfeeding*[f] with 20 action areas
  - The Joint Commission Perinatal Care Voluntary Core Measure, PC-05: *Exclusive Breast Milk Feeding During the Newborn's Entire Hospitalization*[g]

[a] Howell E. Lack of patient preparation for the postpartum period and patients' satisfaction with their obstetric clinicians. Obstet Gynecol 2010;115(2 Pt 1):284–9.
[b] Tyler M, Hellings P. Feeding method and rehospitalization in newborns less than 1 month of age. J Obstet Gynecol Neonatal Nurs 2005;34(1):70–9.
[c] Chren MM, Landefeld CS. Physicians' behavior and their interactions with drug companies. A controlled study of physicians who requested additions to a hospital drug formulary. JAMA 1994;271(9):684–9; Lurie N, Rich EC, Simpson DE, et al. Pharmaceutical representatives in academic medical centers: interaction with faculty and housestaff. J Gen Intern Med. 1990;5:240–3; and Wazana A. Physicians and the pharmaceutical industry: is a gift ever just a gift? JAMA 2000;283(3):373–80.
[d] AHRQ Guide to Clinical Preventive Services, 2010-2011, Primary Care Interventions to Promote Breastfeeding. Available at: http://www.ahrq.gov/clinic/pocketgd1011/gcp10s2e. htm. Accessed September 3, 2012.
[e] Clinical preventive services for women: closing the gaps, released July 19, 2011. Available at: http://www.iom.edu/Reports/2011/Clinical-Preventive-Services-for-Women-Closing-the-Gaps.aspx. Accessed September 3, 2012.
[f] US Department of Health and Human Services. The Surgeon General's call to action to support breastfeeding. Washington, DC: US Department of Health and Human Services, Office of the Surgeon General; 2011.
[g] Specifications Manual for Joint Commission National Quality Measures (v2011A), Available at: http://manual.jointcommission.org/releases/TJC2011A/MIF0170.html. Accessed September 3, 2012.

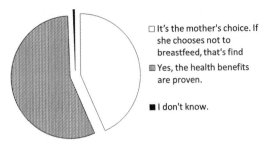

It's the mother's choice. If she chooses not to breastfeed, that's find

Yes, the health benefits are proven.

I don't know.

Fig. 3. Web viewers respond to "should mothers breastfeeding their children" by selecting 1 of 2 nondiscreet questions.

were conveyed as socially unacceptable, making other characters uncomfortable, often within the same story lines that sexualized breasts. These depictions may reinforce myths and discourage women from breastfeeding past the newborn phase or in public. The author of the study noted that these portrayals may help explain why breastfeeding has not yet been culturally normalized, despite an international consensus that it is the best health choice for babies.

Social media and electronic interpersonal communications are having an increasing role on how we view the world. A recent study on social media examined adherence to the WHO *International Code of Marketing of Breast-Milk Substitutes* (the Code), which calls for ethical marketing.[28] The study revealed that infant formula manufacturers have established a social media presence and that violations of the Code as well as promotional practices unforeseen by the Code were common: enabling user-generated content that promotes the use of infant formula, financial relationships between manufacturers and bloggers, and creation of mobile apps for use by parents, further fostered by a lack of transparency in social media-based marketing.

Social marketing may be one way to address the impact of commercial marketing. Social marketing involves the application of commercial marketing principles to advance the public good. Generally, it involves 4 interrelated tasks: audience benefit, target behavior, essence (brand, relevance, positioning), and developing the 4Ps (product, price, place, promotion) marketing mix. A recent review examined the US Department of Agriculture *Loving Support Makes Breastfeeding Work* campaign, launched in 1997 based on social-marketing principles, designed to increase breastfeeding initiation rates and breastfeeding duration among WIC participants.[29] The findings included that it is important to design social-marketing campaigns to target not only mothers but also the influential societal forces (eg, family and friends, health care providers, employers, formula industry, legislators) that affect women's decision and ability to breastfeed. The need to create societal norms brings us to the consideration of political and economic issues, which may not as yet be entirely supportive of breastfeeding.

Economic/Political

Breastfeeding is influenced by economic and political forces. Most women of reproductive age are in the workforce and, in the United States, there is no guaranteed paid maternity leave. Research is showing that there are negative effects of working while pregnant or in the early postpartum period. A nested case-control study in 2002 to 2003 of preterm birth and low birth weight among working women in Southern

California found that provision of maternity leave is associated with about one-fourth of the risk of cesarean delivery, adjusted for covariates (odds ratio, 0.27; 95% confidence interval, 0.08–0.94).[30] Even unpaid leave offered in the United States under the 1993 Family and Medical Leave Act was associated with small increases in birth weight, decreases in the likelihood of a premature birth, and substantial decreases in infant mortality for children of college-educated and married mothers, who were most able to take advantage of unpaid leave.[31] An assessment of the literature on the length of maternity leave and health of mothers and children found a positive ecological association between the length of maternity leave and mother's mental health and duration of breastfeeding, as well as with lower perinatal, neonatal and postneonatal mortality and lower child mortality.[32] Another systematic review found that, taking account of the methodological limitations, there is a statistically significant association between infant mortality and higher income inequality, and infant mortality and other indicators of less redistributive social policy, such as lack of maternity leave.[33] An Australian study found that returning to work in the first 10 months post partum is associated with shorter breastfeeding durations.[34] A Canadian study, which may have contributed to the newly instituted paid maternity leave in that country, noted that nearly 130 countries guarantee working women the right to breastfeed through leave and workplace accommodation to protect the health of infants and mothers alike. The investigators suggest that their country extend policies to ensure adequate maternity leave, legislate a right to breastfeed while working, and adapt workplaces to make this practical.[35]

The more politicoeconomic question then is: can we afford maternity leave? A national survey in the United States revealed many new and unexpected trends.[36] The 2008 National Study of the Changing Workforce, performed by the Family and Work Institute, was a nationally representative study of employees asking about their physical and mental well-being. Following on studies conducted in 1992, 1997, and 2002, the 2008 study allows a look at trends and how current workers differ from workers of the same age in the 1990s. The change, indicated in **Box 2**, is increased economic pressures on families for women to continue work throughout the childbearing years. This situation begs the question as to whether or not society as a whole should support paid leave for maternal and child health, including breastfeeding. Additional study by the Family and Work Institute found that employers reported that investment by firms in paid leave was seen as paying off in the end, or as cost-neutral. The Families and Work Institute survey found that most surveyed firms (84%) viewed the investment in paid leave for maternity, paternity, and serious illness as providing either a positive return on the investment (42%) or as cost-neutral (42%). At a recent Breastfeeding Summit, hosted by the Academy of Breastfeeding Medicine, the economic issues were examined.[37] The conclusion was that although the gains from breastfeeding are at least partially understood, the overall case for breastfeeding remains incomplete economically and many questions remain to be answered to make the economic case for paid maternity leave.

The remaining questions are noted in **Box 3**, with 1 addition: what is the role of government? The United States, along with only Papua New Guinea, Swaziland, Liberia and Lesotho, offers no guaranteed maternity leave, causing the practice of optimal breastfeeding to be an economic challenge. In contrast, Canada has an Employment Insurance Act[38] that offers payment of maternity benefits to biological mothers for up to 15 weeks, with pay equal to 55% of an employee's average insurable earnings for the last 26 weeks. Benefits may begin as early as 8 weeks before the week the baby is due and must generally conclude no later than 17 weeks after the baby is born. If the baby is born prematurely or with a condition that requires hospitalization, this 17-week

---

Box 2
The 2008 National Study of the Changing Workforce: trends in women's and men's roles

- Women in dual-earner couples are contributing more to family income: in 1997, women contributed an average of 39% of annual family income; in 2008, 44%. In addition, there was an increase in the percent of women with earnings at least 10% more than their partners: from 15% in 1997 to 26% in 2008.

- Among those less than 29 years old, women are just as likely as men to want jobs with greater responsibility.

- Women with and without children are equally seeking jobs with more responsibility.

- Men and women are both less likely to embrace traditional gender roles, with only about 40% of each believing that it is better "if the man earns the money and the woman takes care of the home and children."

- Employed fathers are spending more time with children than their age counterparts did 3 decades ago, whereas employed mothers' time has not changed. Young fathers report spending 4.3 hours per workday compared with the 2.4 hours spent by their age counterparts in 1977. Mothers less than 29 years in 2008 average 5.0 hours compared with 4.5 hours in 1977.

- Men are taking more overall responsibility for the care of their children. In 1992, 21% of women said that their spouses or partners were taking as much or more responsibility for the care of their children as they were. By 2008, that percentage has risen to 31%.

From Derogatis K, Sakai K. New study shows significant and surprising changes among men and women at work and at home–first report from 2008 National Study of the Changing Workforce traces the trends in men's and women's attitudes and actions over the past 3 decades. Family and Work Institute; 2009. Available at: http://familiesandwork.org/site/research/reports/main.html; with permission.

---

maximum can be extended by the period of the child's hospitalization up to a maximum of 52 weeks after the week of the date of confinement. In Mexico, Article 123 of the Labor Law provides various protections and guarantees to workers, including an 8-hour workday, a maximum workweek of 6 days, equal pay for equal work, and mandatory

---

Box 3
Research questions that help define the economic argument for paid maternity leave

- What are the incremental benefits from extending breastfeeding month by month?

- How important is exclusivity versus supplemented breastfeeding?

- Which activities or programs increase duration of breastfeeding?

By education, income, and other socioeconomic groups

- What are the total benefits of breastfeeding?

Improved maternal and infant health and social and educational attainment, and sequelae

- What are the full costs of breastfeeding? Labor force, caloric intake, costs to/gains for employers?

- What is the proper role for the health care system and associated financial systems?

- What is the proper role for government?

First 6 bullets from Phelps CE. Economic issues of breastfeeding. Breastfeed Med 2011;6:307–11; with permission.

childbirth and maternity leave: Pregnant employees are entitled to 6 weeks' leave before the approximate date of childbirth and to 6 weeks' leave thereafter with full wages and the right to retained employment.[39] The Mexican Social Security Institute (Instituto Mexicano de Seguridad Social) subsidizes 60% of the female worker's salary; therefore, the employer need only pay the difference. During breastfeeding, mothers are entitled to 2 extra paid half-hour rest periods for nursing their children.

In the United States, women are offered 12 weeks of unpaid leave under the Family and Medical Leave Act, which exempts companies with fewer than 50 paid employees, but in 2011, only 11% of private-sector workers and 17% of public workers reported that they had access to paid maternity leave through their employer.[40] Only about half of first-time mothers can take paid leave when they give birth. This economic deterrent is further compounded in that the US Department of Agriculture offers formula free of cost to about half of all new mothers in the United States through the WIC program. Over the past 20 years, there has been accelerating support for breastfeeding within this system, and the WIC package given to exclusively breastfeeding mothers is greatly expanded, including counseling; follow-up support through peer counselors; eligibility to participate in WIC longer than nonbreastfeeding mothers; an enhanced food package; and pumps, breast shells, or nursing supplementers to help support the initiation and continuation of breastfeeding.[41] In addition, these mothers are not given free formula for at least the first month post partum. As a result of the increasing support, most WIC mothers now initiate breastfeeding. Nonetheless, with this combination of 2 highly unusual programs, mothers in the United States have a double whammy of no paid leave plus free formula for many, creating a double economic advantage in foregoing breastfeeding.

US Congress recently enacted the Patient Protection and Affordable Care Act, which requires employers with 50 or more employees to provide unpaid reasonable break time for mothers of infants to express their milk.[42] It also calls for breastfeeding support, supplies, and counseling to include comprehensive lactation support and counseling, by a trained provider during pregnancy or in the postpartum period, and costs for renting breastfeeding equipment.[43] This development adds urgency to the importance of determining the prevalence of exclusive and periodic milk expression and the consequences of these behaviors, compared with direct breastfeeding, for the health of mothers and their infants. This strategy, as well as the survey data discussed earlier, may open the door for discussion as to whether the United States might consider a form of employment insurance, not unlike disability insurance, to support paid maternity and postpartum leave.

PUBLIC HEALTH

Public health approaches may help in the achievement of population-based health behavior change.[44] Some consider that policy development is a necessary prelude to program intervention. Globally, the major policy approach is the Millennium Development Goals (MDGs) for improving maternal and child health, including gender equity and reproductive justice as underlying needs. The MDGs include 8 goals, all which have implications for breastfeeding. This issue was examined at a global nutrition meeting and is summarized in **Table 2**.

A comprehensive approach, including both clinical and public health considerations, is needed to create an environment and a society that enable optimal breastfeeding success. This need for a comprehensive approach was a major theme of the WHO/UNICEF Global Strategy for Infant and Young Child Feeding[2] launched in 2003, as well as an

Table 2
The role of nutrition and infant and young child feeding in addressing the MDGs

Goal Number and Targets	Contribution of Infant and Young Child Feeding[a]
1. Eradicate extreme poverty and hunger Halve, between 1990 and 2015, the proportion of people: Whose income is less than $1 a day Who suffer from hunger	Breastfeeding significantly reduces early childhood feeding costs, and exclusive breastfeeding halves the cost of breastfeeding.[b] Exclusive breastfeeding and continued breastfeeding for 2 years is associated with reduction in underweight[c] and is an excellent source of high-quality calories for energy
2. Achieve universal primary education Ensure that by 2015, children everywhere, boys and girls alike, will be able to complete a full course of primary education	Breastfeeding and adequate complementary feeding are prerequisites for readiness to learn.[d] Breastfeeding and quality complementary foods significantly contribute to cognitive development
3. Promote gender equality and empower women Eliminate gender disparity in primary and secondary education, preferably by 2005 and in all levels of education no later than 2015	Breastfeeding is the great equalizer, giving every child a fair start in life. Most differences in growth between sexes begin as complementary foods are added into the diet, and gender preference begins to act on feeding decisions. Breastfeeding is uniquely a right of women, and should be supported by society[e]
4. Reduce child mortality Reduce by two-thirds, between 1990 and 2015, under-fives mortality rate	Infant mortality could be readily reduced by about 13% with improved breastfeeding practices alone, and 6% with improved complementary feeding.[f] In addition, about 50%–60% of under-5 mortality is secondary to malnutrition, greatly caused by inadequate complementary foods and feeding following on poor breastfeeding practices[g]
5. Improve maternal health Reduce by three-quarters, between 1990 and 2015, maternal mortality	The activities called for in the global strategy include increased attention to support for the mother's nutritional and social needs. In addition, breastfeeding is associated with decreased maternal postpartum blood loss, decreased breast cancer, ovarian cancer, and endometrial cancer, as well as the probability of decreased bone loss after menopause. Breastfeeding also contributes to the duration of birth intervals, reducing maternal risks of pregnancy too close together
6. Combat HIV/AIDS, malaria and other diseases Have halted by 2015 and begun to reverse the spread of HIV/AIDS	Based on extrapolation from the published literature on the impact of exclusive breastfeeding on MTCT, exclusive breastfeeding in an otherwise untested breastfeeding HIV-infected population could be associated with a significant and measurable reduction in MTCT

(continued on next page)

Table 2
(continued)

Goal Number and Targets	Contribution of Infant and Young Child Feeding[a]
7. Ensure environmental sustainability	Breastfeeding is associated with decreased milk industry waste, pharmaceutical waste, plastics and aluminum tin waste, and excess use of firewood/fossil fuels[h]
8. Develop a global partnership for development	The Global Strategy for Infant and Young Child Feeding fosters multisectoral collaboration and can build on the extant partnerships for support of development through breastfeeding and complementary feeding In terms of future economic productivity, optimal infant feeding has major implications

Abbreviations: HIV, human immunodeficiency virus; MTCT, mother-to-child transmission.

[a] Early and exclusive breastfeeding, continued breastfeeding with complementary feeding and related maternal nutrition.

[b] Bhatnagar S, Jain NP, Tiwari VK. Cost of infant feeding in exclusive and partially breastfed infants. Indian Pediatr 1996;33:655–8.

[c] Dewey KG. Cross-cultural patterns of growth and nutritional status of breast-fed infants. Am J Clin Nutr 1998;67:10–7.

[d] Anderson JW, Johnstone BM, Remley DT. Breast-feeding and cognitive development: a meta-analysis. Am J Clin Nutr 1990;70:525–35.

[e] Labbok M. Breastfeeding: a woman's reproductive right. Int J Gynaecol Obstet 2006;94(3):277–86.

[f] Jones G, Steketee RW, Black RE, et al. How many child deaths can we prevent this year? Lancet 2003;362:65–71.

[g] Pelletier D, Frongillo E. Changes in child survival are strongly associated with changes in malnutrition in developing countries. J Nutr 2003;133:107–19.

[h] Labbok M. Breastfeeding as a women's issue: conclusions and consensus, complementary concerns, and next actions. Int J Gynaecol Obstet 1994;47(Suppl):S55–61.

Courtesy of UN Standing Committee on Nutrition Working Group on breastfeeding/complementary feeding, 2004; with permission.

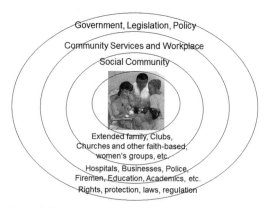

Fig. 4. The socioecological framework includes the broad societal factors that help create a climate in which breastfeeding encouraged or inhibited. These factors include social and cultural norms. Other large societal factors include the health, economic, educational, and social policies that help to maintain economic, social, gender, or racial inequalities between groups in society.

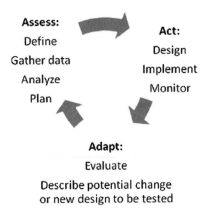

Fig. 5. The triple A approach.

outcome of a 2009 UNICEF expert consultation,[45] and has informed national blueprints. Public health approaches are most effective when they include both prevention and population-level thinking and include both targeted and comprehensive approaches. There are many frameworks, or models, that help clarify the steps in building a public health approach and intervention programming.[44] The socioecological model is perhaps the most frequently cited in public health conceptual thinking and planning, used in many action planning approaches, including the *Surgeon General's Call to Action*.[46] As seen in **Fig. 4**,[47] this framework allows consideration of interventions at many levels: from the individual, to the family, community, societal level, and so on. The CDC and WHO promote a 4-level model to guide research and practice related to effective programs and policies. This model considers the complex interactions between individual, relationship, community, and societal factors. Some models also include an external ring for civil society/government.

Two frequently used constructs for action may be used in clinical or population-level intervention planning. Perhaps the simplest model is the triple A model, suggesting assessment, action, reassessment, and adaptation, in a cyclic approach, as shown in **Fig. 5**. This model might apply to breastfeeding as follows:

Assess: define the health problem through the systematic collection of information about the magnitude, scope, characteristics, and consequences and

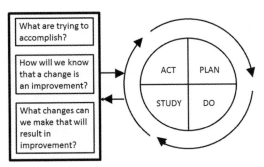

Fig. 6. The PDSA iterative continuous quality improvement approach. (*From* Langley GL, Nolan KM, Nolan TW, et al. The improvement guide: a practical approach to enhancing organizational performance. 2nd edition. San Francisco (CA): Jossey-Bass; 2009; with permission.)

establish the factors that could be modified through interventions. This strategy would be the exploration of the literature and program experience in support of breastfeeding in a setting that affects more than 1 individual.

Action: from the assessment, an intervention may be designed and implemented. This intervention might be in the community or in a clinical outreach or group setting.

Reassessment and adaptation: monitoring the effects of these interventions on risk factors and the target outcome provides information that contributes to the evaluation of their impact and cost-effectiveness. Such evaluation is used to adapt the breastfeeding intervention.

A similar but more targeted iterative approach developed by the Institute for Healthcare Improvement[48] is the plan-do-study-act (PDSA) cycle, which involves testing a change by developing a plan to test it (plan), performing the test (do), observing and learning from the consequences (study), and determining which modifications should be made to the test (act) in an iterative manner, such that a group of workers may try out and discuss small tests of change toward a goal (**Fig. 6**).

No matter which approach is used, the pediatricians and other clinicians are a critical influence for change at every sociopolitical level and in every public health effort. There is no shortage of initial approaches for a coalition of individuals and organizations committed to healthier, happier mothers and babies. The 4 policy pillars as defined by UNICEF and WHO are a solid base for sustainable change (**Box 4, Fig. 7**). These pillars include national/state government commitment, legislation, and policy; health worker training and health system support; communications; and family and community support. A fifth tenet is to address local specific issues, such as the need for exclusive breastfeeding, rather than mixed feeding, in areas endemic for human immunodeficiency virus.[38] As we examine the many potential ways forward, it may be useful to continue to work on these 4 basic areas, initially sparked by the Innocenti Declaration of 1990, as we plan toward the Healthy People goals for 2020.

Box 4
The 4 pillars and possible actions to create a breastfeeding-friendly environment

1. National/governmental commitment: this may be supported using women's and children's rights as arguments for change

2. Legislation/policy for maternity protection and paid leave, health insurance coverage, freedom to breastfeed as children need, and protection against aggressive advertising of infant formula

3. Health training and services improvement; this necessitates cooperation and partnership among state health departments, health professional associations, accrediting organizations, and academic faculties to ensure that preventive medicine, breastfeeding, and attention to women's equity are included in undergraduate training for all health workers

4. Policy in support of family/community: this must include attention to social support for birth spacing and motherhood, as well as the sharing of social marketing and advocacy across sectors; such policy-dictating action would include building with existing socially oriented NGOs, no matter what their primary social goal is

From Labbok M. Transdisciplinary breastfeeding support: creating program and policy synergy across the reproductive continuum. Int Breastfeed J 2008;3:16; with permission.

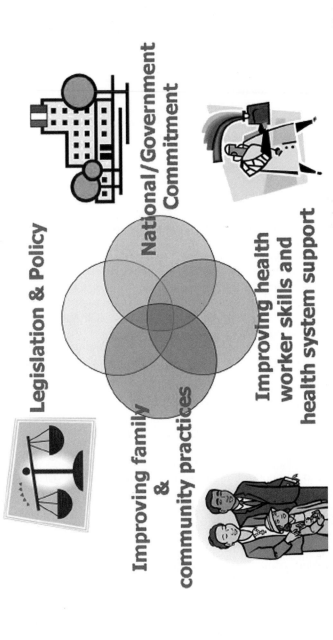

Fig. 7. The 4 pillars: the 4 action areas (pillars) for synergy consideration (figure derived from UNICEF and WHO presentation materials). (*From* Labbok M. Transdisciplinary breastfeeding support: creating program and policy synergy across the reproductive continuum. Int Breastfeed J 2008;3:16; with permission.)

SUMMARY

Clinical support for breastfeeding is essential, but such support has greater impact if it is coupled with public health interventions as well. Clinicians have a vital role to play in ensuring their own skills and knowledge base and that of future clinicians, and they also have a vital role in advocating for comprehensive programming to ensure population-level normalization of optimal breastfeeding for all.

ACKNOWLEDGMENTS

The author wishes to thank the anonymous North Carolina family for supporting the creation of the Carolina Global Breastfeeding Professorship and Institute in the Department of Maternal and Child Health at the University of North Carolina, allowing her to pursue in-depth study of breastfeeding practices and support.

REFERENCES

1. Section on Breastfeeding. AAP policy statement: breastfeeding and the use of human milk. Pediatrics 2012;129(3):e827–41.
2. WHO/UNICEF. Global strategy for infant and young child feeding. Geneva (Switzerland): WHO; 2003.
3. Edmond KM, Zandoh C, Quigley MA, et al. Delayed breastfeeding initiation increases risk of neonatal mortality. Pediatrics 2006;117(3):e380–6.
4. Ip S, Chung M, Raman G, et al. Breastfeeding and maternal and infant health outcomes in developed countries. Evidence Report/Technology Assessment No. 153. AHRQ Publication No. 07–E007. Rockville (MD): Agency for Healthcare Research and Quality; 2007.
5. Horta B, Bahl R, Martines J, et al. Evidence on the long-term effects of breast-feeding systematic reviews and meta-analyses. Geneva (Switzerland): WHO; 2007.
6. Jones G, Steketee RW, Black RE, et al. How many child deaths can we prevent this year? Lancet 2003;362(9377):65–71.
7. Statement by Mr James P. Grant, Executive Director of the United Nations Children's Fund (UNICEF) at the International Conference on Population and Development. Cairo, September 7, 1994.
8. UNICEF. 1990–2005: Celebrating the Innocenti Declaration on the protection, promotion and support of breastfeeding. Florence (Italy): UNICEF/Innocenti Research Centre; 2006.
9. Hill K, You D, Inoue M, et al, Technical Advisory Group of the United Nations Inter-agency Group for Child Mortality Estimation. Child mortality estimation: accelerated progress in reducing global child mortality, 1990-2010. PLoS Med 2012; 9(8):e1001303.
10. Alipui N. Making room for breastfeeding on the worldwide agenda! Breastfeed Med 2012;7:329–31.
11. WHO/UNICEF. Innocenti Declaration on the protection, promotion and support of breastfeeding. Available at: http://www.unicef.org/programme/breastfeeding/innocenti.htm. Accessed September 3, 2012.
12. MacDorman M, Hoyert D, Mathews T. Division of Vital Statistics, National Center for Health Statistics, Centers for Disease Control and Prevention "Data from the National Vital Statistics System" Table 2: Gestational age specific infant mortality rates: US and selected European Countries, 2004. Presentation to the Secretary's

Advisory Committee on Infant Mortality Infant and Maternal Mortality in the US. Washington, DC, August 2, 2011.

13. HealthyPeople.Gov. 2020. Available at: http://www.healthypeople.gov/2020/default. aspx. Accessed September 3, 2012.

14. Lawn J, Cousens S, Zupan J, et al. For the Lancet Neonatal Survival Steering Team*, Neonatal Survival 1: Four Million Neonatal Deaths: When? Where? Why? Lancet 2005;365:891–900.

15. Bertini C. Wikipedia. Available at: http://en.wikipedia.org/wiki/Catherine_Bertini. Accessed September 3, 2012.

16. CDC Breastfeeding Report Card–United States. 2012. Available at: http://www. cdc.gov/breastfeeding/data/reportcard.htm. Accessed September 3, 2012.

17. CDC National Survey of Maternity Practices in Infant Nutrition and Care (mPINC). Available at: http://www.cdc.gov/breastfeeding/data/mpinc/index.htm. Accessed September 3, 2012.

18. Rasmussen K, Geraghty S. The quiet revolution: breastfeeding transformed with the use of breast pumps. Am J Public Health 2011;101(8):1356–9.

19. Labiner-Wolfe J, Fein SB, Shealy KR, et al. Prevalence of breast milk expression and associated factors. Pediatrics 2008;122(Suppl 2):S63–8.

20. Li R, Magadia J, Fein SB, et al. Risk of bottle-feeding for rapid weight gain during the first year of life. Arch Pediatr Adolesc Med 2012;166(5):431–6.

21. Li R, Fein SB, Grummer-Strawn LM. Do infants fed from bottles lack self-regulation of milk intake compared with directly breastfed infants? Pediatrics 2010;125(6):e1386–93.

22. Declercq E, Labbok MH, Sakala C, et al. Hospital practices and women's likelihood of fulfilling their intention to exclusively breastfeed. Am J Public Health 2009;99(5):929–35.

23. DiGirolamo AM, Grummer-Strawn LM, Fein SB. Effect of maternity-care practices on breastfeeding. Pediatrics 2008;122(Suppl 2):S43–9.

24. Taylor E, Nickel N, Labbok M. Implementing the ten steps for successful breastfeeding in hospitals serving low-wealth patients: exploring each step in context. Am J Public Health 2012. [Epub ahead of print].

25. Nickel N, Labbok M, Hudgens M, et al. The extent that noncompliance with the Ten Steps to Successful Breastfeeding impacts breastfeeding duration. JHL. [Accepted for publication].

26. ABM protocols and statements. Available at: http://www.bfmed.org/Resources/ Protocols.aspx. Accessed September 4, 2012.

27. Foss KA. "That's not a beer bong, it's a breast pump!" Representations of breastfeeding in prime-time fictional television. Health Commun 2012. [Epub ahead of print].

28. Abrahams SW. Milk and social media: online communities and the International Code of Marketing of Breast-milk Substitutes. J Hum Lact 2012;28(3): 400–6.

29. Pérez-Escamilla R. Breastfeeding social marketing: lessons learned from USDA's "Loving Support" campaign. Breastfeed Med 2012. [Epub ahead of print].

30. Guendelman S, Pearl M, Graham S, et al. Maternity leave in the ninth month of pregnancy and birth outcomes among working women. Womens Health Issues 2009;19(1):30–7.

31. Rossin M. The effects of maternity leave on children's birth and infant health outcomes in the United States. J Health Econ 2011;30(2):221–39.

32. Staehelin K, Bertea PC, Stutz EZ. Length of maternity leave and health of mother and child–a review. Int J Public Health 2007;52(4):202–9.

33. Spencer N. The effect of income inequality and macro-level social policy on infant mortality and low birthweight in developed countries–a preliminary systematic review. Child Care Health Dev 2004;30(6):699–709.

34. Cooklin AR, Rowe HJ, Fisher JR. Paid parental leave supports breastfeeding and mother-infant relationship: a prospective investigation of maternal postpartum employment. Aust N Z J Public Health 2012;36(3):249–56.

35. Heymann J, Kramer MS. Public policy and breast-feeding: a straightforward and significant solution. Can J Public Health 2009;100(5):381–3.

36. DeRogatis K, Sakai K. First report from 2008 National Study of the Changing Workforce traces the trends in men's and women's attitudes and actions over the past three decades. New York: Family and Work Institute; 2009.

37. Phelps CE. Economic issues of breastfeeding. Breastfeed Med 2011;6(5):307–11.

38. Treasury Board of Canada Secretariat, Maternity and parental benefits. Available at: http://www.tbs-sct.gc.ca/. Accessed September 5, 2012.

39. Human Resources: payroll in Mexico 2012. Available at: http://www.payrollmexico.com/index.php?ID=obligations. Accessed September 5, 2012.

40. The women in public service project. Available at: http://womeninpublicservice.org/2012/06/01/comparing-paid-maternity-leave-around-the-world/. Accessed September 5, 2012.

41. FNS/USDA. Breastfeeding promotion and support in WIC. Available at: http://www.fns.usda.gov/wic/breastfeeding/mainpage.HTM. Accessed September 3, 2012.

42. Patient Protection and Affordable Care Act, Pub L No. 111–148.

43. US Health Resources and Service Administration. Women's preventive services: required health plan coverage guidelines. Available at: http://www.hrsa.gov/womensguidelines/. Accessed September 7, 2012.

44. This section is adapted in part from Labbok M. Chapter 3 Breastfeeding in public health: what is needed for policy and program action?. In: Smith PH, Hausman B, Labbok M, editors. Beyond health, beyond choice. New Brunswick (NJ): Rutgers University Press; 2012.

45. Schultink W, Arabi M. Effective nutrition programming for children and the role of UNICEF: consensus points from an Expert Consultation. Food Nutr Bull 2009; 30(2):189–96 (8).

46. US Department of Health and Human Services. The Surgeon General's call to action to support breastfeeding. Washington, DC: US Department of Health and Human Services, Office of the Surgeon General; 2011.

47. Labbok M. Transdisciplinary breastfeeding support: creating program and policy synergy across the reproductive continuum. Int Breastfeed J 2008;3:16.

48. Langley GL, Nolan KM, Nolan TW, et al. The improvement guide: a practical approach to enhancing organizational performance. 2nd edition. San Francisco (CA): Jossey-Bass; 2009.

Breastfeeding and Health Outcomes for the Mother-Infant Dyad

Christine M. Dieterich, MS, RD, Julia P. Felice, BS,
Elizabeth O'Sullivan, BA, BS,
Kathleen M. Rasmussen, AB, ScM, ScD, RD*

KEYWORDS

- Breastfeeding • Lactation • Postpartum weight retention • Obesity • Maternal health
- Infant health

KEY POINTS

- Most US women do not meet breastfeeding recommendations; a variety of factors determine likelihood of breastfeeding initiation, duration and exclusivity, including socio-demographic and biologic variables, attitudinal characteristics, and the healthcare environment.
- Breastfeeding protects child health and development by reducing risk of infection and Sudden Infant Death Syndrome (SIDS) during infancy and by reducing risk of cancers, improving cognitive outcomes, and promoting appropriate metabolic development through childhood.
- Only one randomized trial, the Promotion of Breastfeeding Intervention Trial (PROBIT) in Belarus, has been conducted to assess the effect of breastfeeding duration and intensity on child health outcomes; results of this trial support many associations identified in epidemiologic studies.
- Breastfeeding protects the health of women by promoting postpartum weight loss and lactational amenorrhea, reducing long-term risk of reproductive cancers, and promoting the return of metabolic profiles to that of the prepregnant state, which may result in decreased risk of later type 2 diabetes and cardiovascular disease.

INTRODUCTION

"Breastfeeding saves lives" and "Breast is best!" are well-known slogans for physicians and women. Putting the newborn to the breast to nurse is now considered "normative" in the United States with 75% of women doing so.[1] Unfortunately, breastfeeding as a way to continue to feed infants is not yet normative. Women do not choose to breastfeed as long nor as exclusively as recommended by health experts[2] and the government,[3] which may result in a missed opportunity for improving infant health and, at the same time, maternal health. The evidence for this possibility is reviewed here.

Division of Nutritional Sciences, 111 Savage Hall, Cornell University, Ithaca, NY 14850, USA
* Corresponding author.
E-mail address: kathleen.rasmussen@cornell.edu

Pediatr Clin N Am 60 (2013) 31–48
http://dx.doi.org/10.1016/j.pcl.2012.09.010
0031-3955/13/$ – see front matter © 2013 Elsevier Inc. All rights reserved.

This article considers some of the known determinants of the duration and exclusivity of breastfeeding and the potential confounders that may be acting at the time of breast-feeding initiation and throughout the breastfeeding period, as some of these factors, such as socioeconomic status and maternal obesity, continue to influence the infant's later health. This article also reviews the latest evidence of relationships between breastfeeding behaviors and health outcomes for both the infant and the mother. The literature covered predominantly refers to feeding the term infant and rarely specifies the mode of feeding breast milk, whether at the breast or from a bottle. Health outcomes associated with feeding breast milk from a bottle compared to at the breast have been minimally explored to date, and are thus not a focus of this article.

DETERMINANTS OF BREASTFEEDING DURATION AND EXCLUSIVITY

Breast milk is recommended as the infant's sole source of nutrition for the first 6 months of life. It is recommended that complementary foods be added to the infant's diet at 6 months of age and that breastfeeding continue for one year or longer as mutually desired by mother and infant.[2] Although women in the United States met the Healthy People 2010 goal for 75% of new mothers to initiate breastfeeding, the duration and exclusivity of breastfeeding remain below national goals. Determinants of breastfeeding duration and exclusivity can be grouped into five broad categories: (1) demographic variables, (2) biologic factors, (3) attitudinal characteristics, (4) hospital practices, and (5) social variables.

Demographic Factors

The demographic determinants of breastfeeding duration are the subject of a large literature and it is widely acknowledged that women who are older, better educated, and of higher income breastfeed longer.[4–6] Black women are less likely to breastfeed than non-black women (**Table 1**).[5] Degree of acculturation also has an impact on breastfeeding; every year of United States residency reduces the odds of breastfeeding to any extent by 4% and breastfeeding to 6 months by 3%.[7] Duration of breastfeeding among participants in the Special Supplemental Nutrition Program for Women, Infants, and Children (WIC) lags behind that of nonparticipants, including those who are WIC-eligible but do not participate.[8] Despite WIC's aim to promote breastfeeding, the distribution of free formula undermines the program's message.

Biologic Factors

A negative relationship between maternal obesity postpartum and breastfeeding duration was first reported in 1992.[9] Since then, the focus has been on maternal obesity at the time of conception, which is negatively associated with both the likelihood of

Table 1 Breastfeeding rates by race or ethnicity			
	Ever Breastfed (%)	BF at 3 Mo (%)	BF at 6 Mo (%)
Hispanic	77.3	57	38.8
Non-Hispanic White	74.9	53.7	40.2
Non-Hispanic Black	51.4	34.5	23.4

Abbreviation: BF, breastfeeding.
Adapted from Li R, Darling N, Maurice E, et al. Breastfeeding rates in the United States by characteristics of the child, mother, or family: the 2002 National Immunization Survey. Pediatrics 2005;115(1):31–7; with permission.

successful initiation of breastfeeding and its duration,[10,11] though one study showed no association among black women.[12] A recent systematic review summarized the potential reasons for the association between maternal obesity and breastfeeding as anatomic/physiologic, medical, sociocultural, and psychological (**Table 2**).[11]

Maternal smoking during pregnancy is strongly negatively associated with breastfeeding duration.[13] A dose-response effect has been shown, with the heaviest smokers having the least likelihood of establishing exclusive breastfeeding.[4] Mothers who smoke have significantly decreased milk production compared with nonsmokers[14]; this association may be partly related to a decreased motivation to breastfeed among smokers.[13]

Insufficient milk supply is consistently reported as a reason for early weaning.[5,6] Although up to 50% of women report that they perceive their milk supply to be insufficient, only about 5% of women suffer from a physiologically insufficient supply.[5,6] In response to the perception of having an insufficient milk supply, many women supplement breastfeeding with infant formula. This reduces demand for breast milk and decreases maternal supply, compounding the problem. This biologic factor has a strong psychological component because low maternal self-efficacy for breastfeeding is associated with perceptions of insufficient milk supply.[6]

Attitudinal Characteristics

High maternal self-efficacy is associated with prolonged breastfeeding.[4,6] A woman's confidence in her breastfeeding ability is positively influenced by her exposure to breastfeeding and her personal breastfeeding experience.[15] In addition, maternal attitudes toward breastfeeding have an impact on duration. Those who perceive breastfeeding to be healthier, easier, and more convenient breastfeed longer than those who perceive that breastfeeding is restrictive, inconvenient, and uncomfortable.[4]

It is not surprising that intended duration of breastfeeding is associated with actual duration of breastfeeding.[4,6] This information is useful for clinicians because it has been suggested that "among women who intend to breastfeed, simply asking how long they plan to do so is an efficient method of identifying prenatally who is at risk for short breastfeeding duration."[16]

Hospital Practices

Hospital practices shown to improve breastfeeding duration and exclusivity include early breastfeeding initiation, infant rooming-in, and providing breast milk only.[4,17] These practices are included in the "10 steps" of the Baby-Friendly Hospital Initiative (BFHI). Hospital participation in the BFHI increases rates of breastfeeding initiation,

Table 2	
Potential reasons why obese women breastfeed for shorter durations	
Anatomic/ physiologic	Delayed lactogenesis Practical difficulties with latch and positioning
Medical	Complications of diabetes or polycystic ovary syndrome causing delayed lactogenesis or low milk supply
Sociocultural	Obese women are more likely to be of lower socioeconomic status, which is a determinant of reduced breastfeeding duration
Psychological	Increased body image dissatisfaction and this increased concern about their bodies makes women less likely to breastfeed

Adapted from Amir L, Donath S. A systematic review of maternal obesity and breastfeeding intention, initiation and duration. BMC Pregnancy Childbirth 2007;7(1):9 PMCID: 1937008.

duration, and exclusivity[18]; however, fewer than 5% of babies in the United States are delivered in hospitals with BFHI certification.[1]

Clinicians may also directly influence maternal breastfeeding behavior. In a prospective cohort study, researchers[19] found that mothers whose pediatricians recommended formula supplementation were significantly more likely to discontinue exclusive breastfeeding by 12 weeks. Moreover, clinicians can also potentially improve women's breastfeeding behavior by making them aware of current national or international goals for breastfeeding duration as suggested in a recent report.[20]

Social Variables

Maternal employment negatively affects breastfeeding behavior.[5] Returning to full-time work outside the home is associated with reduced duration of breastfeeding,[21] whereas length of maternity leave is positively associated with duration of breastfeeding.[4] Many women use breast pumps as a coping strategy for combining breastfeeding and employment.[22]

The impact of professional and lay support on breastfeeding outcomes was assessed in a 2007 Cochrane meta-analysis.[23] All forms of lay and professional support increased the duration of any breastfeeding.[23] However, lay support and combinations of lay and professional support were more effective for continuation of exclusive breastfeeding than professional support alone.[23]

Support from significant others also contributes to breastfeeding success.[5,6] Breastfeeding continuation is associated with the father's knowledge, attitude, and support,[5] and also the support of the maternal grandmother.[6] Fathers who receive breastfeeding information from professionals are more likely to promote and support their partner's breastfeeding efforts.[4]

It is important for clinicians to promote breastfeeding duration and exclusivity to avoid placing infants at risk of the poorer health outcomes that result from being fed infant formula as opposed to being breastfed. To optimize breastfeeding behavior, we must consider which of the determinants discussed are modifiable, when, and by whom. Attitudes, social variables, and health care practices represent a potential target for support and intervention.

PROTECTIVE EFFECTS FOR INFANTS
How Breast Milk Confers Its Benefits

Breast milk has evolved to provide the best nutrition, immune protection, and regulation of growth, development, and metabolism for the human infant.[24] Breast milk is critical in compensating for developmental delays in immune function in the neonate and is responsible for reducing permeability of the intestine to prepare it for extrauterine life.[25]

The predominant antibody in breast milk, secretory IgA (sIgA), confers its immunoprotection by inhibiting the adherence to or penetration of the gastrointestinal (GI) tract by pathogens and by phagocytosis or cytotoxicity of pathogens.[26] sIgA is higher in colostrum than mature milk, is present in a form resistant to digestion, and provides key temporal and ubiquitous immunoprotection.[27,28] Additional, acquired secretory antibodies, such as IgM and IgG, depend on prior maternal exposure to pathogens and provide the infant with environment-specific immunoprotection.[27]

The favorable gut microbiome that results from breastfeeding protects the infant from pathogenic bacteria and has been associated with reduced asthma and reduced obesity rates in children.[29] This microbiome is a function of the interaction between human milk's microbiota, such as *Bifidobacteria* and *Lactobacilli*, and the oligosaccharides which serve as fuel for these bacteria; these components resist digestion and have important antimicrobial activity.[27,30] The healthy microbiome promotes integrity of the intestinal barrier and competitively inhibits pathogen binding, thereby preventing inflammatory responses.[25,27] Additionally, the gut microbiota contribute to regulation of the expression of genes that affect fat metabolism and deposition.[31]

This healthy microbiome is one of many examples of the functional efficiency of breast milk because it provides immunoprotection and nutrients by synthesizing several essential micronutrients, namely vitamins B_{12}, B_6, folate, and vitamin K.[31] Lactoferrin is another key example of functional efficiency because it aids in iron absorption, provides a significant proportion of digested amino acids, and provides immunoprotection by promoting epithelial growth and restricting bacterial access to iron.[27,28] Digested milk fat globules yield monoglycerides and medium- and long-chain fatty acids with additive antimicrobial properties,[32] and undigested milk fat globules function as vehicles for small proportions of sIgA.[33]

Finally, breast milk contains hormones, neuropeptides, and growth factors that may affect growth, development, and self-regulation of food intake, contributing to the differences observed between breastfed and formula-fed infants.[34] Leptin suppresses appetite and the breastfed infant's serum leptin is positively correlated with maternal concentrations. Ghrelin, which stimulates appetite, is found in higher concentrations in foremilk than in hindmilk.[35] This concentration difference may also contribute to the better self-regulation of intake in breastfed infants compared to formula-fed infants, and is, thus, a potential explanation for increased bottle-emptying behavior that is observed among bottle-fed infants.[36]

Breastfeeding and Infant Health Outcomes

It is well-known that breastfeeding saves and improves the quality of lives even in relatively clean, industrialized contexts. In an analysis of data from the 2005 National Immunization Survey, researchers calculated that if 90% of infants were exclusively breastfed for 6 months, 911 deaths would be prevented.[37] In an earlier analysis of the costs of formula-feeding, other investigators[38] found that, compared with 1000 infants exclusively breastfed for 3 months, 1000 infants never breastfed required 2033 more office visits, 212 more days in the hospital, and 609 more prescriptions in the first year.

The associations between breastfeeding behaviors and infant health outcomes are the subject of a large literature that, despite limitations, establishes breastfeeding as the "gold standard" against which alternative feeds should be evaluated (**Box 1**). Most evidence is observational because of the ethical difficulties in randomizing individuals to breastfeeding or formula-feeding. Only one large-scale experimental trial exists in a developed country: the Promotion of Breastfeeding Intervention Trial (PROBIT) in Belarus, in which hospitals were randomized to promotion of breastfeeding or standard care.[39] As a result, the intervention and control arms of the trial comprise infants from hospitals with increased breastfeeding rates compared with infants at hospitals with baseline breastfeeding rates, and illustrate the benefits of improving breastfeeding behaviors. Because associations between breastfeeding behaviors and infant health outcomes are confounded by socioeconomic and psychosocial factors, this experimental design offers the best available evidence of causal relationships between breastfeeding and health outcomes. Moreover, among PROBIT participants, breastfeeding was nearly universal in both the intervention and control arms and illness rates were low, reducing the investigators' power to detect a benefit of breastfeeding. Nonetheless, between-group differences were observed, and for these

---

Box 1
Strength of evidence for improved health outcomes among breastfed infants and breastfeeding mothers

Infant Health Outcomes

Strong or Causal Evidence:
  GI tract infections
  Upper- and lower-respiratory tract infections
  Otitis media
  Acute lymphoblastic leukemia
  Sudden Infant Death Syndrome

Evidence in Development:
  Cognitive development
  Atopic allergies
  Asthma
  Other pediatric cancers
  Childhood obesity

Maternal Health Outcomes

Strong or Causal Evidence:
  Postpartum weight loss
  Lactational amenorrhea
  Breast cancer

Evidence in Development:
  Ovarian cancer
  Type 2 diabetes
  Cardiovascular disease
  Bonding

---

outcomes a clear causal relationship can be inferred—particularly because biologic evidence supports these effects and suggests mechanisms by which these effects may occur. The evidence from PROBIT is supplemented by many systematic reviews and meta-analyses (summarized in **Table 3** with associated effect measures) that, although subject to the same confounding factors, unequivocally support breastfeeding for optimal infant health.

Infections and illnesses

Infants who are not breastfed, or who are breastfed for short periods or at low intensity, have a higher risk of infection and illness than those who are breastfed optimally. In the PROBIT trial, the standard-care group experienced more GI tract infections than the intervention group. These between-group differences were clear despite diminished power, as described above.[39] In the United States, where daycare is widespread and infection rates are higher than in Belarus,[40] a greater effect would be expected. These findings are supported in the observational studies reviewed recently,[41,42] with breastfed infants 64% less likely to contract a GI infection.

PROBIT investigators were unable to confirm a similar protective effect of breastfeeding against respiratory ailments and otitis media with experimental data, but the unexpectedly high breastfeeding rates and low incidence of these infections may not have allowed adequate power to do so.[39] In their recent meta-analysis of studies from 1980 to 2001, Bachrach and colleagues[43] found that breastfed infants had a 72% lower risk of hospitalization for respiratory infections. In addition, investigators of a subsequent prospective cohort in the Netherlands found evidence to support a protective role for breastfeeding against GI and upper- and lower-respiratory tract infections. In the Netherlands cohort, only infants who were breastfed for at least 6 months had lower risk for GI and respiratory-tract infections than controls who were not breastfed.[44] Moreover, the protective effects of breastfeeding persisted after cessation, although they diminished over time.[41,42]

In addition to sufficient breastfeeding duration, it is important to provide breast milk exclusively to reduce the risk of infection and illness because this behavior reduces the infant's exposure to illness-causing agents. Among PROBIT infants who were exclusively breastfed for at least 3 months, those who continued to be exclusively breastfed were one-third less likely to have 1 or more GI infections in the first year than infants who were partially breastfed thereafter.[45] In a recent meta-analysis of cohorts from 1989 to 1997, the investigators found that although infants ever breastfed were three-quarters as likely to contract otitis media than those never breastfed, infants exclusively breastfed for at least 3 months were half as likely.[41] In a subsequent prospective cohort, infants exclusively breastfed for 4 months were at greater risk of contracting an upper-respiratory tract infection than those exclusively breastfed for a full 6 months.[44]

Neurologic outcomes
Breastfed and formula-fed babies differ in neurologic outcomes, but this association is confounded by socioeconomic status, parental education, parental intelligence, and the home environment.[41,46] The experimental design of the PROBIT provides strong evidence of an effect independent of these confounders; at 6.5 years follow-up, children who were in the intervention arm had higher IQ scores and teacher ratings than those in the control arm.[47] Although Der and colleagues[46] did not find support for the association between breastfeeding and cognitive outcomes in their recent prospective cohort and meta-analysis of prior studies through 2004, their sibling analysis in the cohort and the observational design of studies included in the meta-analysis may not have sufficiently controlled for confounding.

Sudden infant death syndrome
Although sudden infant death syndrome (SIDS) deaths have declined substantially in 20 years,[48] SIDS remains the leading cause of postneonatal death in the United States.[49] PROBIT was not statistically powered to detect differences in mortality, yet investigators found a nonsignificant trend in reduction of SIDS risk in the intervention group ($P = .12$).[39] The American Academy of Pediatrics (AAP)[48] recommends breastfeeding to further reduce SIDS risk because, although this association is not well-understood, it has been recently shown to be independent of infant sleeping position.[50] In two recent meta-analyses, the investigators found a protective effect of ever breastfeeding.[41,51] Hauck and colleagues[51] analyzed studies conducted during 1966 to 2009 and found that, compared with formula-fed infants, those who were ever breastfed had a 45% reduction in SIDS risk, those breastfed at least 2 months had a 62% reduction, and those exclusively breastfed for any duration had a 73% reduction. Breastfed infants are more easily aroused from sleep than formula-fed infants, which may explain these findings.[52] This evidence and the AAP recommendation support the incorporation of breastfeeding promotion into the United States SIDS-reduction campaign.

Asthma and atopic allergies
Although it is commonly thought that breastfeeding behavior is associated with risk of asthma and allergies, there was no difference in allergy risk between PROBIT groups.[53] Meta-analyses and reviews of observational evidence have been unable to clarify this association because of lack of power, inconsistent diagnostic criteria, and unresolved confounding. Meta-analyses have found protective effects of breastfeeding, particularly when family history for allergic rhinitis,[54] atopic allergies,[55] and asthma[41] was present. However, there is some evidence from cohort studies that breastfed infants have increased risk of asthma[56] and similar or increased risk of allergy.[56,57]

Pediatric cancers
Despite a large literature, including recent meta-analyses,[41,58] evidence linking breastfeeding and risk of childhood cancers is limited. This results from limited exploration of

Table 3
Evidence supporting protective effects of breastfeeding on infant health

Health Outcome	Strongest Evidence	Source	Comparison Groups	Odds ratio[a]	(Amount)-Fold Risk[b]
GI tract infection (0–12 mo)	Experimental (hospital BF promotion vs standard care)	Kramer et al,[39] 2001	Intervention vs control (baseline breastfeeding vs increased breastfeeding)	0.6	1.67
GI tract infection (3–6 mo)	Experimental (hospital BF promotion vs standard care)	Kramer et al,[45] 2003	Exclusively BF at 3 mo and partially BF ≥6 mo vs exclusively BF ≥6 mo	0.35	2.86
	Meta-analysis of cohorts	Chien et al,[42] 2001	Ever-BF vs never-BF	0.36	2.78
Respiratory infection	Cohort	Duijts et al,[44] 2010	Exclusively BF at 4 mo and partially BF thereafter vs never-BF	URTI: 0.65 LRTI: 0.50	URTI: 1.54 LRTI: 2.00
			Exclusively BF ≥6 mo vs never-BF	URTI: 0.37 LRTI: 0.33	URTI: 2.70 LRTI: 3.03
Hospitalization for respiratory infection	Meta-analysis	Bachrach et al,[43] 2003	Ever-BF vs never-BF	0.26	3.85
Otitis Media	Meta-analysis of cohorts	Ip et al,[41] 2009	Ever-BF vs never-BF	0.77	1.30
			Exclusively BF ≥3 mo vs never-BF	0.5	2.00

	Experimental (hospital BF promotion vs standard care)		Intervention vs control (ie, baseline breastfeeding vs increased breastfeeding)	+5.9 points on full-scale IQ	N/A
Cognitive Development		Kramer et al,[47] 2008		+5.9 points on full-scale IQ	N/A
Sudden Infant Death Syndrome	Meta-analysis	Hauck et al,[51] 2011	Ever-BF vs never-BF BF ≥2 mo vs never-BF Exclusively BF any duration vs never-BF	0.55 0.38 0.27	1.82 2.63 3.70
Acute Lymphoblastic Leukemia	Meta-analysis	Ip et al,[41] 2009	BF >6 mo vs never-BF	0.81	1.23
Obesity	Meta-analysis	Arenz et al,[63] 2004	Ever-BF vs never-BF	0.79	1.27
	Meta-analysis	Owen et al,[62] 2005	Ever-BF vs never-BF	0.87	1.15
	Meta-analysis	Harder et al,[64] 2005	BF duration 1–3 mo vs never-BF BF duration 4–6 mo vs never-BF BF duration 7–9 mo vs never-BF	0.81 0.76 0.67	1.23 1.32 1.49

Abbreviations: BF, breastfed; LRTI, lower respiratory tract infection; URTI, upper respiratory tract infection.

[a] Odds ratios reported by original investigators, in which the less-ideal behavior (the second comparison group listed) is used as the referent. The OR thus represents the benefit conferred by breastfeeding.

[b] (Amount)-fold-risk as recalculated by the authors, in which the more-ideal breastfeeding behavior (the first comparison group listed) is used as the referent, reflecting the authors' suggestion that breastfeeding be considered the normative standard. The (amount)-fold-risk represents the increase in morbidity and mortality associated with formula-feeding.

certain cancers, small sample sizes, reliance on long-term recall, conflicting or null results, and between-study design heterogeneity. However, there is some evidence that breastfeeding may reduce risk of acute lymphoblastic leukemia, and duration of breastfeeding may be important. Studies have reported that infants breastfed greater than 6 months had a 24%[58] and 19%[41] reduction in risk of acute lymphoblastic leukemia compared with those not breastfed, whereas those breastfed less than or equal to 6 months had a 12% reduction.[58]

Childhood obesity

The two major mechanisms by which breastfeeding may protect against obesity in the child are through the components or composition of human milk and behaviors related to infant feeding (**Fig. 1**). In addition to the effects of breast milk components and the microbiome described above, its lower protein concentration may help to protect the infant against later adiposity.[59] Behaviors of the caregiver may also contribute to the higher obesity rates observed among formula-fed than breastfed infants. Caregivers who encourage bottle-fed infants to empty the bottle may override the infants' internal satiety cues, which may result in poor infant self-regulation of intake. A study by Li and colleagues[36] supports this notion because infants fed more often from a bottle (vs at the breast) were more likely to finish a bottle at a feeding.

The association between breastfeeding and obesity is controversial. Data from the 6.5-year follow-up of PROBIT provide the only experimental evidence with which to determine whether or not formula-feeding instead of breastfeeding increases the risk of childhood obesity.[60] No differences were observed between the intervention and standard-care groups in overweight or obesity. It is possible that the difference between *some* breastfeeding in the control versus *more* breastfeeding in the intervention groups was not large enough to observe an effect on child obesity because most mothers in both groups initiated and were still breastfeeding at 3 months postpartum. Additionally, the investigators advise caution when generalizing these findings to contexts in which the obesity epidemic is rampant because the proportions of children in PROBIT who were greater than or equal to the 85th (13%) or the 95th (5%) percentiles for BMI were substantially lower than those in the United States (33% and 18%, respectively).[61]

In meta-analyses of observational studies of breastfeeding and the risk of childhood obesity there were small, yet consistent, reductions in obesity risk of 13%[62] and 22%[63] for breastfed compared with formula-fed infants. In another meta-analysis,[64] a dose-response relationship was identified; there was a 4% reduction in obesity risk for each month of breastfeeding. In contrast, mean body mass index (BMI) was only minimally lower among breastfed compared with formula-fed individuals in a quantitative review of published and unpublished studies, which the investigators attributed to confounding factors.[65]

The importance of breastfeeding for growth may depend on the child's existing adiposity. In one recent study, it seemed that breastfeeding resulted in a healthier BMI distribution overall[66] as fewer children were either underweight or obese.

Infants born to obese mothers are at high risk of developing obesity for several reasons. These infants may have inherited a genetic predisposition to obesity, are exposed to an obesogenic environment in utero, are likely to be breastfed for a shorter period than infants of normal-weight mothers, and may be exposed to an obesogenic family food environment. Infants of heavier Danish mothers who were breastfed for longer periods gained 11% less in their first year of life than those who were breastfed for shorter periods.[67] In a study of US infants, Li and colleagues[68] found that children of obese mothers who never breastfed had a sixfold higher odds of becoming

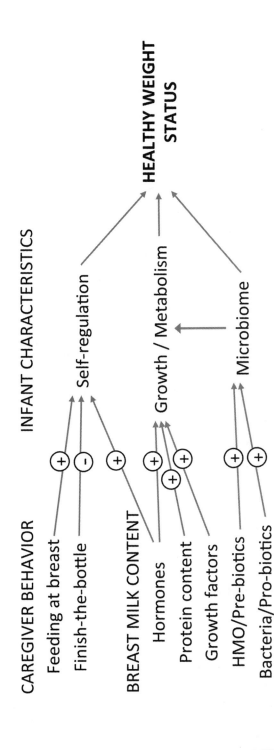

Fig. 1. Possible mechanisms, beneficial effects (+) and detrimental effect (−), through which breastfeeding promotes healthy infant weight status. Caregiver behaviors and the contents of human milk have effects on the breastfed infant's self-regulation of intake, growth and metabolism, and the intestinal microbiome, which, in turn, promote development of healthy weight. HMO, human milk oligosaccharides.

overweight compared with children of normal-weight mothers that breastfed for at least 4 months. Based on this evidence, mothers who are obese and children of obese mothers are a key group to target for breastfeeding assistance, and effective interventions are needed to help this population.[69]

Cardiovascular and metabolic disease risk

Effects of breastfeeding on risk factors for cardiovascular and other metabolic diseases have also been examined in observational studies. In a meta-analysis of seven studies, breastfeeding decreased the risk of type 2 diabetes by nearly 40% compared with formula-feeding.[70] Fasting insulin values in later life were 3% lower among those who were breastfed, indicating an association with improved insulin-sensitivity. Breastfeeding may also decrease later risk of type 1 diabetes[41] and blood pressure in adulthood,[71] although evidence for these outcomes are less conclusive because of potential problems of confounding and publication bias.

MATERNAL HEALTH OUTCOMES OF BREASTFEEDING

The advantages of breastfeeding for mothers are not as well studied as those for infants, but there is adequate evidence to state that women who breastfeed are likely to have improved health in the short-term, and are at lower risk of developing future diseases (**Box 2**).[72]

Immediate and Early Benefits to the Mother

Postpartum weight loss

Childbearing is associated with long-term weight gain,[73] and postpartum weight retention has been associated with adverse outcomes in later pregnancies.[74]

Box 2
Maternal benefits of breastfeeding

Breastfeeding may confer immediate and long-term benefits to mothers, especially if recommendations for exclusivity and duration are met. Such benefits may strengthen motivation or commitment to breastfeeding

- Reasons to initiate breastfeeding
  - Reduce maternal bleeding after delivery
  - Involute uterus
  - Facilitate positive metabolic changes
  - Facilitate postpartum weight loss
  - Reduce stress
  - Delay ovulation
- Reasons to continue breastfeeding
  - Increase postpartum weight loss
  - Prolong lactational amenorrhea
  - Decrease visceral adiposity
  - Reduce type 2 diabetes risk
  - Reduce cardiovascular risk
  - Reduce breast cancer risk
  - Reduce ovarian cancer risk

Breastfeeding, conversely, is associated with postpartum weight loss.[75,76] In a large prospective cohort study, Baker and colleagues[76] showed that greater intensity (exclusivity) and duration of breastfeeding was associated with greater weight loss at 6 and 18 months postpartum in women of all BMI categories. This is not surprising since exclusive breastfeeding has a maternal energy cost of about 500 kcal per day. However, it must not be overlooked that increases in maternal caloric intake or decreases in physical activity can attenuate the weight loss effects of lactation.[77]

Bonding

Breastfeeding is often mentioned as a facilitator of mother-infant bonding[78] and bonding is reported by women as a reason for breastfeeding.[79] Although potential hormonal and social mechanisms exist that may promote bonding, a systematic review by Jansen and colleagues[80] found that the empirical evidence is limited. Subsequently, evidence for a biologic link between breastfeeding and bonding is emerging. Higher brain responses to their own infants' cry and more sensitive behavior were exhibited by breastfeeding mothers than by formula-feeding mothers.[81]

Lactational amenorrhea

Breastfeeding exclusively has the natural effect of suppressing ovulation, thereby acting as a natural birth control for up to 6 months (or as long as the woman is exclusively breastfeeding and her menses have not returned).[72] Lactation must be used with caution for family planning among women to do not breastfeed exclusively or only do so for a brief period.

Long-Term Maternal Benefits of Breastfeeding

Diabetes, metabolic, and cardiovascular risk

Pregnancy is associated with changes in glucose and lipid metabolism that support the growing fetus; however, these changes can be deleterious to the mother's health. Breastfeeding, on the other hand, is associated with favorable metabolic changes. The "Reset Hypothesis"[77] proposes that the favorable metabolic changes in lactation persist after weaning, resulting in the observed long-term decreases in chronic disease risk among women who have breastfed. All of the current evidence for this comes from observational studies, so confounding and selection bias cannot be ruled out.

Pregnancy is an insulin-resistant state, which results from the effects on the mother of placental hormones with anti-insulin effects. These metabolic changes can cause gestational diabetes, and may increase the risk of type 2 diabetes later in life. Conversely, during lactation, insulin-sensitivity improves and may have lasting effects[77] because a 4% to 12% reduction in the risk of type 2 diabetes was observed for every 12 months of lifetime lactation.[82] Breastfeeding intensity may also be also important because a 50% higher risk of developing type 2 diabetes was observed among women who never exclusively breastfed compared with those who exclusively breastfed for 1 to 3 months.[83]

Pregnancy is also a hyperlipidemic state, with increased concentrations of blood cholesterol and triglycerides; conversely, lactation promotes favorable effects on maternal blood lipids.[77] Research has found that lactation is associated with lower risk of longer-term metabolic risk factors and cardiovascular disease.[84,85] Women who breastfed their children have been less likely to have developed hypertension, diabetes, hyperlipidemia, and cardiovascular disease when controlling for multiple important socio-demographic and lifestyle variables.[84] Conversely, some studies have found no association of breastfeeding and disease risk.[86] A systematic review is warranted to assess the totality of this growing literature.

Reproductive cancers

A decrease in risk for reproductive cancers has been observed among women who have breastfed, possibly due to their reduced lifetime exposure to hormones such as estrogen. According to a 2002 meta-analysis, women with breast cancer were less likely to have breastfed, and they had a shorter average lifetime duration of breastfeeding than did women who had not developed this disease.[87] Furthermore, the risk of breast cancer decreased by 4.3% for each year of breastfeeding, which indicates that longer breast-feeding duration may increase protection against breast cancer. In another meta-analysis, there was a 28% lower risk of developing ovarian cancer among women who breastfed for at least 12 months compared with women who never breastfed.[41]

Together, the evidence of effects of breastfeeding on maternal health suggest that breastfeeding protects the mother from many short- and long-term health problems, and that breastfeeding exclusively and for longer durations results in the most optimal maternal health.

SUMMARY

As this overview makes clear, there is persuasive evidence available to support recommendations by the health authorities[2,3,88] and to support national goals for breastfeeding duration. These recommendations and goals treat breastfeeding as the optimal way to feed infants during their first year of life, along with the timely addition of complementary foods. Moreover, there is a growing body of evidence that supports breastfeeding as a way to improve a woman's health after pregnancy because it may help her to return to a normal metabolic profile and to lose the weight she gained during pregnancy — among other benefits. Indeed "breast is best!" for mothers as well as their babies.

REFERENCES

1. Centers for Disease Control, Prevention. Breastfeeding report card—United states 2011. Atlanta (GA): Centers for Disease Control and Prevention; 2011. Available at: www.cdc.gov/breastfeeding/pdf/2011breastfeedingreportcard.pdf. Accessed August 8, 2012.
2. Eidelman AI, Schanler RJ, Johnston M, et al. Breastfeeding and the use of human milk. Pediatrics 2012;129(3):e827–41.
3. US Department of Health and Human Services. Healthy People 2020. Washington, DC. Available at: www.healthypeople.gov/2020/topicsobjectives2020/objectiveslist.aspx?topicid=26. Accessed August 8, 2012.
4. Dennis CL. Breastfeeding initiation and duration: a 1990–2000 literature review. J Obstet Gynecol Neonatal Nurs 2002;31(1):12–32.
5. Thulier D, Mercer J. Variables associated with breastfeeding duration. J Obstet Gynecol Neonatal Nurs 2009;38(3):259–68.
6. Meedya S, Fahy K, Kable A. Factors that positively influence breastfeeding duration to 6 months: a literature review. Women Birth 2010;23(4):135–45.
7. Gibson-Davis CM, Brooks-Gunn J. Couples' immigration status and ethnicity as determinants of breastfeeding. Am J Public Health 2006;96(4):641–6.
8. Li R, Darling N, Maurice E, et al. Breastfeeding rates in the United States by characteristics of the child, mother, or family: the 2002 National Immunization Survey. Pediatrics 2005;115(1):31–7.
9. Rutishauser IH, Carlin JB. Body mass index and duration of breast feeding: a survival analysis during the first six months of life. J Epidemiol Community Health 1992;46(6):559–65.

10. Rasmussen KM. Association of maternal obesity before conception with poor lactation performance. Annu Rev Nutr 2007;27(1):103–21.
11. Amir LH, Donath S. A systematic review of maternal obesity and breastfeeding intention, initiation and duration. BMC Pregnancy Childbirth 2007;7(1):9 PMCID: 1937008.
12. Kugyelka JG, Rasmussen KM, Frongillo EA. Maternal obesity is negatively associated with breastfeeding success among Hispanic but not Black women. J Nutr 2004;134(7):1746–53.
13. Donath SM, Amir LH. The relationship between maternal smoking and breastfeeding duration after adjustment for maternal infant feeding intention. Acta Paediatr 2004;93(11):1514–8.
14. Hopkinson JM, Schanler RJ, Fraley JK, et al. Milk production by mothers of premature infants: influence of cigarette smoking. Pediatrics 1992;90(6):934–8.
15. Blyth R, Creedy D, Dennis C, et al. Effect of maternal confidence on breastfeeding duration: an application of breastfeeding self-efficacy theory. Birth 2002; 29(4):278–84.
16. O'Campo P, Faden RR, Gielen AC, et al. Prenatal factors associated with breastfeeding duration: recommendations for prenatal interventions. Birth 1992;19(4):195–201.
17. Murray EK, Ricketts S, Dellaport J. Hospital practices that increase breastfeeding duration: results from a population-based study. Birth 2007;34(3):202–11.
18. Philipp BL, Merewood A. The baby-friendly way: the best breastfeeding start. Pediatr Clin North Am 2004;51(3):761–83.
19. Taveras EM, Li R, Grummer-Strawn L, et al. Opinions and practices of clinicians associated with continuation of exclusive breastfeeding. Pediatrics 2004;113(4): 283–90.
20. Wen LM, Simpson JM, Rissel C, et al. Awareness of breastfeeding recommendations and duration of breastfeeding: findings from the Healthy Beginnings Trial. Breastfeed Med 2012;7:223–9.
21. Ryan AS, Zhou W, Arensberg MB. The effect of employment status on breastfeeding in the United States. Womens Health Issues 2006;16(5):243–51.
22. Fein SB, Mandal B, Roe BE. Success of strategies for combining employment and breastfeeding. Pediatrics 2008;122(Suppl 2):s56–62.
23. Britton C, McCormick FM, Renfrew MJ, et al. Support for breastfeeding mothers. Cochrane Database Syst Rev 2007;(1):CD001141.
24. Goldman AS. Evolution of immune functions of the mammary gland and protection of the infant. Breastfeed Med 2012;7(3):132–42.
25. Goldman AS. Modulation of the gastrointestinal tract of infants by human milk. Interfaces and interactions. An evolutionary perspective. J Nutr 2000;130(Suppl 2): 426s–31s.
26. Brandtzaeg P. Mucosal immunity: integration between mother and the breast-fed infant. Vaccine 2003;21(24):3382–8.
27. Newburg DS, Walker WA. Protection of the neonate by the innate immune system of developing gut and of human milk. Pediatr Res 2007;61(1):2–8.
28. Chirico G, Marzollo R, Cortinovis S, et al. Antiinfective properties of human milk. J Nutr 2008;138(9):1801s–6s.
29. Isolauri E. Development of healthy gut microbiota early in life. J Paediatr Child Health 2012;48(Suppl 3):1–6.
30. Newburg DS, Ruiz-Palacios GM, Morrow AL. Human milk glycans protect infants against enteric pathogens. Annu Rev Nutr 2005;25(1):37–58.
31. Kau AL, Ahern PP, Griffin NW, et al. Human nutrition, the gut microbiome and the immune system. Nature 2011;474(7351):327–36.

32. Isaacs CE. Antimicrobial lipids in milk. In: Thormar H, editor. Lipids and essential oils as antimicrobial agents. Chichester (West Sussex): Wiley; 2011. p. 81–97.
33. Schroten H, Bosch M, Nobis-Bosch R, et al. Anti-infectious properties of the human milk fat globule. In: Newburg D, editor. Bioactive components of human milk. New York: Plenum Publishers; 2001. p. 189–92.
34. Savino F, Liguori SA. Update on breast milk hormones: leptin, ghrelin and adiponectin. Clin Nutr 2008;27(1):42–7.
35. Karatas Z, Durmus Aydogdu S, Dinleyici EC, et al. Breastmilk ghrelin, leptin, and fat levels changing foremilk to hindmilk: Is that important for self-control of feeding? Eur J Pediatr 2011;170(10):1273–80.
36. Li R, Grummer-Strawn LM, Fein SB. Do infants fed from bottles lack self-regulation of milk intake compared with directly breastfed infants? Pediatrics 2010;125(6):e1386–93.
37. Bartick M, Reinhold A. The burden of suboptimal breastfeeding in the United States: a pediatric cost analysis. Pediatrics 2010;125(5):e1048–56.
38. Ball TM, Wright AL. Health care costs of formula-feeding in the first year of life. Pediatrics 1999;103(4):870–6.
39. Kramer MS, Chalmers B, Hodnett ED, et al. Promotion of Breastfeeding Intervention Trial (PROBIT): a randomized trial in the Republic of Belarus. JAMA 2001; 285(4):413–20.
40. Singleton RJ, Holman RC, Folkema AM, et al. Trends in lower respiratory tract infection hospitalizations among American Indian/Alaska Native children and the general US child population. J Pediatr 2012;161(2):296–302.e2.
41. Ip S, Chung M, Raman G, et al. A summary of the agency for healthcare research and quality's evidence report on breastfeeding in developed countries. Breastfeed Med 2009;4(1):S17–30.
42. Chien PF, Howie PW. Breast milk and the risk of opportunistic infection in infancy in industrialized and non-industrialized settings. Adv Nutr Res 2001; 10:69–104.
43. Bachrach VR, Schwarz E, Bachrach LR. Breastfeeding and the risk of hospitalization for respiratory disease in infancy: a meta-analysis. Arch Pediatr Adolesc Med 2003;157(3):237–43.
44. Duijts L, Jaddoe VW, Hofman A, et al. Prolonged and exclusive breastfeeding reduces the risk of infectious diseases in infancy. Pediatrics 2010;126(1):e18–25.
45. Kramer MS, Guo T, Platt RW, et al. Infant growth and health outcomes associated with 3 compared with 6 mo of exclusive breastfeeding. Am J Clin Nutr 2003;78(2):291–5.
46. Der G, David BG, Deary IJ. Effect of breast feeding on intelligence in children: prospective study, sibling pairs analysis, and meta-analysis. BMJ 2006; 333(7575):945.
47. Kramer MS, Aboud F, Mironova E, et al. Breastfeeding and child cognitive development: new evidence from a large randomized trial. Arch Gen Psychiatry 2008; 65(5):578–84.
48. Task Force on Sudden Infant Death Syndrome. SIDS and other sleep-related infant deaths: expansion of recommendations for a safe infant sleeping environment. Pediatrics 2011;128(5):e1341–67.
49. Heron M. Deaths: leading causes for 2004. National Vital Statistics Reports; vol56, no5. Hyattsville (MD): National Center for Health Statistics; 2007.
50. Vennemann MM, Brinkmann B, Yucesan K, et al. Does breastfeeding reduce the risk of sudden infant death syndrome? Pediatrics 2009;123(3):e406–10.
51. Hauck FR, Thompson JM, Tanabe KO, et al. Breastfeeding and reduced risk of sudden infant death syndrome: a meta-analysis. Pediatrics 2011;128(1):103–10.

52. Horne RS, Parslow PM, Harding R. Respiratory control and arousal in sleeping infants. Paediatr Respir Rev 2004;5(3):190–8.
53. Kramer MS, Matush L, Vanilovich I, et al. Effect of prolonged and exclusive breast feeding on risk of allergy and asthma: cluster randomised trial. BMJ 2007; 335(7624):815.
54. Mimouni Bloch A, Mimouni D, Mimouni M, et al. Does breastfeeding protect against allergic rhinitis during childhood? A meta-analysis of prospective studies. Acta Paediatr 2002;91(3):275–9.
55. Gdalevich M, Mimouni D, David M, et al. Breast-feeding and the onset of atopic dermatitis in childhood: a systematic review and meta-analysis of prospective studies. J Am Acad Dermatol 2001;45(4):520–7.
56. Sears M, Greene J, Willan A, et al. Long-term relation between breastfeeding and development of atopy and asthma in children and young adults: a longitudinal study. Lancet 2002;360(9337):901–7.
57. Wegienka G, Ownby D, Havstad S, et al. Breastfeeding history and childhood allergic status in a prospective birth cohort. Ann Allergy Asthma Immunol 2006; 97(1):78–83.
58. Kwan M, Buffler P, Abrams B, et al. Breastfeeding and the risk of childhood leukemia: a meta-analysis. Public Health Rep 2004;119(6):521–35.
59. Singhal A, Lanigan J. Breastfeeding, early growth and later obesity. Obes Rev 2007;8(Suppl 1):51–4.
60. Kramer MS, Matush L, Vanilovich I, et al. Effects of prolonged and exclusive breast-feeding on child height, weight, adiposity, and blood pressure at age 6.5 y: evidence from a large randomized trial. Am J Clin Nutr 2007;86(6):1717–21.
61. Ogden CL, Carroll MD, Kit BK, et al. Prevalence of obesity and trends in body mass index among us children and adolescents, 1999-2010. JAMA 2012; 307(5):483–90.
62. Owen CG, Martin RM, Whincup PH, et al. Effect of infant feeding on the risk of obesity across the life course: a quantitative review of published evidence. Pediatrics 2005;115(5):1367–77.
63. Arenz S, Ruckerl R, Koletzko B, et al. Breast-feeding and childhood obesity—a systematic review. Int J Obes Relat Metab Disord 2004;28(10):1247–56.
64. Harder T, Bergmann R, Kallischnigg G, et al. Duration of breastfeeding and risk of overweight: a meta-analysis. Am J Epidemiol 2005;162(5):397–403.
65. Owen CG, Martin RM, Whincup PH, et al. The effect of breastfeeding on mean body mass index throughout life: a quantitative review of published and unpublished observational evidence. Am J Clin Nutr 2005;82(6):1298–307.
66. Beyerlein A, Von Kries R, Toschke AM. Breastfeeding and childhood obesity: shift of the entire BMI distribution or only the upper parts? Obesity 2008;16(12): 2730–3.
67. Baker JL, Michaelsen KF, Rasmussen KM, et al. Maternal prepregnant body mass index, duration of breastfeeding, and timing of complementary food introduction are associated with infant weight gain. Am J Clin Nutr 2004;80(6):1579–88.
68. Li C, Kaur H, Choi WS, et al. Additive interactions of maternal prepregnancy BMI and breast-feeding on childhood overweight. Obes Res 2005;13(2):362–71.
69. Rasmussen KM, Dieterich CM, Zelek ST, et al. Interventions to increase the duration of breastfeeding in obese mothers: the Bassett improving breastfeeding study. Breastfeed Med 2011;6(2):69–75.
70. Owen CG, Martin RM, Whincup PH, et al. Does breastfeeding influence risk of type 2 diabetes in later life? A quantitative analysis of published evidence. Am J Clin Nutr 2006;84(5):1043–54.

71. Owen CG, Whincup PH, Cook DG. Symposium II: infant and childhood nutrition and disease: breast-feeding and cardiovascular risk factors and outcomes in later life: evidence from epidemiological studies. Proc Nutr Soc 2011;70(4): 478–84.

72. Godfrey JR, Lawrence RA. Toward optimal health: the maternal benefits of breast-feeding. J Womens Health 2010;19(9):1597–602.

73. Wolfe WS, Sobal J, Olson CM, et al. Parity-associated weight gain and its modification by sociodemographic and behavioral factors: a prospective analysis in US women. Int J Obes Relat Metab Disord 1997;21(9):802–10.

74. Villamor E, Cnattingius S. Interpregnancy weight change and risk of adverse pregnancy outcomes: a population-based study. Lancet 2006;368(9542): 1164–70.

75. Dewey KG, Heinig MJ, Nommsen LA. Maternal weight-loss patterns during prolonged lactation. Am J Clin Nutr 1993;58(2):162–6.

76. Baker JL, Gamborg M, Heitmann BL, et al. Breastfeeding reduces postpartum weight retention. Am J Clin Nutr 2008;88(6):1543–51.

77. Stuebe AM, Rich-Edwards JW. The reset hypothesis: lactation and maternal metabolism. Am J Perinatol 2009;26(1):81–8.

78. Leung AK, Sauve RS. Breast is best for babies. J Natl Med Assoc 2005;97(7): 1010–9.

79. Arora S, McJunkin C, Wehrer J, et al. Major factors influencing breastfeeding rates: mother's perception of father's attitude and milk supply. Pediatrics 2000; 106(5):e67.

80. Jansen J, de Weerth C, Riksen-Walraven JM. Breastfeeding and the mother-infant relationship—a review. Dev Rev 2008;28(4):503–21.

81. Kim P, Feldman R, Mayes LC, et al. Breastfeeding, brain activation to own infant cry, and maternal sensitivity. J Child Psychol Psychiatry 2011;52(8):907–15.

82. Stuebe AM, Rich-Edwards JW, Willett WC, et al. Duration of lactation and incidence of type 2 diabetes. JAMA 2005;294(20):2601–10.

83. Schwarz EB, Brown JS, Creasman JM, et al. Lactation and maternal risk of type 2 diabetes: a population-based study. Am J Med 2010;123(9):863–6.

84. Schwarz EB, Ray RM, Stuebe AM, et al. Duration of lactation and risk factors for maternal cardiovascular disease. Obstet Gynecol 2009;113(5):974–82.

85. Natland ST, Nilsen TIL, Midthjell K, et al. Lactation and cardiovascular risk factors in mothers in a population-based study: the HUNT-study. Int Breastfeed J 2012;7:8.

86. Stuebe A, Kleinman K, Gillman MW, et al. Duration of lactation and maternal metabolism at 3 years postpartum. J Womens Health 2010;19(5):941–50.

87. Collaborative Group on Hormonal Factors in Breast Cancer. Breast cancer and breastfeeding: collaborative reanalysis of individual data from 47 epidemiological studies in 30 countries, including 50,302 women with breast cancer and 96,973 women without the disease. Lancet 2002;360(9328):187–95.

88. World Health Organization. Global strategy for infant and young child feeding. Geneva (Switzerland): WHO and UNICEF; 2003.

Human Milk Composition
Nutrients and Bioactive Factors

Olivia Ballard, JD[a],*, Ardythe L. Morrow, PhD, MSc[b]

KEYWORDS

- Human milk composition • Breastfeeding • Infant nutrition • Pasteurization
- Bioactive factors

KEY POINTS

- Human milk composition provides the standard for human infant nutrition, including the bioactive components that safeguard infant growth and development.
- The composition of human milk is variable within feeds, diurnally, over lactation, and between mothers and populations. This variability has benefits for infant health and survival, but for high-risk infants requiring close nutritional oversight, strategies for managing the variability of human milk feeds are needed.
- The composition of human milk can be altered with treatment of expressed milk, including its storage and pasteurization. Therefore, attention to management of expressed milk is important.

INTRODUCTION

Exclusive human milk feeding for the first 6 months of life, with continued breastfeeding for 1 to 2 years of life or longer, is recognized as the normative standard for infant feeding.[1,2] Human milk is uniquely suited to the human infant, both in its nutritional composition and in the nonnutritive bioactive factors that promote survival and healthy development.[3] This article briefly reviews the nutritional composition of human milk

Disclosures: Dr Morrow has grant funding from Mead Johnson Nutrition, Inc. to study the composition of human milk. This work was supported in part by grants to Dr Morrow from the National Institute of Child Health and Human Development (P01 HD 13021 "The role of human milk in infant nutrition and health") to study bioactive factors in human milk and from Mead Johnson Nutrition, Inc to conduct a comprehensive study of human milk factors ("The Global Exploration of Human Milk [GEHM] Study").
a Division of Immunobiology, Center for Interdisciplinary Research in Human Milk and Lactation, Cincinnati Children's Hospital Medical Center, 3333 Burnet Avenue, MLC 7009, Cincinnati, OH 45229, USA; b Center for Interdisciplinary Research in Human Milk and Lactation, Perinatal Institute, Cincinnati Children's Hospital Medical Center, 3333 Burnet Avenue, MLC 7009, Cincinnati, OH 45229, USA
* Corresponding author.
E-mail address: Olivia.Ballard@cchmc.org

and provides an overview of its varied bioactive factors, which include cells, anti-infectious and anti-inflammatory agents, growth factors, and prebiotics. Unlike infant formula, which is standardized within a very narrow range of composition, human milk composition is dynamic, and varies within a feeding, diurnally, over lactation, and between mothers and populations. Influences on compositional differences of human milk include maternal and environmental factors and the expression and management of milk (eg, its storage and pasteurization). Understanding human milk composition provides an important tool for the management of infant feeding, particularly of fragile, high-risk infants, and for understanding the potential impact of storage and pasteurization on milk components. Furthermore, some bioactive components found in human milk are being developed and tested for potential medical applications as prophylactic or therapeutic agents.

STAGES OF LACTATION

The first fluid produced by mothers after delivery is colostrum, which is distinct in volume, appearance, and composition. Colostrum, produced in low quantities in the first few days postpartum, is rich in immunologic components such as secretory immunoglobulin (Ig)A, lactoferrin, leukocytes, and developmental factors such as epidermal growth factor (EGF).[4–6] Colostrum also contains relatively low concentrations of lactose, indicating its primary functions to be immunologic and trophic rather than nutritional. Levels of sodium, chloride, and magnesium are higher and levels of potassium and calcium are lower in colostrum than in later milk.[5,6] As tight junction closure occurs in the mammary epithelium, the sodium to potassium ratio declines and lactose concentration increases, indicating secretory activation and the production of transitional milk. The timing of secretory activation (lactogenesis stage II) varies among women, but typically occurs over the first few days postpartum. Delayed onset of lactogenesis, defined as onset greater than 72 hours after delivery, appears to occur more often with preterm delivery and maternal obesity and may be predicted by markers of metabolic health.[7,8] Biochemical markers in early milk for onset of secretory activation include its sodium content, the sodium to potassium ratio, citrate, and lactose.[9]

Transitional milk shares some of the characteristics of colostrum but represents a period of "ramped up" milk production to support the nutritional and developmental needs of the rapidly growing infant, and typically occurs from 5 days to 2 weeks postpartum, after which milk is considered largely mature. By 4 to 6 weeks postpartum, human milk is considered fully mature. In contrast to the dramatic shift in composition observed in the first month of life, human milk remains relatively similar in composition, although subtle changes in milk composition do occur over the course of lactation.

STUDIES OF HUMAN MILK COMPOSITION

A Medline search using only the phrase "human milk composition" reveals a steady increase in publications since the 1960s, with new components still being identified in human milk and the functionality of those components under active investigation in many laboratories worldwide. Many studies of human milk composition have been conducted in diverse populations using varied collection, storage, and testing methods. The gold standard of milk collection involves sampling of all milk expressed over 24 hours, with collection on multiple occasions from the same individuals over time.[10,11] This method, however, can be costly, limiting the number of participants. Alternatively, studies of milk composition can standardize collection at a specific time of day (eg, morning) by emptying the entire breast, avoiding collection from a breast that was used for nursing within the past 2 to 3 hours, with collection on multiple occasions from the same individuals over time.[12] However, most published studies involve nonstandardized collection from donors to milk banks whose milk is collected at different times of day, at different timings within a feed, or at diverse stages of lactation. Studies of human milk composition also vary in their attention to storage or treatment conditions, such as the number of freeze-thaw cycles, duration of storage, or pasteurization, which may sometimes explain differing study results.

NUTRITIONAL COMPONENTS OF HUMAN MILK

The nutritional components of human milk derive from 3 sources: some of the nutrients of milk originate by synthesis in the lactocyte, some are dietary in origin, and some originate from maternal stores. Overall the nutritional quality of human milk is highly conserved, but attention to maternal diet is important for some vitamins and the fatty acid composition of human milk (see article elsewhere in this issue by Valentine and Wagner).

Macronutrients

The macronutrient composition of human milk varies within mothers and across lactation but is remarkably conserved across populations despite variations in maternal nutritional status.[13] As shown in **Table 1**, the mean macronutrient composition of mature, term milk is estimated to be approximately 0.9 to 1.2 g/dL for protein, 3.2 to 3.6 g/dL for fat, and 6.7 to 7.8 g/dL for lactose. Energy estimates range from 65 to 70 kcal/dL, and are highly correlated with the fat content of human milk. Macronutrient composition differs between preterm and term milk, with preterm milk tending to be higher in protein and fat (see **Table 1**). A study in Davis, California examined the association between maternal characteristics and the composition of human milk macronutrients[10] and found that after 4 months postpartum, the macronutrient concentrations of human milk are associated with 1 or more of the following factors: maternal body weight for height, protein intake, parity, return of menstruation, and nursing frequency. This study also found that mothers who produce higher quantities of milk tend to have lower milk concentrations of fat and protein but higher concentrations of lactose.

The proteins of human milk are divided into the whey and casein fractions or complexes, each comprising a remarkable array of specific proteins and peptides.[14,15] The most abundant proteins are casein, α-lactalbumin, lactoferrin, secretory IgA (sIgA), lysozyme, and serum albumin.[16,17] Nonprotein nitrogen-containing compounds, including urea, uric acid, creatine, creatinine, amino acids, and nucleotides, comprise approximately 25% of human milk nitrogen. The protein content of milk obtained from mothers who deliver preterm is significantly higher than that of mothers who deliver at term (see **Table 1**). Protein levels decrease in human milk over the first 4 to 6 weeks or more of life regardless of timing of delivery (**Fig. 1**).[11] For feeding preterm infants, the lower level of total protein and specific amino acids from donor (typically, term, late lactation) milk alone is limiting, and requires additional supplementation (see article elsewhere in this issue by Underwood).[18] Concentration of human milk protein is not affected by maternal diet, but increases with maternal body weight for height, and decreases in mothers producing higher amounts of milk.[10]

Human milk fat is characterized by high contents of palmitic and oleic acids, the former heavily concentrated in the 2-position and the latter in the 1- and 3-positions of the triglycerides. Fat is the most highly variable macronutrient of milk. Hindmilk, defined as the last milk of a feed, may contain 2 to 3 times the concentration of milk

Table 1
Macronutrient (g/dL) and energy (kcal/dL) composition of human milk from specified references

Authors[Ref.] (year), N	Protein Mean (±2 SD)	Fat Mean (±2 SD)	Lactose Mean (±2 SD)	Energy Mean (±2 SD)
Term infants, 24-h collection, mature milk				
Nommsen et al[10,a] (1991), N = 58	1.2 (0.9, 1.5)	3.6 (2.2, 5.0)	7.4 (7.2, 7.7)	70 (57, 83)
Donor human milk samples				
Wojcik et al[167,b] (2009), N = 415	1.2 (0.7, 1.7)	3.2 (1.2, 5.2)	7.8 (6.0, 9.6)	65 (43, 87)
Michaelsen et al[26,c] (1990), N = 2553	0.9 (0.6, 1.4)[d]	3.6 (1.8, 8.9)[d]	7.2 (6.4, 7.6)[d]	67 (50,115)[d]
Representative values of mature milk, term infants				
Reference standard[e]	0.9	3.5	6.7	65 to 70
Preterm, 24-h collection, first 8 wk of life				
Bauer and Gerss[11,f] (2011)				
Born <29 wk, n = 52	2.2 (1.3, 3.3)	4.4 (2.6, 6.2)	7.6 (6.4, 8.8)	78 (61, 94)
Born 32–33 wk, n = 20	1.9 (1.3, 2.5)	4.8 (2.8, 6.8)	7.5 (6.5, 8.5)	77 (64, 89)
Preterm donor milk				
Landers and Hartmann[g] (2012), N = 47	1.4 (0.8, 1.9)	4.2 (2.4, 5.9)	6.7 (5.5, 7.9)	70 (53, 87)

[a] Davis, California: mothers at 3 months postpartum.
[b] United States milk bank donors.
[c] Danish milk bank donors.
[d] Median (lower 2.5 percentile, upper 97.5 percentile).
[e] Based on expert review: *Pediatric Nutrition Handbook*, 6th edition, Table C-1, p. 1201 (mature milk).
[f] Preterm infants 23 to 33 weeks' gestational age.
[g] Australian donor mothers of preterm infants (see article elsewhere this issue by Landers and Hartmann).

fat found in foremilk, defined as the initial milk of a feed.[19] A study of milk from 71 mothers over a 24-hour period found that the milk fat content was significantly lower in night and morning feedings compared with afternoon or evening feedings.[20] Another study found that approximately 25% of the variation in lipid concentration between mothers' milk may be explained by maternal protein intake.[10]

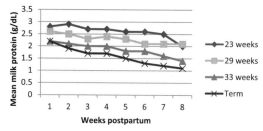

Fig. 1. Milk protein concentrations, comparing milk from mothers who delivered preterm and term, by gestational age at delivery and weeks postpartum. (*Data from* Bauer J, Gerss J. Longitudinal analysis of macronutrients and minerals in human milk produced by mothers of preterm infants. Clin Nutr 2011;30(2):215–20.)

The fatty acid profile of human milk varies in relation to maternal diet, particularly in the long-chain polyunsaturated fatty acids (LCPUFAs). LCPUFA intake in the Western world is skewed toward the ω-6 fatty acids, with suboptimal intake of ω-3 fatty acids. The docosahexaenoic acid (DHA) composition of human milk is particularly low in North American populations; supplementation should be considered for breastfeeding North American women with DHA-limited diets.[18,21,22]

The principal sugar of human milk is the disaccharide lactose. The concentration of lactose in human milk is the least variable of the macronutrients, but higher concentrations of lactose are found in the milk of mothers producing higher quantities of milk.[10] The other significant carbohydrates of human milk are the oligosaccharides, which comprise approximately 1 g/dL in human milk, depending on stage of lactation and maternal genetic factors.[23–25] The oligosaccharides are among the nonnutritive bioactive factors discussed later.

The mean values for macronutrients provided here, while valid, belie the observed variability of individual milk samples, particularly in their fat and protein content. Individual donor milk samples from term mothers range at least from 0.6 to 1.4 g/dL for total protein, 1.8 to 8.9 g/dL for fat, 6.4 to 7.6 g/dL for lactose, and 50 to 115 kcal/dL for energy.[26] Furthermore, the typical composition of preterm milk differs from that of term milk (see **Table 1**). Thus, nutritional management of high-risk infants using human milk requires individualized, adaptive or targeted, strategies for fortification, based on measurement of milk composition and growth monitoring.[27]

Micronutrients

Human milk provides the normative standard for infant nutrition. Nevertheless, many micronutrients vary in human milk depending on maternal diet and body stores (see article elsewhere in this issue by Valentine and Wagner), including vitamins A, B1, B2, B6, B12, D, and iodine. The maternal diet is not always optimal, so continuing multivitamins during lactation is recommended.[28,29] Regardless of maternal diet, Vitamin K is extremely low in human milk and thus, the American Academy of Pediatrics recommends an injection of this vitamin to avoid hemorrhagic disease of the newborn.[28] Vitamin D also occurs in low quantity in human milk, particularly with low maternal exposure to sunshine, a circumstance now common in populations worldwide.[30] While the impact of maternal supplementation with vitamin D on milk composition is under investigation, current pediatric recommendations target postnatal vitamin D supplementation of breastfed infants. Detailed review of the micronutrient composition of human milk is not possible here, but reviews and composition tables are available elsewhere.[28,29,31]

BIOACTIVE COMPONENTS AND THEIR SOURCES

Bioactive components of food are defined as elements that "affect biological processes or substrates and hence have an impact on body function or condition and ultimately health."[32] Bioactive components in human milk come from a variety of sources; some are produced and secreted by the mammary epithelium, some are produced by cells carried within the milk,[33] whereas others are drawn from maternal serum and carried across the mammary epithelium by receptor-mediated transport. Furthermore, the secretion of the milk fat globule (MFG) into milk by the mammary epithelium carries with it a diverse collection of membrane-bound proteins and lipids into the milk.[34] Together these methods produce the variety of bioactive components in human milk. For example, in lactating women, antigen-specific B cells home to the mammary gland, where polymeric immunoglobulin receptors (pIgR) transport sIgA into the lumen of the duct.[35] An alternative example is vascular endothelial growth factor (VEGF), which is found at concentrations significantly higher in milk than in maternal serum, indicating a mammary gland source.[36,37] Understanding the sources of bioactive components of milk also helps to explain the variability in milk concentrations that are observed following maternal use of specific medications (see article elsewhere in this issue by Rowe and colleagues).

What are the clinical implications of research on bioactive factors in human milk? The depth of scientific evidence is such that in patient or public education, it is valid to clarify that human milk is not "merely nutrition." Rather, human milk contains a variety of factors with medicinal qualities that have a profound role in infant survival and health. Thus, safe donor milk substitutes are needed for infants at medical risk when a mother's own milk is not available. Proteomic analysis has discovered thematic distinctions in the proteins that compose milk at differing stages of lactation, as well as differences between term and preterm milks.[14,15] These studies suggest that when donor milk is needed, it should be matched to the developmental stage of the infant whenever feasible, although this is often difficult in practice. Furthermore, recognition of potent, bioactive human milk factors indicates the importance of preserving their biological activity, to the extent possible, through the process of milk collection, storage, and pasteurization. Finally, recognition of the unique mechanisms by which human milk protects and enhances development provides models for new preventive and therapeutic approaches in medicine.

A complete characterization of bioactive factors of human milk is beyond the scope of this review. Here the focus is on a selected set of bioactive factors that vary between mothers of term and preterm infants, or over the course of lactation, and thus represent responsiveness to the changing needs of the infant (**Table 2**). Many of these factors act synergistically, such that consumption of human milk is superior to supplementation with individual factors or their combinations.[38]

GROWTH FACTORS

Human milk contains numerous growth factors that have wide-ranging effects on the intestinal tract, vasculature, nervous system, and endocrine system.

Intestinal Maturation and Repair: Epidermal Growth Factor

Found in both amniotic fluid and breast milk,[38–40] EGF is critical to the maturation and healing of the intestinal mucosa. EGF is resistant to low pH and digestive enzymes, allowing it to pass through the stomach to the intestine, where it stimulates the enterocyte to increase DNA synthesis, cell division, absorbance of water and glucose, and protein synthesis.[41,42] There are multiple protective mechanisms of action for EGF in the infant intestine, including inhibition of programmed cell death, and correcting alterations in intestinal and liver tight junction proteins induced by proinflammatory tumor necrosis factor (TNF)-α.[43] Heparin-binding EGF (HB-EGF) is a member of the EGF family, and the primary growth factor responsible for damage resolution following hypoxia, ischemia-reperfusion injury, hemorrhagic shock/resuscitation injury, and necrotizing enterocolitis.[44] EGF is highest in early milk and decreases over lactation.[45,46] The average EGF level in colostrum is 2000-fold higher and in mature milk is 100-fold higher than in maternal serum.[41] Furthermore, preterm milk contains higher levels of EGF than does term milk.[45,46]

Growth and Development of the Enteral Nervous System: Neuronal Growth Factors

The immaturity of the newborn intestine extends to the enteral nervous system, which requires brain-derived neurotrophic factor (BDNF) and glial cell-line derived

Table 2
Major bioactive factors in human milk

Component	Function	References
Cells		
Macrophages	Protection against infection, T-cell activation	Jarvinen,[87] 2002; Yagi,[93] 2010; Ichikawa,[99] 2003
Stem cells	Regeneration and repair	Indumathi,[90] 2012
Immunoglobulins		
IgA/sIgA	Pathogen binding inhibition	Van de Perre,[35] 2003; Cianga,[168] 1999; Brandtzaeg,[124] 2010; Kadaoui,[125] 2007; Corthésy,[126] 2009; Hurley,[127] 2011; Agarwal,[94] 2011; Castellote,[4] 2011
IgG	Antimicrobial, activation of phagocytosis (IgG1, IgG2, IgG3); anti-inflammatory, response to allergens (IgG4)	Cianga,[168] 1999; Agarwal,[94] 2011
IgM	Agglutination, complement activation	Brandtzaeg,[124] 2010; Van de Perre,[169] 1993; Agarwal,[94] 2011
Cytokines		
IL-6	Stimulation of the acute phase response, B-cell activation, proinflammatory	Ustundag,[111] 2005; Meki,[115] 2003; Mizuno,[119] 2012; Agarwal,[94] 2011; Castellote,[4] 2011
IL-7	Increased thymic size and output	Aspinall,[110] 2011; Ngom,[109] 2004
IL-8	Recruitment of neutrophils, proinflammatory	Claud,[74] 2003; Ustundag,[111] 2005; Meki,[115] 2003; Maheshwari,[116] 2002; Maheshwari,[118] 2003; Maheshwari,[117] 2004; Hunt,[120] 2012; Agarwal,[94] 2011; Castellote,[4] 2011; Mehta,[170] 2011
IL-10	Repressing Th1-type inflammation, induction of antibody production, facilitation of tolerance	Meki,[115] 2003; Agarwal,[94] 2011; Castellote,[4] 2011; Mehta,[170] 2011
IFN-γ	Proinflammatory, stimulates Th1 response	Hrdý,[121] 2012; Agarwal,[94] 2011
TGF-β	Anti-inflammatory, stimulation of T-cell phenotype switch	Penttila,[97] 2010; Kalliomäki,[98] 1999; Saito,[99] 1993; Nakamura,[100] 2009; Letterio,[101] 1994; Ando,[102] 2007; Ozawa,[103] 2009; Donnet-Hughes,[104] 2000; Verhasselt,[171] 2008; Verhasselt,[172] 2010; Penttila,[173] 2003; Mosconi,[174] 2010; Okamoto,[175] 2005; Penttila,[176] 2006; Peroni,[160] 2009; McPherson,[177] 2001; Ewaschuk,[162] 2011; Castellote,[4] 2011

(continued on next page)

Table 2
(continued)

Component	Function	References
TNF-α	Stimulates inflammatory immune activation	Rudloff,[178] 1992; Ustundag,[111] 2005; Erbağci,[114] 2005; Meki,[115] 2003; Agarwal,[94] 2011; Castellote,[4] 2011
Chemokines		
G-CSF	Trophic factor in intestines	Gilmore,[105] 1994; Gersting,[106] 2003; Calhoun,[107] 2003; Gersting,[108] 2004
MIF	Prevents macrophage movement, increases antipathogen activity of macrophages	Magi,[179] 2002; Vigh,[180] 2011
Cytokine Inhibitors		
TNFR I and II	Inhibition of TNF-α, anti-inflammatory	Buescher,[112] 1998; Buescher,[113] 1996; Meki,[115] 2003; Castellote,[4] 2011
Growth Factors		
EGF	Stimulation of cell proliferation and maturation	Patki,[37] 2012; Kobata,[36] 2008; Hirai,[38] 2002; Wagner,[40] 2008; Dvorak,[45] 2003; Dvorak,[46] 2004; Chang,[42] 2002; Khailova,[43] 2009; Coursodon,[181] 2012; Clark,[182] 2004; Castellote,[4] 2011; Untalan,[183] 2009
HB-EGF	Protective against damage from hypoxia and ischemia	Radulescu,[44] 2011
VEGF	Promotion of angiogenesis and tissue repair	Loui,[64] 2012; Ozgurtas,[184] 2011
NGF	Promotion of neuron growth and maturation	Rodrigues,[47] 2011; Boesmans,[48] 2008; Sánchez,[49] 1996; Fichter,[51] 2011
IGF	Stimulation of growth and development, increased RBCs and hemoglobin	Chellakooty,[185] 2006; Blum,[52] 2002; Burrin,[53] 1997; Philipps,[54] 2002; Milsom,[55] 2008; Prosser,[56] 1996; Elmlinger,[57] 2007; Peterson,[58] 2000; Murali,[59] 2005; Corpeleijn,[60] 2008; Baregamian,[186] 2006; Baregamian,[187] 2012; Büyükkayhan,[61] 2003; Philipps,[62] 2000; Kling,[63] 2006
Erythropoietin	Erythropoiesis, intestinal development	Carbonell-Estrany,[69] 2000; Juul,[188] 2003; Kling,[70] 2008; Miller-Gilbert,[189] 2001; Pasha,[71] 2008; Soubasi,[68] 1995; Shiou,[72] 2011; Arsenault,[73] 2010; Miller,[190] 2002; Untalan,[183] 2009

	Function	References
Hormones		
Calcitonin	Development of enteric neurons	Struck,[75] 2002; Wookey,[76] 2012
Somatostatin	Regulation of gastric epithelial growth	Rao,[77] 1999; Gama,[78] 1996
Antimicrobial		
Lactoferrin	Acute phase protein, chelates iron, antibacterial, antioxidant	Adamkin,[129] 2012; Sherman,[134] 2004; Manzoni,[133] 2009; Hirotani,[191] 2008; Buccigrossi,[192] 2007; Velona,[128] 1999
Lactadherin/MFG E8	Antiviral, prevents inflammation by enhancing phagocytosis of apoptotic cells	Stubbs,[135] 1990; Kusunoki,[140] 2012; Aziz,[138] 2011; Shi,[139] 2004; Chogle,[141] 2011; Baghdadi,[142] 2012; Peterson,[136] 1998; Newburg,[137] 1998; Shah,[193] 2012; Miksa,[194] 2006; Komura,[195] 2009; Miksa,[196] 2009; Wu,[197] 2012; Matsuda,[198] 2011; Silvestre,[199] 2005
Metabolic hormones		
Adiponectin	Reduction of infant BMI and weight, anti-inflammatory	Martin,[80] 2006; Newburg,[79] 2010; Woo,[81] 2009; Woo,[200] 2012; Ley,[201] 2011; Dundar,[202] 2010; Ozarda,[203] 2012; Savino,[83] 2008; Weyermann,[204] 2007
Leptin	Regulation of energy conversion and infant BMI, appetite regulation	Savino,[83] 2008; Savino,[82] 2012; Palou,[84] 2009; Weyermann,[204] 2007
Ghrelin	Regulation of energy conversion and infant BMI	Savino,[83] 2008; Savino,[82] 2012; Dundar,[85] 2010
Oligosaccharides & glycans		
HMOS	Prebiotic, stimulating beneficial colonization and reducing colonization with pathogens; reduced inflammation	Newburg,[23] 2005; Morrow,[24] 2005; DeLeoz,[153] 2012; Marcoba,[205] 2012; Kunz,[206] 2012; Ruhaak,[207] 2012; Bode,[152] 2012
Gangliosides	Brain development; anti-infectious	Wang B,[208] 2012
Glycosaminoglycans	Anti-infectious	Coppa,[209] 2012; Coppa,[210] 2011
Mucins		
MUC1	Blocks infection by viruses and bacteria	Ruvoen-Clouet,[146] 2006; Liu,[151] 2012; Sando,[211] 2009; Saeland,[148] 2009; Yolken,[149] 1992
MUC4	Blocks infection by viruses and bacteria	Ruvoen-Clouet,[146] 2006; Liu,[151] 2012; Chaturvedi,[212] 2008

Abbreviations: BMI, body mass index; EGF, epidermal growth factor; G-CSF, granulocyte-colony stimulating factor; HB-EGF, heparin-binding epidermal growth factor; HMOS, human milk oligosaccharides; IFN, interferon; Ig, immunoglobulin; IGF, insulin-like growth factor; IL, interleukin; MFG, milk fat globule; MIF, macrophage migratory inhibitory factor; MUC, mucin; NGF, nerve growth factor; RBCs, red blood cells; sIg, secretory Ig; TGF, transforming growth factor; Th1, T-helper cell 1; TNF, tumor necrosis factor; TNFR, tumor necrosis factor receptor; VEGF, vascular endothelial growth factor.

neurotrophic factor (GDNF) for its development.[47] BDNF can enhance peristalsis, a function frequently impaired in the preterm gut.[48] Rodents that lack GDNF display a profound loss of neurons in the enteral nervous system.[49] BDNF, GDNF, and a related protein, ciliary neurotrophic factor (CNTF), are detected in human milk up to 90 days after birth.[50,51] In human cells, breast milk–derived GDNF increases neuron survival and outgrowth.[51]

Tissue Growth: the Insulin-Like Growth Factor Superfamily

Insulin-like growth factor (IGF)-I and IGF-II, as well as IGF binding proteins and IGF-specific proteases, are found in human milk.[52–54] Levels are highest in colostrum, and steadily decline over the course of lactation.[55,56] There are no significant differences between preterm and term milk, with the exception of IGF binding protein 2, which is higher in preterm milk.[52,57] In rodents, administration of human IGF-I during surgical stress/total parental nutrition causes increased tissue growth[58] and attenuates intestinal atrophy,[59] although no human trial has been conducted.[60] IGF-1 may also play a role in the survival of enterocytes following intestinal damage from oxidative stress.[57] Breastfed infants have higher circulating IGF-I in the serum.[61] IGF can be taken up in a bioactive form by intestines and transported into the blood.[54,62] The function of absorbed IGF has not been fully detailed, but enteral administration of physiologic levels of IGF-I stimulates erythropoiesis and increases hematocrit.[63]

Regulation of the Vascular System: Vascular Endothelial Growth Factor

Angiogenesis is regulated primarily by the relative expression of VEGF and its antagonists. VEGF concentration is highest in colostrum in both preterm and term human milk, with preterm milk containing less VEGF than term milk.[64] In retinopathy of prematurity (ROP), it is thought that pulmonary immaturity, supplemental oxygen, and negative regulation of VEGF lead to dysregulated vascularization of the retina,[65,66] suggesting a mechanism by which human milk may help reduce the burden of ROP.

Intestinal Development and Prevention of Anemia: Erythropoietin

Milk contains significant quantities of erythropoietin (Epo), which is the primary hormone responsible for increasing red blood cells (RBCs). Blood loss, intestinal pathology, and immaturity of the hematopoietic system all contribute to anemia of prematurity, which profoundly affects growth and development.[67] Thus some suggest that Epo may help prevent anemia of prematurity,[68] but administration of Epo has shown mixed results.[69] Administration of Epo in conjunction with iron, however, may increase hemoglobin and hematocrit levels.[70] A small trial of enteral Epo in preterm infants showed increased serum and reticulocyte levels.[71] In addition, Epo is an important trophic factor and tightens intestinal junctions.[72] There is some evidence that Epo may help protect against mother-to-child transmission of human immunodeficiency virus (HIV),[73] and may reduce the risk of necrotizing enterocolitis.[72,74]

Growth-Regulating Hormones: Calcitonin and Somatostatin

Calcitonin and its precursor procalcitonin are present in large quantities in milk.[75] Enteric neurons express the calcitonin receptor immunoreactivity from late gestation into infancy.[76] Somatostatin is rapidly degraded in the jejunum and is not transferred through the intestinal wall, but delivery with milk protects it from degradation and maintains bioactivity within the lumen.[77] Somatostatin normally inhibits growth factors, but its role in human milk remains unclear.[78]

Regulating Metabolism and Body Composition: Adiponectin and Other Hormones

Adiponectin is a large, multifunctional hormone that actively regulates metabolism and suppresses inflammation. Found in large quantities in human milk, adiponectin can cross the intestinal barrier, and appears to modify infant metabolism.[79,80] Levels of adiponectin in milk correlate inversely with infant weight and body mass index while exclusively breastfeeding, leading to the proposal by some that adiponectin in human milk may contribute to reduced incidence of overweight and obesity in later life, although this remains to be determined.[79,81] Other metabolism-regulating hormones found in effective quantities in human milk are leptin, resistin, and ghrelin, which appear to play an important role in regulating energy conversion, body composition, and appetite control.[82-85]

IMMUNOLOGIC FACTORS

Feeding human milk protects against infection and inflammation,[86] and early milk is enriched in immune factors that help to ensure infant survival.[15] The specific protective components of human milk are so numerous and multifunctional that science is just beginning to understand their functions.

Transfer of Living Protection and Programming: Cells of Human Milk

Human milk contains a variety of cells, including macrophages, T cells, stem cells, and lymphocytes.[87-93] In early lactation, the breastfed infant may consume as many as 10^{10} maternal leukocytes per day. The relative quantity of these cells differs among mothers and is reported to differ in the milk of infants who develop allergy.[87] About 80% of the cells in early milk are breast milk macrophages, which originate as peripheral blood monocytes that exit the bloodstream and migrate into milk through the mammary epithelium. Phagocytosis of human milk components transforms these monocytes into potent breast milk macrophages with unique functional features, including the ability to differentiate into dendritic cells that stimulate infant T-cell activity.[89,93] This capability provides broadly powerful protection against pathogens while stimulating development of the infant's own immune system. In women infected with HIV-1 and human T-lymphotropic virus 1; however, the activity of these cells unfortunately enables mother-to-infant viral transmission (see article elsewhere in this issue by Lawrence). Stem cells have also been identified in human milk[88,90]; their function is under investigation.

Communication Between Cells: Cytokines and Chemokines

Cytokines are multifunctional peptides that act in an autocrine/paracrine fashion.[33] Chemokines are a special class of chemotactic cytokines that induce movement of other cells. Human milk cytokines can cross the intestinal barrier, where they "communicate" with cells to influence immune activity. While many cytokines and chemokines have multiple functions, milk-borne cytokines may be grouped broadly into those that enhance inflammation or defend against infection, and those that reduce inflammation. A complete review of the cytokines of human milk is available elsewhere.[33,94-96]

The transforming growth factor (TGF)-β family constitute the most abundant cytokines of human milk and consist of 3 isoforms, of which TGF-β2 predominates.[97-99] Milk-borne TGF-β regulates inflammation and wound repair, and helps prevent allergic diseases. TGF-β is converted to its active form by the low pH of the stomach.[100] Only 15 minutes after TGF-β1–deficient mouse pups are suckled by heterozygous dams, TGF-β1 is measurable in the pup's serum and tissue.[101] Milk TGF-β has tolerance-enhancing activity in the intestinal tract,[100,102–104] a proposed mechanism for its antiallergenic effects.

Granulocyte-colony stimulating factor (G-CSF), identified in human milk decades ago,[105] has beneficial effects on intestinal development and the treatment of sepsis. While milk-borne G-CSF survives transit through the stomach, it is not appreciably absorbed and acts at the intestinal surface,[106,107] where it increases villi, crypt depth, and cell proliferation.[108] Other regulatory cytokines found in milk are interleukin (IL)-10 and IL-7[109]; milk-borne IL-7 is known to cross the intestinal wall and influence thymic development.[110]

Proinflammatory cytokines TNF-α, IL-6, IL-8, and interferon (IFN)-γ are also found in mother's milk, generally at lower levels and decreasing over lactation.[4,111] The levels of these cytokines in milk are also associated with the timing of delivery.[4,111] Intriguingly, soluble TNF receptors I and II, which neutralize TNF-α, also are found in human milk.[112] thus, most TNF-α may be bound and not freely active in milk.[113] Both IL-8 and TNF-α are modestly increased in mature milk of mothers who have had preeclampsia.[114] Levels of TNF-α correlate positively with those of other inflammatory cytokines.[115] IL-6 is associated with systemic inflammation and fever.[115] The role of the inflammatory cytokines found in human milk remains under investigation, but they are known to be engaged in the recruitment of neutrophils and to enhance intestinal development, while IL-8 may help protect against TNF-α–mediated damage.[116–118] Higher levels of IL-6 and IL-8 occur in mastitis, with higher cytokine levels confined to only the affected lobes.[119,120] IFN-γ has also been widely studied because of its proinflammatory role; IFN-γ enhances the T-helper (Th)1/inflammation response while suppressing the Th2/allergic response.[94] The colostrum of allergic mothers contains lower IFN-γ but higher Th2 cytokines IL-4 and IL-13 compared with the colostrum of nonallergic mothers.[121]

Protection from Infection: Acquired and Innate Factors

A recent study in Nepal found a 9-fold increase in risk of diarrhea in children who were not breastfed,[122] consistent with previous global studies.[123] Infants are born with immature adaptive immunity, and rely on maternal antibodies for defense against pathogens.[124] Human milk sIgA-antigen complexes are taken up and processed by intestinal dendritic cells, which allows for antigen recognition while maintaining a noninflammatory environment.[125] While sIgA is the predominant antibody of human milk, milk also contains IgM and IgG, the latter becoming more abundant in later lactation.[15] A comprehensive review of human milk immunoglobulins is available elsewhere.[124,126,127]

A set of innate, multifunctional molecules known as defensins also provide significant protection against infection. These molecules are typically highest in colostrum, and decrease over lactation. Among the most abundant of these is lactoferrin, an iron-binding glycoprotein belonging to the transferrin family,[128,129] which is effective against many different bacteria, viruses, and fungi.[130–134] Another glycoprotein, lactadherin, was initially identified in the MFG.[135] Milk-borne lactadherin survives transit through the stomach[136] and prevents rotaviral infection in the newborn.[137] Following infection or damage, lactadherin mediates phagocytic uptake of apoptotic cells[138,139] and stimulates a signaling cascade that results in decreased inflammation via blockade of toll-like receptor 4 and nuclear factor κB signaling.[138,140] Lactadherin promotes healing during intestinal inflammation[140,141] and a tolerogenic phenotype in intestinal dendritic cells and macrophages,[138,142] which is important in maintaining gut health. Another multifunctional protein, bile salt–stimulating lipase (BSSL),[143] is a highly glycosylated enzyme that breaks down milk fats, thereby releasing their energy for infant metabolism. Milk-borne BSSL also protects infants from viral infection, including Norwalk virus and HIV. BSSL binds to dendritic cells, preventing HIV transinfection of CD4$^+$ T cells.[144,145] The bioactive region of BSSL is modified by the glycans present, which change with maternal genetics and over lactation.[143,146]

The MFG contains mucins (MUC1, MUC4, and potentially others) derived from the maternal plasma membrane.[147] These mucins are multifunctional, but most importantly protect infants from infection. For example, MUC1 blocks infection by HIV and rotavirus[148,149] and both MUC1 and MUC4 block infection by *Salmonella enterica* serovar *typhimurium* and Norwalk virus.[146,150,151]

Selection for the Growth of Beneficial Organisms: Oligosaccharides

The human milk oligosaccharides (HMOS) range from 3 to 32 sugars in size, and differ in composition from those of any other mammal.[23,24] Though nonnutritive to the infant, HMOS constitute a remarkable quantity of human milk, similar to the quantity of total protein. These structures are synthesized glycosyltransferases, enzymes that also synthesize similar structures in other human secretions and on mucosal surfaces. The HMOS are prebiotic agents that selectively encourage the growth of beneficial (probiotic) organisms. In addition, the HMOS and their protein conjugates are recognized as pathogen-binding inhibitors that function as soluble "decoy" receptors for pathogens that have an affinity for binding to oligosaccharide receptors expressed on the infant's intestinal surface. Mothers vary in the specific structures of HMOS in their milk as a result of genetic differences similar to blood group types.[23–25] This variation in HMOS composition, unlike blood group types, does not create incompatibility, so that all mothers may be considered "universal donors." Rather, the variation in HMOS composition among mothers is thought to promote human survival, as pathogens differ in their affinity for binding to specific oligosaccharides. Protection by some forms of HMOS but not others has been shown in relation to diarrhea caused by specific pathogens[23,24] and HIV.[152] The apparent differences in lactose and HMOS composition of preterm milk requires further investigation.[25,153]

It was long believed that human milk was sterile, but it is now recognized that human milk harbors a microbial community, the composition of which appears to change with maternal characteristics and over the course of lactation.[154,155] The HMOS influence intestinal colonization and may also influence the composition of the bacterial community in milk.

IMPACT OF STORAGE AND PASTEURIZATION ON MILK COMPONENTS

Increasingly, human milk feeding occurs apart from feeding at the mother's breast. Most lactating women in North America now express and store their milk at some time.[156] Varying degrees of nutrient loss occurs, depending on the nutrient and the storage methods. For vitamin C loss occurs rapidly, even during the process of feeding freshly expressed human milk by bottle.[155] For multiple human milk components, however, significant degradation may occur only with long-term storage and freeze-thaw cycles, which tend to reduce bactericidal capacity. The Academy of Breastfeeding Medicine protocol for home storage of human milk can be used to guide mothers in these activities to optimize the integrity of expressed and stored milk (see article elsewhere in this issue by Chantry and Howard).

Another major movement has been the development of milk sharing via donor human milk banks or alternatively via Internet milk sharing (see article elsewhere in this issue by Landers and Hartmann). Because of the perceived risk of transmitting pathogens via human milk, a variety of protocols have been developed for pasteurization of donor milk, including: high-temperature short-time (HTST) heating (72°C for

15 seconds); Holder pasteurization (62.5°C for 30 minutes, a low-temperature long-time [LTLT] method); and flash heating (a low-tech HTST method that involves heating a jar of milk in a water bath, which is rapidly brought to a rolling boil, before milk is removed and rapidly cooled). Flash heating was developed with the goal of achieving effective pasteurization in a home environment in resource-poor areas of the world to prevent transmission of HIV.

Each pasteurization method has been investigated for its ability to eliminate pathogens while preserving as many bioactive components and nutrients as possible.[157–159] Unfortunately, heat treatment of human milk reduces the concentration and functionality of its bioactive components, particularly in protein composition and function. Significant reductions have been demonstrated after pasteurization in sIgA, lysozyme, BSSL, cytokines, lipases, TGF-β, and adiponectin, among other proteins.[160–162] Pasteurization damages some proteins more than others,[162] but is particularly damaging when paired with the multiple freeze-thaw cycles that can occur with donated milk.[163] The degree of impact appears to vary by pasteurization method. Boiling is likely the most damaging, while Holder pasteurization, the method used by the milk banks associated with the Human Milk Banking Association of North America, may be more destructive than HTST (see article elsewhere in this issue by Landers and Hartmann). Though a low-tech method, flash-heat treatment appears to preserve the bacteriostatic activity of human milk.[158] Much work remains to be done regarding the bioactivity of human milk components following milk treatment.[162]

HUMAN MILK COMPONENTS IN RELATION TO INFANT HEALTH
Management or Augmentation of Human Milk Factors

Recognition of the dynamic variability of human milk is important to the management of human milk feeding. For example, mothers of term infants are commonly advised to empty an entire breast before feeding from the other breast. As hindmilk is more energy dense because of its higher lipid content, this recommendation ensures that infant satiety and energy needs for growth are well met. Hindmilk has been successfully used to improve growth of very premature infants, and is recommended for their nutritional management.[164] Furthermore, understanding the dynamic variability of human milk, donor milk banks have established protocols for pooling different milk donations to achieve more uniform milk for distribution.

Some milk factors can be modified through dietary intake or exposures to optimize infant growth and health. For example, maternal diet influences the DHA content of milk, which is below recommended levels in many populations. Valentine[164] has shown that maternal supplementation with 1 g of preformed DHA daily significantly increases milk DHA levels, which thereby improves the dietary DHA of breastfed infants. Another approach to modification of human milk is through maternal immunization, which is being actively pursued as a public health strategy. Trials of maternal immunization have demonstrated significant increases in the level of protective immunoglobulins in milk and have dramatically reduced influenza in mothers and infants.[165]

Potential Novel Therapeutics Based on Human Milk Components

The important maternal act of breastfeeding provides many bioactive components to infants. Some of these components have been proposed as novel medical agents for prevention or treatment of disease, including lactoferrin, lactadherin, EGF, Epo, and HMOS. While various human milk components have demonstrated significant biological activity in *vitro* or in *vivo*, only a few have been tested in human clinical trials to improve specific health outcomes. One of the most studied of these factors is lactoferrin. Testing lactoferrin as a novel medical agent has been advanced by the use of recombinant bovine lactoferrin, owing to its high homology with human lactoferrin. An Italian study of preterm infants found that supplementation with bovine lactoferrin, alone or in combination with *Lactobacillus casei* subsp *rhamnosus*, significantly reduced the risk of late-onset sepsis.[133,134] A current phase 1/2 trial is evaluating the safety and efficacy of an oral lactoferrin solution to prevent infection in preterm infants.[161] Many other individual milk components may be tested in future for specific applications, but human milk remains the unique and potent standard for feeding infants.

SUMMARY

Human milk is a dynamic, multifaceted fluid containing nutrients and bioactive factors needed for infant health and development. Its composition varies by stage of lactation and between term and preterm infants. While many studies of human milk composition have been conducted, components of human milk are still being identified. Standardized, multipopulation studies of human milk composition are sorely needed to create a rigorous, comprehensive reference inclusive of nutrients and bioactive factors. Nevertheless, knowledge of human milk composition is increasing, leading to greater understanding of the role of human milk in infant health and development.[166]

ACKNOWLEDGMENTS

The authors gratefully acknowledge Donna Wuest for assistance with manuscript preparation.

REFERENCES

1. Section on Breastfeeding. Breastfeeding and the use of human milk. Pediatrics 2012;129(3):e827–41.
2. WHO. Infant and young child nutrition. Geneva (Switzerland): WHO; 2003.
3. Oftedal OT. The evolution of milk secretion and its ancient origins. Animal 2012; 6(3):355–68.
4. Castellote C, Casillas R, Ramirez-Santana C, et al. Premature delivery influences the immunological composition of colostrum and transitional and mature human milk. J Nutr 2011;141(6):1181–7.
5. Pang WW, Hartmann PE. Initiation of human lactation: secretory differentiation and secretory activation. J Mammary Gland Biol Neoplasia 2007;12(4):211–21.
6. Kulski JK, Hartmann PE. Changes in human milk composition during the initiation of lactation. Aust J Exp Biol Med Sci 1981;59(1):101–14.
7. Henderson JJ, Hartmann PE, Newnham JP, et al. Effect of preterm birth and antenatal corticosteroid treatment on lactogenesis II in women. Pediatrics 2008;121(1):e92–100.
8. Nommsen-Rivers LA, Dolan LM, Huang B. Timing of stage II lactogenesis is predicted by antenatal metabolic health in a cohort of primiparas. Breastfeed Med 2012;7(1):43–9.
9. Cregan MD, De Mello TR, Kershaw D, et al. Initiation of lactation in women after preterm delivery. Acta Obstet Gynecol Scand 2002;81(9):870–7.
10. Nommsen LA, Lovelady CA, Heinig MJ, et al. Determinants of energy, protein, lipid, and lactose concentrations in human milk during the first 12 mo of lactation: the DARLING Study. Am J Clin Nutr 1991;53(2):457–65.

11. Bauer J, Gerss J. Longitudinal analysis of macronutrients and minerals in human milk produced by mothers of preterm infants. Clin Nutr 2011;30(2):215–20.

12. Geraghty SR, Davidson BS, Warner BB, et al. The development of a research human milk bank. J Hum Lact 2005;21(1):59–66.

13. Prentice A. Regional variations in the composition of human milk. In: Jensen RG, editor. Handbook of milk composition. San Diego (CA): Academic Press, Inc; 1995. p. 919.

14. Liao Y, Alvarado R, Phinney B, et al. Proteomic characterization of human milk whey proteins during a twelve-month lactation period. J Proteome Res 2011; 10(4):1746–54.

15. Gao X, McMahon RJ, Woo JG, et al. Temporal changes in milk proteomes reveal developing milk functions. J Proteome Res 2012;11(7):3897–907.

16. Lonnerdal B. Human milk proteins: key components for the biological activity of human milk. Adv Exp Med Biol 2004;554:11–25.

17. Jensen RG. Handbook of milk composition. San Diego (CA): Academic Press, Inc; 1995.

18. Valentine CJ, Morrow G, Fernandez S, et al. Docosahexaenoic acid and amino acid contents in pasteurized donor milk are low for preterm infants. J Pediatr 2010;157(6):906–10.

19. Saarela T, Kokkonen J, Koivisto M. Macronutrient and energy contents of human milk fractions during the first six months of lactation. Acta Paediatr 2005;94(9): 1176–81.

20. Kent JC, Mitoulas LR, Cregan MD, et al. Volume and frequency of breastfeedings and fat content of breast milk throughout the day. Pediatrics 2006;117(3):e387–95.

21. Valentine CJ, Morrow G, Pennell M, et al. Randomized controlled trial of docosahexaenoic acid supplementation in midwestern U.S. Human milk donors. Breastfeed Med 2012. http://dx.doi.org/10.1089/bfm.2011.0126.

22. Martin MA, Lassek WD, Gaulin SJ, et al. Fatty acid composition in the mature milk of Bolivian forager-horticulturalists: controlled comparisons with a US sample. Matern Child Nutr 2012;8(3):404–18.

23. Newburg DS, Ruiz-Palacios GM, Morrow AL. Human milk glycans protect infants against enteric pathogens. Annu Rev Nutr 2005;25:37–58.

24. Morrow AL, Ruiz-Palacios GM, Jiang X, et al. Human-milk glycans that inhibit pathogen binding protect breast-feeding infants against infectious diarrhea. J Nutr 2005;135(5):1304–7.

25. Gabrielli O, Zampini L, Galeazzi T, et al. Preterm milk oligosaccharides during the first month of lactation. Pediatrics 2011;128(6):e1520–31.

26. Michaelsen KF, Skafte L, Badsberg JH, et al. Variation in macronutrients in human bank milk: influencing factors and implications for human milk banking. J Pediatr Gastroenterol Nutr 1990;11(2):229–39.

27. Arslanoglu S, Moro GE, Ziegler EE, The WAPM Working Group on Nutrition. Optimization of human milk fortification for preterm infants: new concepts and recommendations. J Perinat Med 2010;38(3):233–8.

28. Greer FR. Do breastfed infants need supplemental vitamins? Pediatr Clin North Am 2001;48(2):415–23.

29. Allen LH. B vitamins in breast milk: relative importance of maternal status and intake, and effects on infant status and function. Adv Nutr 2012;3(3):362–9.

30. Dawodu A, Zalla L, Woo JG, et al. Heightened attention to supplementation is needed to improve the vitamin D status of breastfeeding mothers and infants when sunshine exposure is restricted. Matern Child Nutr 2012. http://dx.doi.org/ 10.1111/j.1740-8709.2012.00422.x.

31. American Academy of Pediatrics. Pediatric nutrition handbook. 6th edition. Elk Gove Village (IL): American Academy of Pediatrics; 2009.
32. Schrezenmeir J, Korhonen H, Williams C, et al. Foreword. Br J Nutr 2000;84(S1):1.
33. Garofalo R. Cytokines in human milk. J Pediatr 2010;156(Suppl 2):S36–40.
34. Cavaletto M, Giuffrida MG, Conti A. The proteomic approach to analysis of human milk fat globule membrane. Clin Chim Acta 2004;347(1–2):41–8.
35. Van de Perre P. Transfer of antibody via mother's milk. Vaccine 2003;21(24): 3374–6.
36. Kobata R, Tsukahara H, Ohshima Y, et al. High levels of growth factors in human breast milk. Early Hum Dev 2008;84(1):67–9.
37. Patki S, Patki U, Patil R, et al. Comparison of the levels of the growth factors in umbilical cord serum and human milk and its clinical significance. Cytokine 2012;59(2):305–8.
38. Hirai C, Ichiba H, Saito M, et al. Trophic effect of multiple growth factors in amniotic fluid or human milk on cultured human fetal small intestinal cells. J Pediatr Gastroenterol Nutr 2002;34:524–8.
39. Chailler P, Menard D. Ontogeny of EGF receptors in the human gut. Front Biosci 1999;4:87–101.
40. Wagner CL, Taylor SN, Johnson D. Host factors in amniotic fluid and breast milk that contribute to gut maturation. Clin Rev Allergy Immunol 2008;34: 191–204.
41. Read LC, Upton FM, Francis GL, et al. Changes in the growth-promoting activity of human milk during lactation. Pediatr Res 1984;18(2):133–9.
42. Chang CJ, Chao JC. Effect of human milk and epidermal growth factor on growth of human intestinal caco-2 cells. J Pediatr Gastroenterol Nutr 2002;34: 394–401.
43. Khailova L, Dvorak K, Arganbright KM, et al. Changes in hepatic cell junctions structure during experimental necrotizing enterocolitis: effect of EGF treatment. Pediatr Res 2009;66(2):140–4.
44. Radulescu A, Zhang H-Y, Chen C-L, et al. Heparin-binding EGF-like growth factor promotes intestinal anastomotic healing. J Surg Res 2011;171:540–50.
45. Dvorak B, Fituch CC, Williams CS, et al. Increased epidermal growth factor levels in human milk of mothers with extremely premature infants. Pediatr Res 2003;54(1):15–9.
46. Dvorak B, Fituch CC, Williams CS, et al. Concentrations of epidermal growth factor and transforming growth factor-alpha in preterm milk. Advances in experimental medicine and biology 2004;554:407–9.
47. Rodrigues D, Li A, Nair D, et al. Glial cell line-derived neurotrophic factor is a key neurotrophin in the postnatal enteric nervous system. Neurogastroenterol Motil 2011;23:e44–56.
48. Boesmans W, Gomes P, Janssens J, et al. Brain-derived neurotrophic factor amplifies neurotransmitter responses and promotes synaptic communication in the enteric nervous system. Gut 2008;57:314–22.
49. Sánchez M, Silos-Santiago I, Frisén J, et al. Renal agenesis and the absence of enteric neurons in mice lacking GDNF. Nature 1996;382(6586):70–3.
50. Li R, Xia W, Zhang Z, et al. S100B protein, brain-derived neurotrophic factor, and glial cell line-derived neurotrophic factor in human milk. PLoS One 2011;6(6): e21663.
51. Fichter M, Klotz M, Hirschberg DL, et al. Breast milk contains relevant neurotrophic factors and cytokines for enteric nervous system development. Mol Nutr Food Res 2011;55:1592–6.

52. Blum JW, Baumrucker CR. Colostral and milk insulin-like growth factors and related substances: mammary gland and neonatal (intestinal and systemic) targets. Domest Anim Endocrinol 2002;23:101–10.

53. Burrin DG. Is milk-borne insulin-like growth factor-I essential for neonatal development? J Nutr 1997;127:975S–9S.

54. Philipps AF, Kling PJ, Grille JG, et al. Intestinal transport of insulin-like growth factor-I (IGF-I) in the suckling rat. J Pediatr Gastroenterol Nutr 2002;35:539–44.

55. Milsom SR, Blum WF, Gunn AJ. Temporal changes in insulin-like growth factors I and II and in insulin-like growth factor binding proteins 1, 2, and 3 in human milk. Horm Res 2008;69:307–11.

56. Prosser CG. Insulin-like growth factors in milk and mammary gland. J Mammary Gland Biol Neoplasia 1996;1(3):297–306.

57. Elmlinger MW, Hochhaus F, Loui A, et al. Insulin-like growth factors and binding proteins in early milk from mothers of preterm and term infants. Horm Res 2007; 68:124–31.

58. Peterson CA, Gillingham MB, Mohapatra NK, et al. Enterotrophic effect of insulin-like growth factor-I but not growth hormone and localized expression of insulin-like growth factor-I, insulin-like growth factor binding protein-3 and -5 mRNAs in jejunum of parenterally fed rats. JPEN J Parenter Eternal Nutr 2000;24(5):288–95.

59. Murali SG, Nelson DW, Draxler AK, et al. Insulin-like growth factor-I (IGF-I) attenuates jejunal atrophy in association with increased expression of IGF-I binding protein-5 in parenterally fed mice. J Nutr 2005;135(11):2553–9.

60. Corpeleijn WE, van Vliet I, de Gast-Bakker DA, et al. Effect of enteral IGF-1 supplementation on feeding tolerance, growth, and gut permeability in enterally fed premature neonates. J Pediatr Gastroenterol Nutr 2008;46:184–90.

61. Büyükkayhan D, Tanzer F, Erselcan T, et al. Umbilical serum insulin-like growth factor 1 (IGF-1) in newborns: effects of gestational age, postnatal age, and nutrition. Int J Vitam Nutr Res 2003;73(5):343–6.

62. Philipps AF, Dvorak B, Kling PJ, et al. Absorption of milk-borne insulin-like growth factor-I into portal blood of suckling rats. J Pediatr Gastroenterol Nutr 2000;31:128–35.

63. Kling PJ, Taing KM, Dvorak B, et al. Insulin-like growth factor-I stimulates erythropoiesis when administered enterally. Growth Factors 2006;24(3):218–23.

64. Loui A, Eilers E, Strauss E, et al. Vascular endothelial growth factor (VEGF) and soluble VEGF Receptor 1 (Sflt-1) levels in early and mature human milk from mothers of preterm versus term infants. J Hum Lact 2012;28(4):522–8.

65. Reynolds JD. The management of retinopathy of prematurity. Paediatr Drugs 2001;3(4):263–72.

66. DiBiasie A. Evidence-based review of retinopathy of prematurity prevention in VLBW and ELBW infants. Neonatal Netw 2006;25(6):393–403.

67. Kett JC. Anemia in infancy. Pediatr Rev 2012;33(4):186–7.

68. Soubasi V, Kremenopoulos G, Diamanti E, et al. Follow-up of very low birth weight infants after erythropoietin treatment to prevent anemia of prematurity. J Pediatr 1995;127:291–7.

69. Carbonell-Estrany X, Figueras-Aloy J, Alvarez E. Erythropoietin and prematurity—where do we stand? J Perinat Med 2005;33:277–86.

70. Kling PJ, Willeitner A, Dvorak B, et al. Enteral erythropoietin and iron stimulate erythropoiesis in suckling rats. J Pediatr Gastroenterol Nutr 2008;46:202–7.

71. Pasha YZ, Ahmadpour-Kacho M, Hajiahmadi M, et al. Enteral erythropoietin increases plasma erythropoietin level in preterm infants: a randomized controlled trial. Indian Pediatr 2008;45:25–8.

72. Shiou SR, Yu Y, Chen S, et al. Erythropoietin protects intestinal epithelial barrier function and lowers the incidence of experimental neonatal necrotizing enterocolitis. J Biol Chem 2011;286(14):12123–32.

73. Arsenault JE, Webb AL, Koulinska IN, et al. Association between breast milk erythropoietin and reduced risk of mother-to-child transmission of HIV. J Infect Dis 2010;202(3):370–3.

74. Claud EC, Savidge T, Walker WA. Modulation of human intestinal epithelial cell IL-8 secretion by human milk factors. Pediatr Res 2003;53:419–25.

75. Struck J, Pd Almeida, Bergmann A, et al. High concentrations of procalcitonin but not mature calcitonin in normal human milk. Horm Metab Res 2002;34:460–5.

76. Wookey PJ, Turner K, Furness JB. Transient expression of the calcitonin receptor by enteric neurons of the embryonic and early post-natal mouse. Cell Tissue Res 2012;347:311–7.

77. Rao RK, Davis TP, Williams C, et al. Effect of milk on somatostatin degradation in suckling rat jejunum in vivo. J Pediatr Gastroenterol Nutr 1999;28(1):84–94.

78. Gama P, Alvares EP. LHRH and somatostatin effects on the cell proliferation of the gastric epithelium of suckling and weaning rats. Regul Pept 1996;63:73–8.

79. Newburg DS, Woo JG, Morrow AL. Characteristics and potential functions of human milk adiponectin. J Pediatr 2010;156(Suppl 2):S41–6.

80. Martin LJ, Woo JG, Geraghty SR, et al. Adiponectin is present in human milk and is associated with maternal factors. Am J Clin Nutr 2006;83:1106–11.

81. Woo JG, Guerrero ML, Guo F, et al. Human milk adiponectin affects infant weight trajectory during the second year of life. J Pediatr Gastroenterol Nutr 2012;54(4):532–9.

82. Savino F, Sorrenti M, Benetti S, et al. Resistin and leptin in breast milk and infants in early life. Early Hum Dev 2012;88:779–82.

83. Savino F, Liguori SA. Update on breast milk hormones: leptin, ghrelin and adiponectin. Clin Nutr 2008;27:42–7.

84. Palou A, Sánchez J, Picó C. Nutrient–gene interactions in early life programming: leptin in breast milk prevents obesity later on in life. Advances in experimental medicine and biology 2009;646:95–104.

85. Dündar NO, Dündar B, Cesur G, et al. Ghrelin and adiponectin levels in colostrum, cord blood and maternal serum. Pediatr Int 2010;52:622–5.

86. Goldman AS. Modulation of the gastrointestinal tract of infants by human milk. Interfaces and interactions. An evolutionary perspective1. J Nutr 2000;130:426S–31S.

87. Jarvinen KM, Suomalainen H. Leucocytes in human milk and lymphocyte subsets in cow's milk-allergic infants. Pediatr Allergy Immunol 2002;13(4):243–54.

88. Patki S, Kadam S, Chandra V, et al. Human breast milk is a rich source of multipotent mesenchymal stem cells. Hum Cell 2010;23(2):35–40.

89. Ichikawa M, Sugita M, Takahashi M, et al. Breast milk macrophages spontaneously produce granulocyte-macrophage colony-stimulating factor and differentiate into dendritic cells in the presence of exogenous interleukin-4 alone. Immunology 2003;108(2):189–95.

90. Indumathi S, Dhanasekaran M, Rajkumar JS, et al. Exploring the stem cell and non-stem cell constituents of human breast milk. Cytotechnology 2012. [Epub ahead of print].

91. Riskin A, Almog M, Peri R, et al. Changes in immunomodulatory constituents of human milk in response to active infection in the nursing infant. Pediatr Res 2012;71(2):220–5.

92. Sabbaj S, Ibegbu CC, Kourtis AP. Cellular immunity in breast milk: implications for postnatal transmission of HIV-1 to the infant. Adv Exp Med Biol 2012;743: 161–9.

93. Yagi Y, Watanabe E, Watari E, et al. Inhibition of DC-SIGN-mediated transmission of human immunodeficiency virus type 1 by Toll-like receptor 3 signalling in breast milk macrophages. Immunology 2010;130(4):597–607.

94. Agarwal S, Karmaus W, Davis S, et al. Immune markers in breast milk and fetal and maternal body fluids: a systematic review of perinatal concentrations. J Hum Lact 2011;27(2):171–86.

95. Groer MW, Beckstead JW. Multidimensional scaling of multiplex data: human milk cytokines. Biol Res Nurs 2011;13(3):289–96.

96. Kverka M, Burianova J, Lodinova-Zadnikova R, et al. Cytokine profiling in human colostrum and milk by protein array. Clin Chem 2007;53(5):955–62.

97. Penttila IA. Milk-derived transforming growth factor-b and the infant immune response. J Pediatr 2010;156:S21–5.

98. Kalliomäki M, Ouwehand A, Arvilommi H, et al. Transforming growth factor-β in breast milk: a potential regulator of atopic disease at an early age. J Allergy Clin Immunol 1999;104:1251–7.

99. Saito S, Yoshida M, Ichijo M, et al. Transforming growth factor-beta (TGF-β) in human milk. Clin Exp Immunol 1993;94:220–4.

100. Nakamura Y, Miyata M, Ando T, et al. The latent form of transforming growth factor-β administered orally is activated by gastric acid in mice. J Nutr 2009; 139:1463–8.

101. Letterio JJ, Geiser AG, Kulkarni Ashok B, et al. Maternal rescue of transforming growth factor-β1 null mice. Science 1994;264:1936–8.

102. Ando T, Hatsushika K, Wako M, et al. Orally administered TGF-β is biologically active in the intestinal mucosa and enhances oral tolerance. J Allergy Clin Immunol 2007;120:916–23.

103. Ozawa T, Miyata M, Nishimura M, et al. Transforming growth factor-β activity in commercially available pasteurized cow milk provides protection against inflammation in mice. J Nutr 2009;139:69–75.

104. Donnet-Hughes A, Duc N, Serrant P, et al. Bioactive molecules in milk and their role in health and disease: the role of transforming growth factor-β. Immunol Cell Biol 2000;78:74–9.

105. Gilmore W, McKelvey-Martin V, Rutherford S, et al. Human milk contains granulocyte colony stimulating factor. Eur J Clin Nutr 1994;48(3):222–4.

106. Gersting JA, Kotto-Komeb CA, Dua Y, et al. Bioavailability of granulocyte colony-stimulating factor administered enterally to suckling mice. Pharmacol Res 2003; 48:643–7.

107. Calhoun DA, Maheshwari A, Christensen RD. Recombinant granulocyte colony-stimulating factor administered enterally to neonates is not absorbed. Pediatrics 2003;112(2):421–3.

108. Gersting JA, Christensen RD, Calhoun DA. Effects of enterally administering granulocyte colony-stimulating factor to suckling mice. Pediatr Res 2004; 55(5):802–6.

109. Ngom P, Collinson A, Pido-Lopez J, et al. Improved thymic function in exclusively breastfed infants is associated with higher interleukin 7 concentrations in their mothers' breast milk. Am J Clin Nutr 2004;80(3):722–8.

110. Aspinall R, Prentice AM, Ngom PT. Interleukin 7 from maternal milk crosses the intestinal barrier and modulates T-cell development in offspring. PLoS One 2011;6(6):e20812.

111. Ustundag B, Yilmaz E, Dogan Y, et al. Levels of cytokines (IL-1beta, IL-2, IL-6, IL-8, TNF-alpha) and trace elements (Zn, Cu) in breast milk from mothers of preterm and term infants. Mediators Inflamm 2005;2005(6):331–6.
112. Buescher ES, McWilliams-Koeppen P. Soluble tumor necrosis factor-α (TNF-α) receptors in human colostrum and milk bind to TNF-α and neutralize TNF-α bioactivity. Pediatr Res 1998;44:37–42.
113. Buescher E, Malinowska I. Soluble receptors and cytokine antagonists in human milk. Pediatr Res 1996;40(6):839–44.
114. Erbağci A, Cekmen M, Balat O, et al. Persistency of high proinflammatory cytokine levels from colostrum to mature milk in preeclampsia. Clin Biochem 2005; 38(8):712–6.
115. Meki AR, Saleem TH, Al-Ghazali MH, et al. Interleukins -6, -8 and -10 and tumor necrosis factor alpha and its soluble receptor I in human milk at different periods of lactation. Nutr Res 2003;23:845–55.
116. Maheshwari A, Lu W, Lacson A, et al. Effects of Interleukin-8 on the developing human intestine. Cytokine 2002;20(6):256–67.
117. Maheshwari A, Lacson A, Lu W, et al. Interleukin-8/CXCL8 forms an autocrine loop in fetal intestinal mucosa. Pediatr Res 2004;56(2):240–9.
118. Maheshwari A, Christensen RD, Calhoun DA. ELR+ CXC chemokines in human milk. Cytokine 2003;24:91–102.
119. Mizuno K, Hatsuno M, Aikawa K, et al. Mastitis is associated with IL-6 Levels and milk fat globule size in breast milk. J Hum Lact 2012;28(4):529–34.
120. Hunt KM, Williams JE, Shafii B, et al. Mastitis is associated with increased free fatty acids, somatic cell count, and interleukin-8 concentrations in human milk. Breastfeed Med 2012. [Epub ahead of print].
121. Hrdý J, Novotná O, Kocourková I, et al. Cytokine expression in the colostral cells of healthy and allergic mothers. Folia Microbiol (Praha) 2012;57(3):215–9.
122. Strand TA, Sharma PR, Gjessing HK, et al. Risk factors for extended duration of acute diarrhea in young children. PLoS One 2012;7(5):e36436.
123. Lamberti LM, Walker CLF, Noiman A, et al. Breastfeeding and the risk for diarrhea morbidity and mortality. BMC Public Health 2011;11(Suppl 3):S15.
124. Brandtzaeg P. The mucosal immune system and its integration with the mammary glands. J Pediatr 2010;156(Suppl 2):S8–15.
125. Kadaoui KA, Corthésy B. Secretory IgA mediates bacterial translocation to dendritic cells in mouse Peyer's patches with restriction to mucosal compartment. J Immunol 2007;179:7751–7.
126. Corthesy B. Secretory immunoglobulin a: well beyond immune exclusion at mucosal surfaces. Immunopharmacol Immunotoxicol 2009;31(2):174–9.
127. Hurley WL, Theil PK. Perspectives on immunoglobulins in colostrum and milk. Nutrients 2011;3(4):442–74.
128. Velona T, Abbiati L, Beretta B, et al. Protein profiles in breast milk from mothers delivering term and preterm babies. Pediatr Res 1999;45(5):658–63.
129. Adamkin DH. Mother's milk, feeding strategies, and lactoferrin to prevent necrotizing enterocolitis. JPEN J Parenter Enteral Nutr 2012;36:25S–9S.
130. Beljaars L, van der Strate BW, Bakker HI, et al. Inhibition of cytomegalovirus infection by lactoferrin in vitro and in vivo. Antiviral Res 2004;63(3):197–208.
131. Kuipers ME, de Vries HG, Eikelboom MC, et al. Synergistic fungistatic effects of lactoferrin in combination with antifungal drugs against clinical *Candida* isolates. Antimicrob Agents Chemother 1999;43(11):2635–41.
132. Leitch EC, Willcox MD. Lactoferrin increases the susceptibility of *S. epidermidis* biofilms to lysozyme and vancomycin. Curr Eye Res 1999;19(1):12–9.

133. Manzoni P, Rinaldi M, Cattani S, et al. Bovine lactoferrin supplementation for prevention of late-onset sepsis in very low-birth-weight neonates: a randomized trial. JAMA 2009;302(13):1421–8.

134. Sherman MP, Bennett SH, Hwang FF, et al. Neonatal small bowel epithelia: enhancing anti-bacterial defense with lactoferrin and Lactobacillus GG. Biometals 2004;17(3):285–9.

135. Stubbs J, Lekutis C, Singer K, et al. cDNA cloning of a mouse mammary epithelial cell surface protein reveals the existence of epidermal growth factor-like domains linked to factor VIII-like sequences. Proc Natl Acad Sci U S A 1990; 87(21):8417–21.

136. Peterson J, Hamosh M, Scallan C, et al. Milk fat globule glycoproteins in human milk and in gastric aspirates of mother's milk-fed preterm infants. Pediatr Res 1998;44(4):499–506.

137. Newburg D, Peterson J, Ruiz-Palacios G, et al. Role of human-milk lactadherin in protection against symptomatic rotavirus infection. Lancet 1998;351(9110):1160–4.

138. Aziz M, Jacob A, Matsuda A, et al. Review: milk fat globule-EGF factor 8 expression, function and plausible signal transduction in resolving inflammation. Apoptosis 2011;16:1077–86.

139. Shi J, Heegaard CW, Rasmussen JT, et al. Lactadherin binds selectively to membranes containing phosphatidyl-l-serine and increased curvature. Biochim Biophys Acta 2004;1667:82–90.

140. Kusunoki R, Ishihara S, Aziz M, et al. Roles of milk fat globule-epidermal growth factor 8 in intestinal inflammation. Digestion 2012;85:103–7.

141. Chogle A, Bu H-F, Wang X, et al. Milk fat globule-EGF factor 8 is a critical protein for healing of dextran sodium sulfate-induced acute colitis in mice. Mol Med 2011;17(5):502–7.

142. Baghdadi M, Chiba S, Yamashina T, et al. MFG-E8 regulates the immunogenic potential of dendritic cells primed with necrotic cell-mediated inflammatory signals. PLoS One 2012;7(6):e39607.

143. Landberg E, Huang Y, Stromqvist M, et al. Changes in glycosylation of human bile-salt-stimulated lipase during lactation. Arch Biochem Biophys 2000;377(2): 246–54.

144. Stax MJ, Naarding MA, Tanck MWT, et al. Binding of human milk to pathogen receptor DC-SIGN varies with bile salt-stimulated lipase (BSSL) gene polymorphism. PLoS One 2011;6(2):e17316.

145. Naarding MA, Dirac AM, Ludwig IS, et al. Bile salt-stimulated lipase from human milk binds DC-SIGN and inhibits human immunodeficiency virus type 1 transfer to CD4+ T cells. Antimicrob Agents Chemother 2006;50(10):3367–74.

146. Ruvoen-Clouet N, Mas E, Mariounneau S, et al. Bile-salt-stimulated lipase and mucins from milk of 'secretor' mothers inhibit the binding of Norwalk virus capsids to their carbohydrate ligands. Biochem J 2006;393:627–34.

147. Hettinga K, van VH, de VS, et al. The host defense proteome of human and bovine milk. PLoS One 2011;6(4):e19433.

148. Saeland E, de Jong MA, Nabatov AA, et al. MUC1 in human milk blocks transmission of human immunodeficiency virus from dendritic cells to T cells. Mol Immunol 2009;46:2309–16.

149. Yolken RH, Peterson JA, Vonderfecht SL, et al. Human milk mucin inhibits rotavirus replication and prevents experimental gastroenteritis. J Clin Invest 1992; 90:1984–7.

150. Parker P, Sando L, Pearson R, et al. Bovine Muc1 inhibits binding of enteric bacteria to Caco-2 cells. Glycoconj J 2010;27:89–97.

151. Liu B, Yu Z, Chen C, et al. Human milk mucin 1 and mucin 4 inhibit *Salmonella enterica* serovar *typhimurium* invasion of human intestinal epithelial cells in vitro. J Nutr 2012;142:1504–9.

152. Bode L, Kuhn L, Kim HY, et al. Human milk oligosaccharide concentration and risk of postnatal transmission of HIV through breastfeeding. Am J Clin Nutr 2012; 96(4):831–9.

153. De Leoz ML, Gaerlan SC, Strum JS, et al. Lacto-N-tetraose, fucosylation, and secretor status are highly variable in human milk oligosaccharides from women delivering preterm. J Proteome Res 2012;11(9):4662–72.

154. Hunt KM, Foster JA, Forney LJ, et al. Characterization of the diversity and temporal stability of bacterial communities in human milk. PLoS One 2011; 6(6):e21313.

155. Cabrera-Rubio R, Collado MC, Laitinen K, et al. The human milk microbiome changes over lactation and is shaped by maternal weight and mode of delivery. Am J Clin Nutr 2012;96(3):544–51.

156. Rasmussen KM, Geraghty SR. The quiet revolution: breastfeeding transformed with the use of breast pumps. Am J Public Health 2011;101(8):1356–9.

157. Baro C, Giribaldi M, Arslanoglu S, et al. Effect of two pasteurization methods on the protein content of human milk. Front Biosci (Elite Ed) 2011;3:818–29.

158. Chantry CJ, Wiedeman J, Buehring G, et al. Effect of flash-heat treatment on antimicrobial activity of breastmilk. Breastfeed Med 2011;6(3):111–6.

159. Israel-Ballard K, Donovan R, Chantry C, et al. Flash-heat inactivation of HIV-1 in human milk: a potential method to reduce postnatal transmission in developing countries. J Acquir Immune Defic Syndr 2007;45(3):318–23.

160. Peroni D, Piacentini G, Bodini A, et al. Transforming growth factor-β1 is elevated in unpasteurized cow's milk. Pediatr Allergy Immunol 2009;20:42–4.

161. Agennix. Phase 1/2 study of talactoferrin oral solution for nosocomial infection in preterm infants: Available at: http://clinicaltrials.gov/ct2/show/NCT00854633. Accessed August 23, 2012.

162. Ewaschuk JB, Unger S, O'Connor DL, et al. Effect of pasteurization on selected immune components of donated human breast milk. J Perinatol 2011;31(9): 593–8.

163. Akinbi H, Meinzen-Derr J, Auer C, et al. Alterations in the host defense properties of human milk following prolonged storage or pasteurization. J Pediatr Gastroenterol Nutr 2010;51(3):347–52.

164. Valentine CJ. Optimizing human milk fortification for the preterm infant. PNPG Building Block for Life 2011;34(4):9–11.

165. Steinhoff MC, Omer SB. A review of fetal and infant protection associated with antenatal influenza immunization. Am J Obstet Gynecol 2012;207(Suppl 3): S21–7.

166. Neville MC, Anderson SM, McManaman JL, et al. Lactation and neonatal nutrition: defining and refining the critical questions. J Mammary Gland Biol Neoplasia 2012;17(2):167–88.

167. Wojcik KY, Rechtman DJ, Lee ML, et al. Macronutrient analysis of a nationwide sample of donor breast milk. Journal of the American Dietetic Association 2009; 109(1):137–40.

168. Cianga P, Medesan C, Richardson JA, et al. Identification and function of neonatal Fc receptor in mammary gland of lactating mice. Eur J Immunol 1999;29:2515–23.

169. VandePerre P, Simonon A, Karita E, et al. Infective and anti-infective properties of breastmilk from HIV-1-infected women. The Lancet 1993;341:914–8.

170. Mehta R, Petrova A. Very preterm gestation and breastmilk cytokine content during the first month of lactation. Breastfeeding Med 2011;6(1):21–4.

171. Verhasselt V, Milcent V, Cazareth J, et al. Breast milk–mediated transfer of an antigen induces tolerance and protection from allergic asthma. Nat Med 2008;14(2):170–5.

172. Verhasselt V. Neonatal tolerance under breastfeeding influence: The presence of allergen and transforming growth factor-b in breast milk protects the progeny from allergic asthma. J Pediatr 2010;156:S16–20.

173. Penttila IA, Flesch IEA, McCue AL, et al. Maternal milk regulation of cell infiltration and interleukin 18 in the intestine of suckling rat pups. Gut 2003;52: 1579–86.

174. Mosconi E, Rekima A, Seitz-Polski B, et al. Breast milk immune complexes are potent inducers of oral tolerance in neonates and prevent asthma development. Nat Mucos Immun 2010;3(5):461–74.

175. Okamoto A, Kawamura T, Kanbe K, et al. Suppression of serum IgE response and systemic anaphylaxis in a food allergy model by orally administered high-dose TGF-b. Int Immunol 2005;17(6):705–12.

176. Penttila I. Effects of transforming growth factor-beta and formula feeding on systemic immune responses to dietary b-lactoglobulin in allergy-prone rats. Pediatr Res 2006;59(5):650–5.

177. McPherson R, Wagner C. The effect of pasteurization on transforming growth factor alpha and transforming growth factor beta 2 concentrations in human milk. Adv Exp Med Biol 2001;501:559–66.

178. Rudloff HE, Schmalstieg FC, Mushtaha A, et al. Tumor Necrosis Factor-a in human milk. Pediatr Res 1992;31(1):29–33.

179. Magi B, Ietta F, Romagnoli R, et al. Presence of macrophage migration inhibitory factor in human milk: evidence in the aqueous phase and milk fat globules. Pediatr Res 2002;51(5):619–24.

180. Vigh É, Bódis J, Garai J. Longitudinal changes in macrophage migration inhibitory factor in breast milk during the first three months of lactation. J Reprod Immunol 2011;89:92–4.

181. Coursodon CF, Dvorak B. Epidermal growth factor and necrotizing enterocolitis. Curr Opinion Pediatr 2012;24:160–4.

182. Clark JA, Lane RH, et al. Epidermal growth factor reduces intestinal apoptosis in an experimental model of necrotizing enterocolitis. Am J Physiol Gastrointest Liver Physiol 2004;288:G755–62.

183. Untalan PB, Keeney SE, Palkowetz KH, et al. Heat susceptibility of interleukin-10 and other cytokines in donor human milk. Breastfeeding Med 2009;4(3):137–44.

184. Ozgurtas T, Aydin I, Turan O, et al. Soluble Vascular Endothelial Growth Factor Receptor 1 in Human Breast Milk. Horm Res Paediatr 2011;76:17–21.

185. Chellakooty M, Juul A, Boisen KA, et al. A prospective study of serum insulin-like growth factor I (IGF-I) and IGF-binding protein-3 in 942 healthy infants: associations with birth weight, gender, growth velocity, and breastfeeding. J Clin Endocrin & Metab 2006;91(3):820–6.

186. Baregamian N, Song J, Jeschke MG, et al. IGF-1 protects intestinal epithelial cells from oxidative stress-induced apoptosis. J Surg Res 2006;136:31–7.

187. Baregamian N, Song J, Chung DH. Effects of oxidative stress on intestinal type I insulinlLike growth factor receptor expression. Eur J Ped Surg 2012;22(1): 97–104.

188. Juul SE, Christensen RD. Absorption of enteral recombinant human erythropoietin by neonates. Ann Pharmocother 2003;37:782–6.

189. Miller-Gilbert AL, Dubuque SH, Dvorak B, et al. Enteral absorption of erythropoietin in the suckling rat. Pediatr Res 2001;50(2):261–7.
190. Miller M, Iliff P, Stoltzfus RJ, et al. Breastmilk erythropoietin and mother-to-child HIV transmission through breastmilk. The Lancet 2002;360:1246–8.
191. Hirotani Y, Ikeda K, Kato R, et al. Protective effects of lactoferrin against intestinal mucosal damage induced by lipopolysaccharide in human intestinal Caco-2 cells. Yakugaku Zasshi 2008;128(9):1363–8.
192. Buccigrossi V, Marco Gd, Bruzzese E, et al. Lactoferrin induces concentration-dependent functional modulation of intestinal proliferation and differentiation. Pediatr Res 2007;61(4):410–4.
193. Shah KG, Wu R, Jacob A, et al. Recombinant human milk fat globule-EGF factor 8 produces dose-dependent benefits in sepsis. Intensive Care Med 2012;38:128–36.
194. Miksa M, Wu R, Dong W, et al. Dendritic cell derived exosomes containing Milk Fat Globule-Epidermal Growth Factor VIII attenuate proinflammatory responses in sepsis. Shock 2006;25(6):586–93.
195. Komura H, Miksa M, Wu R, et al. Milk Fat Globule Epidermal Growth Factor-Factor VIII is down-regulated in sepsis via the lipopolysaccharide-CD14 pathway. J Immunol 2009;182:581–7.
196. Miksa M, Wu R, Dong W, et al. Immature dendritic cell-derived exosomes rescue septic animals via Milk Fat Globule Epidermal Growth Factor VIII. J Immunol 2009;183:5983–90.
197. Wu R, Dong W, Wang Z, et al. Enhancing apoptotic cell clearance mitigates bacterial translocation and promotes tissue repair after gut ischemia-reperfusion injury. Int J Mol Med 2012;30(3):593–8.
198. Matsuda A, Jacob A, Wu R, et al. Milk Fat Globule-EGF Factor VIII in sepsis and ischemia-reperfusion injury. Mol Med 2011;17:126–33.
199. Silvestre J-S, Théry C, Hamard G, et al. Lactadherin promotes VEGF-dependent neovascularization. Nature Med 2005;11(5):499–506.
200. Woo JG, Guerrero ML, Guo F, et al. Human milk adiponectin affects infant weight trajectory during the second year of life. JPGN 2012;54:532–9.
201. Ley SH, Hanley AJ, Stone D, et al. Effects of pasteurization on adiponectin and insulin concentrations in donor human milk. Pediatr Res 2011;70(3):278–81.
202. Dündar NO, Dündar B, Cesur G, et al. Ghrelin and adiponectin levels in colostrum, cord blood and maternal serum. Pediatr Int 2010;52:622–5.
203. Ozarda Y, Gunes Y, Tuncer GO. The concentration of adiponectin in breast milk is related to maternal hormonal and inflammatory status during 6 months of lactation. Clin Chem Lab Med 2012;50(5):911–7.
204. Weyermann M, Brenner H, Rothenbacher D. Adipokines in human milk and risk of overweight in early childhood: a prospective cohort study. Epidemiol 2007; 18(6):722–9.
205. Marcobal A, Sonnenburg JL. Human milk oligosaccharide consumption by intestinal microbiota. Clin Microbiol Infect 2012;18(Suppl 4):12–5.
206. Rudloff S, Kunz C. Milk oligosaccharides and metabolism in infants. Adv Nutr 2012;3(3):398S–405S.
207. Ruhaak LR, Lebrilla CB. Analysis and role of oligosaccharides in milk. BMB Rep 2012;45(8):442–51.
208. Wang B. Molecular mechanism underlying sialic acid as an essential nutrient for brain development and cognition. Adv Nutr 2012;3(3):465S–72S.
209. Coppa GV, Gabrielli O, Zampini L, et al. Glycosaminoglycan content in term and preterm milk during the first month of lactation. Neonatology 2012;101(1): 74–6.

210. Coppa GV, Gabrielli O, Buzzega D, et al. Composition and structure elucidation of human milk glycosaminoglycans. Glycobiology 2011;21(3):295–303.

211. Sando L, Pearson R, Gray C, et al. Bovine Muc1 is a highly polymorphic gene encoding an extensively glycosylated mucin that binds bacteria. J Dairy Sci 2009;92:5276–91.

212. Chaturvedi P, Singh AP, Batra SK. Structure, evolution, and biology of the MUC4 mucin. FASEB J 2008;22:966–81.

Clinical Protocols for Management of Breastfeeding

Caroline J. Chantry, MD[a],*, Cynthia R. Howard, MD, MPH[b]

KEYWORDS

- Clinical guidelines • Protocols • Evidence-based • Breastfeeding • Management
- Academy of Breastfeeding Medicine

KEY POINTS

- Clinical breastfeeding guidelines are systematically developed statements about specific clinical situations to assist health care professionals provide evidence-based care.
- The Academy of Breastfeeding Medicine's clinical protocols are summarized, including purpose, content overview, level of evidence, and research gaps.
- Wide research gaps exist in many areas of breastfeeding medicine, including many of the situations addressed by the ABM protocols.

INTRODUCTION

Physicians and other health care providers often face uncertainty in diagnosis and management of patients and must rely on the scientific literature in addition to their own knowledge and experience; yet, a careful literature review can be difficult and time-consuming. Clinical practice guidelines, also called clinical guidelines or protocols, have been developed in medicine to address this widespread issue, and are defined as "systematically developed statements to assist practitioners with appropriate health care for specific circumstances."[1] As health care becomes more complex, there is increased focus on use of evidence-based guidelines to optimize quality, safety, and cost.

A number of national and international organizations have issued breastfeeding guidelines, including the American Academy of Pediatrics (AAP),[2] the American Academy of Family Physicians (AAFP),[3] the American Congress of Obstetrics and Gynecology (ACOG),[4] and the World Health Organization (WHO).[5] Typically these are comprehensive policy statements intended primarily for member physicians which review the health implications of breastfeeding; endorse exclusive breastfeeding for

Authors have nothing to disclose.
[a] Department of Pediatrics, University of California Davis Medical Center, Ticon II, Suite 334, 2516 Stockton Boulevard, Sacramento, CA 95817, USA; [b] University of Rochester, Rochester General Hospital, 1425 Portland Avenue, Rochester, NY 14621, USA
* Corresponding author.
E-mail address: caroline.chantry@ucdmc.ucdavis.edu

6 months; and discuss the recommended minimum breastfeeding duration, physician education, role of physicians in promoting, protecting and supporting the breastfeeding dyad, and a variety of common clinical scenarios (eg, contraindications, maternal medication and substance use, and special infant and maternal conditions, such as preterm infants). These widely read statements are valuable tools that establish standards. The International Lactation Consultant Association has developed guidelines written by lactation consultants to guide care provided by nurses and allied health care professionals[6]; practice guidelines specifically for nurses are also available.[7] Additionally, WHO has produced clinical guidelines on more specific topics (eg, HIV and infant feeding,[8] medical indications for formula use,[9] and mastitis[10]). In fact, the WHO/United Nations Children's Fund (UNICEF) Ten Steps to Successful Breastfeeding (**Box 1**) are undoubtedly the most widely used clinical guidelines in breastfeeding medicine.

Institution-specific clinical practice guidelines in breastfeeding are also available on the Internet. For example, the Royal Women's Hospital in Victoria, Australia, publishes evidence-based guidelines used by health care professionals in their setting on a variety of specific breastfeeding topics [eg, mastitis, galactagogues, nipple and breast pain (www.thewomens.org.au/BreastfeedingClinicalPracticeGuidelines). Limited information, however, is available from these sources on the process used to develop, review, and update guidelines.

The Academy of Breastfeeding Medicine (ABM), a worldwide, multidisciplinary organization of physicians dedicated to promotion, protection, and support of breastfeeding and human lactation, was established in the early 1990s and immediately recognized the need for a variety of more specialized clinical practice guidelines for physicians managing breastfeeding dyads. ABM currently has 25 different clinical protocols that address a variety of clinical circumstances (**Table 1**). Development of ABM protocols in breastfeeding medicine remains a prominent priority within the organization, specifically maintaining and increasing the number, circulation, usefulness, international

---

Box 1
WHO/UNICEF Ten Steps to successful breastfeeding

Every facility providing maternity services and care for newborn infants should

1. Have a written breastfeeding policy that is routinely communicated to all health care staff.
2. Train all health care staff in skills necessary to implement this policy.
3. Inform all pregnant women about the benefits and management of breastfeeding.
4. Help mothers initiate breastfeeding within half an hour of birth.
5. Show mothers how to breastfeed, and how to maintain lactation, even if they should be separated from their infants.
6. Give newborn infants no food or drink other than breast milk, unless medically indicated.
7. Practice rooming-in (ie, allow mothers and infants to remain together 24 hours a day).
8. Encourage breastfeeding on demand.
9. Give no artificial teats or pacifiers (also called dummies or soothers) to breastfeeding infants.
10. Foster the establishment of breastfeeding support groups and refer mothers to them on discharge from the hospital or clinic.

Data from: Protecting, Promoting and Supporting Breastfeeding: The Special Role of Maternity Services, a joint WHO/UNICEF statement published by the World Health Organization. Available at: http://whqlibdoc.who.int/publications/9241561300.pdf. Accessed September 14, 2012.

Table 1
Academy of Breastfeeding Medicine clinical protocols: summary of reviewed evidence levels and salient research gaps

Protocol[a]	Levels of Evidence					Research Gaps[b]
	I	II-1	II-2	II-3	III	
1. Hypoglycemia (2006)						• Well-controlled studies evaluating plasma glucose concentrations, symptoms and outcomes to better understand appropriate thresholds for intervention
Total Annotated	1	0	21	21	49	• More reliable point-of-care tests
Review	0	0	0	0	13	• Clearer understanding of glucose-sparing fuels and methods to measure them clinically to assist with treatment decisions
Metabolism	0	0	4	1	6	
Incidence/Definition	0	0	9	3	5	
Long-term outcomes	1	0	4	6	5	
Risk factors	0	0	4	1	3	
Manifestations	0	0	0	2	0	
Management	0	0	0	0	15	
Point-of-care tests	0	0	0	8	2	
2. Going Home (2008)						• Interventions to reduce number of women who perceive inadequate milk supply and thus supplement with formula impacting duration and exclusivity. A better understanding of the effect of culture, ethnicity, and race on this perception is lacking
Total Annotated	11	0	2	15	39	• The effect of length of hospital stay and effect on the development/resolution of BF problems
BF effectiveness/perceived need to supplement	0	0	0	2	4	• Maternal advanced age and technologically induced pregnancies and effect on BF
Maternal/infant risk factors for BF problems	0	0	0	3	3	• Cost benefit analyses on providing pumps to mothers who are separated from their infants and long-term health outcomes in infants
Interventions to improve breastfeeding rates	0	0	1	1	9	
Commercial formula discharge bags and pacifiers—effect on BF	6	0	1	5	3	
Breast pump access and BF management in NICU setting or with maternal-infant separation	0	0	0	0	5	
BF and return to work or school	0	0	0	0	6	
Peer counseling and BF duration	3	0	0	2	2	
Timing of hospital discharge on BF	1	0	0	1	4	
Skin-to-skin and mom baby separation	1	0	0	1	3	

(continued on next page)

Table 1
(continued)

Protocol[a]	Levels of Evidence					Research Gaps[b]
	I	II-1	II-2	II-3	III	
3. Supplementation (2008)						• Appropriate supplementation volumes/intervals; if and how these should vary by specific conditions, indications, infant weight, and choice of supplemental feeds
Total Annotated	14	8	26	23	26	
Review articles	0	1	3	0	1	
Benefits of exclusive BF	0	0	1	0	2	• Optimal method(s) of supplementation and if this is condition and age specific, specifically with regard to least interference of successfully establishing direct and exclusive BF
Newborn transitional physiology	3	2	6	1	5	
Risks of inappropriate supplementation	5	3	10	15	6	
Inappropriate reasons for supplementation	1	0	3	5	2	
Valid medical indications for supplementation	1	0	1	0	4	
Recommendations	0	0	0	0	4	
Quality and quantity of supplementation	1	2	2	1	1	
Methods of supplementation	3	0	0	1	1	
4. Mastitis (2007)						• Need controlled trials to guide most appropriate antibiotic use – when antibiotics should be used, which agents should be first line, appropriate duration;
Total Annotated	8	3	20	0	11	
Prevalence of mastitis	0	0	7	0	0	
Pathophysiology	0	0	0	0	4	• Role of probiotics in prevention and treatment
Microbiology	0	0	7	0	3	
Causes of mastitis	0	0	4	0	0	
Management: nonpharmacologic	1	0	0	0	0	
Management: pharmacologic	0	0	0	0	0	
Prevention of mastitis	6	3	0	0	0	
Breast abscess: incidence	0	0	2	0	0	
Breast abscess: management	0	0	0	4	4	

Category						Future research directions
5. Peripartum Breastfeeding Management (2008)						• Better understanding of the effect of intrapartum analgesia on breastfeeding success (especially epidural analgesia composition and dosage) • Effect of maternal peripartum complications (eg, diabetes, preeclampsia) on breastfeeding • Optimization of postpartum support services and referrals from hospitals, including for different ethnicities and cultures
Total Annotated	7	0	0	7	0	8
Background/hospital policies	0	0	1	1	0	2
Prenatal education	1	0	0	0	0	1
Labor and delivery	2	0	0	0	0	1
Immediate postpartum period	2	0	1	1	0	2
Discharge policies	1	0	0	0	0	0
Expressing breast milk	0	0	0	0	0	0
Background	0	0	0	0	0	1
Bed-sharing and infant mortality	0	0	5	5	0	1
6. Cosleeping (2008)						• Significant flaws in methodology used to determine SIDS cases in published literature (eg, lack of death scene investigations and gaps in data collection, categorization of infant deaths). Need for population-based research using impartial, prospective protocols with standardized, well-defined data-collection methods, relevant control groups • Identification of dangerous, modifiable factors associated with bed sharing (couch, recliner use; smoking; alcohol or drug use by cosleeping parent, obesity in parent, more than one cosleeping adult or child) • Attention to issues of ethnic diversity and cultural practices • Impact of cosleeping on infant behavior, physiology, SIDS, and breastfeeding
Total Annotated	4	5	9	1		28
Background	0	0	0	0		1
Bed-sharing and infant mortality	0	0	5	0		1
Ethnic diversity	4	5	4	1		26
7. Model Hospital Policy (2010)						• Identification of effective "spread" strategies to increase implementation of Baby-Friendly practices in the hospital setting • Effective techniques to ensure staff adherence to hospital's breastfeeding policy • Investigating other practices that may enhance hospital support of breastfeeding mothers in addition to the Ten Steps
Total Annotated	5	6	7	3		26
Organizational statements in support of BF or Ten Steps	0	0	0	0		19
Pacifiers/alternative feeding methods	3	0	0	0		0
Breastfeeding analgesia	1	0	6	0		0
Ten Steps effects	1	6	6	3		0
Skin-to-skin and delivery room practice	0	2	0	1		0
Miscellaneous	0	0	1	0		7

(continued on next page)

Table 1
(continued)

Protocol[a]	Levels of Evidence					Research Gaps[b]
	I	II-1	II-2	II-3	III	
8. Human Milk Storage (2010)						• Larger, high-quality studies evaluating human milk storage in a variety of circumstances (eg, freezing, high ambient "room" temperatures) to better understand safe storage durations
Total Annotated	1	34	2	0	12	• How milk quality is affected during storage and implications for child health
Bacterial growth	1	12	1	0	3	• Observational trials that define "safe" levels of bacterial growth and loss of antimicrobial properties
Nutrient content	0	5	0	0	0	
Containers	0	4	0	0	4	
Milk quality	0	16	1	0	1	
Review/recommendations	0	0	0	0	4	
Thawing/heating	0	2	0	0	0	
9. Galactogogues (2009)						• Well-designed, adequately powered RCT in both mothers of preterm and term infants employing maximal lactation support, varying doses of galactagogues with well-measured relevant clinical outcomes including weight gain, volume of artificial milk use, measures of breastmilk production, and drug side effects
Total Annotated	31	3	5	21	28	
Background and reviews	2	0	1	6	8	
Milk expression and rate of synthesis	3	0	2	3	3	
Metoclopromide	8	1	0	7	2	
Domperidone	5	1	1	2	6	
Thyrotropin-releasing hormone	2	0	1	0	0	
Sulpiride	3	0	0	0	0	
Human growth hormone	5	0	0	0	0	
Herbals	2	1	0	2	9	
Studies examining multiple medications	1	0	0	1	0	

10. Breastfeeding the Late Preterm Infant (2010)	10	8	82	24	45
Total Annotated	10	8	82	24	45
Physiologic vulnerabilities					
Definition	0	0	0	0	1
Physiologic maturation	0	0	3	1	3
Mortality	0	0	8	0	1
Morbidity	0	0	16	1	4
Length of stay and readmission	0	0	10	0	0
Respiratory	0	0	13	0	0
Jaundice	0	0	8	1	2
Feeding	0	0	3	0	0
Developmental outcome	0	3	14	0	3
Evidence regarding management					
Obstetric practice/late preterm	0	0	13	1	2
Gestational age assessment	0	0	0	0	1
Breastfeeding assessment	0	0	0	6	2
Feeding techniques					
Cup feeding	6	2	1	2	5
Nipple shields	0	0	1	5	4
Finger feeding	0	0	0	0	1
Pumping	1	0	0	2	0
Test weights	0	0	1	4	0
Skin-to-skin	3	2	0	0	1
General review: Management	0	1	2	0	11
Hyperbilirubinemia	0	0	1	1	5
11. Ankyloglossia (2012) *(expired under revision)*					
Total Annotated	2	0	4	13	7
Breastfeeding and frenulotomy	2	0	1	9	0
Epidemiology	0	0	0	1	0
Assessment of ankyloglossia	0	0	0	2	0
Mechanisms of normal feeding (as relevant to ankyloglossia)	0	0	3	0	0
Adverse outcomes associated with tongue tie	0	0	0	1	0
Editorials	0	0	0	0	2
Reviews, policy statements	0	0	0	0	5

Notes for section 10:
- Need evidence to support best practices for monitoring early physiologic stability that optimize mother-infant interactions and BF initiation (currently practices institution-specific and without evidence to support specific recommendations)
- Best methods for BF assessment in this population
- Evidence to develop late preterm-specific supplementation guidelines (indications, volume, and method)
- Data in late preterms to develop evidence-based guidelines for optimal use of nipple shields, routine guidelines for breastmilk expression, and criteria for discharge

Notes for section 11:
- Longer-term randomized, investigator-blinded trials identifying risks, benefits of frenulotomy, particularly with mild to moderate ankyloglossia—need descriptions of length of incision, physical breast characteristics in addition to frenulum
- Predictors of benefit from intervention in mild/moderate ankyloglossia
- Critical need for tools to assess degree of ankyloglossia, function of tongue and BF performance
- Best methods for assessing and treating posterior ankyloglossia

(continued on next page)

Table 1
(continued)

Protocol[a]	Levels of Evidence					Research Gaps[b]
	I	II-1	II-2	II-3	III	
12. NICU Grad (expired under revision)	Annotated bibliography in process.					To be defined in revised protocol.
13. Contraception (2005) (expired under revision)						• Studies of estrogen on the quantity of breastmilk were conducted with women on higher doses of estrogen; the risk of decreased milk supply with ultra-low-dose estrogen on breastfeeding is not known
Total Annotated	6	1	3	6	6	
Progestin-only methods	2	0	1	0	2	
Estrogen-containing contraceptives	2	0	1	0	1	• Vaginal ring and the contraceptive patch, which contain low-dose estrogen warrant study
Intrauterine devices	2	1	0	6	1	• Significant controversy exists about the effects of immediate postpartum (2–5 d) vs later (6 wk) depoprovera use on breastmilk production and breastfeeding duration (exclusive and any)
General and comparative information	0	0	1	0	2	
14. Breastfeeding-Friendly Physicians' Office (2006) (expired under revision)						• Studies demonstrating the effectiveness of specific educational interventions related to breastfeeding (eg, distribution of handouts, counseling by the primary care provider, group counseling, counseling by nurse) during pediatric preventive care visits
Total Annotated	7	0	1	0	14	
Systems evaluation	1	0	0	0	2	
Influence on infant feeding choice	0	0	0	0	1	
Support of breastfeeding in practice setting	0	0	1	0	1	• Effects of specific office practices on breastfeeding initiation, exclusivity, and maintenance
Lactation consultant/peer counselor support effect on BF	1	0	0	0	0	• Studies on the short-term and long-term effectiveness of educational programs for physicians are needed
Organizational statements in support of BF or Ten Steps	0	0	0	0	4	• Research on specific challenges to providing support in the outpatient setting
Staff/physician education	0	0	0	0	2	• Cost-effectiveness of steps related to making an outpatient practice BF friendly are lacking
WIC/peer counselor support/family	1	0	0	0	3	
Discharge bags/commercial formula promotion effects	3	0	0	0	1	
Miscellaneous	1	0	0	0	0	

						Comments
15. Analgesia and Anesthesia for the Breastfeeding Mother (2006)						• Limited evidence of BF outcomes with labor analgesia and anesthesia—widespread epidural use makes this a high priority
Total Annotated	10	0	10	0	14	• Data regarding effects of intravenous fluid administration during labor and effect on breast engorgement, milk supply, neonatal weight loss from birth are needed for appropriate guidance as to early infant feeding assessment and management of infant weight loss postpartum (eg, indications for supplemental feeds)
BF outcomes and anesthesia/analgesia	2	0	0	0	0	
Postpartum analgesia and BF	0	0	0	0	1	
Outcomes and infant behavior	1	0	1	0	0	
Other forms of pharmacologic anesthesia/analgesia	2	0	1	0	2	• Studies of special needs of premature and unstable babies, including ability to metabolize maternal anesthetic and analgesic drugs and how they vary from their healthy counterparts
Labor-related anesthesia/analgesia and secondary effect on BF	1	0	0	0	2	
Studies of infant outcomes of anesthesia for cesarean section	2	0	0	0	1	
Review of alternative methods of labor pain relief management	2	0	0	0	2	
Drug choice for analgesia in labor	0	0	0	0	2	
Anesthesia in BF women (outside immediate postpartum period)	0	0	8	0	4	
Infant outcomes of anesthesia for cesarean section	2	0	0	0	1	
16. Breastfeeding the Hypotonic Infant (2006)						• Methods of assessing and optimizing suck and milk transfer in hypotonic infants needs further study
Total Annotated	0	0	11	1	9	• Use of pacifiers during gavage feeds as "practice" feeds, which can assist premature infants transition to breastfeeds, merits study in hypotonic infants
BF outcomes and maturation: Down syndrome	0	0	2	0	1	
BF with sucking, swallowing and neurologic disorders	0	0	0	0	3	
BF and clinical outcomes	0	0	9	0	0	• Physiologic stability and efficiency during different types of feeding should be studied to optimize methods of supplementation
Maternal experiences	0	0	0	0	1	
Other	0	0	0	1	0	
Review	0	0	0	0	4	

(continued on next page)

Table 1
(continued)

Protocol[a]	Levels of Evidence					Research Gaps[b]
	I	II-1	II-2	II-3	III	
17. Breastfeeding Infants with Cleft Lip, Cleft Palate, or Cleft Lip and Palate (2007)						• Health care providers currently face a lack of evidence on BF in these infants on which to base clinical decision making. Well-designed studies in well-described populations are needed which document BF success rates and management strategies and associated infant outcomes
Total Annotated	5	1	8	3	31	
Feeding difficulties	0	0	2	0	15	
Outcomes with BF	0	0	4	0	0	
Syndromes	0	0	0	0	2	
Support	0	0	0	0	2	
Weight gain and growth	0	1	1	0	1	
Postoperative feeding	0	0	1	2	2	
Devices	2	0	1	0	9	
Review	3	0	0	0	0	
18. Use of Antidepressants in Nursing Mothers (2008)						• General lack of empiric evidence in this area • Glaring lack of long-term neurobehavioral and developmental follow-up of infants exposed to antidepressants in human milk during a time of rapid central nervous system development. Despite many publications empiric evidence lacks both inclusiveness and consistency of findings for clinicians and mothers to make confident clinical decisions about individual medications. Trials often report no adverse effects but fail to state how adverse effects were determined • There is a lack of any RCT in lactating women for any class of antidepressant (and all 6 controlled studies with methodologic flaws) • Case reports confounded by in utero exposure, infant age ranges, and inconsistent pharmacokinetic measures, and so forth
Total Annotated	0	0	5	6	17	
Background	0	0	0	0	4	
Meta-analysis	0	0	1	0	0	
Multiple drug studies	0	0	3	0	0	
Tricyclic antidepressants	0	0	1	0	1	
Selective serotonin reuptake inhibitors	0	0	0	5	11	
Miscellaneous	0	0	0	1	1	

19. Breastfeeding Promotion in the Prenatal Setting (2008)					
Total Annotated	6	1	4	3	2
Primary care interventions	3	0	3	1	0
Resources for providers	0	0	0	0	1
Organizational statements or protocols	0	0	0	0	1
Group teaching/care in prenatal setting	1	0	0	0	0
WIC education/peer counseling	2	1	0	1	0
Social/family support	0	0	1	0	0
Miscellaneous	0	0	0	1	0

- Evidence regarding physician-only interactions in support of BF during prenatal visits
- Studies that delineate effects of prenatal interventions alone vs in combination with continuum support
- Cost-effectiveness about prenatal interventions
- Effect of different prenatal interventions on socioeconomically, ethnically, racially, culturally diverse populations are lacking
- Specific challenges to providing prenatal BF support

20. Engorgement (2009)					
Total Annotated	4	4	9	2	25
Management strategies in lactating ± nonlactating women	3	2	3	1	6
Management strategies for suppression of lactation and management in nonlactating women	1	2	6	1	19

- Physiology of engorgement
- Well-designed prevention and treatment trials
- Evidence to develop and validate a uniform tool for measuring severity could standardize assessment—would allow better evaluation of predictors and cross-study comparison of prevention/treatment strategies

21. Breastfeeding and the Drug-Dependent Woman (2010)					
Total Annotated	0	1	7	0	13
Reviews of medication use during BF including drugs of abuse	0	0	0	0	5
Maternal drugs of abuse other than methadone	0	0	1	0	3
Methadone use in BF	0	1	6	0	2
BF effect of neonatal NAS scores	0	0	0	0	0
Buprenorphine	0	0	0	0	3

- Case-controlled studies evaluating buprenorphine and breastfeeding (eg, transfer to human milk, and neurobehavioral effects on the infant)
- Long-term RCT evaluations of infant exposure via human milk to methadone vs buprenorphine to include infant developmental assessment
- Evaluations of maternal milk and plasma and infant plasma pharmacokinetic data regarding prescription opioids use during lactation
- Long-term prospective cohort evaluations of infants exposed to marijuana via human milk including infant developmental outcomes

22. Jaundice (2006)					
Total Annotated	8	7	15	3	1
Breastmilk jaundice	2	1	7	0	1
Breastfeeding and serum bilirubin	4	3	0	2	0
Related hospital practices	2	3	8	1	0

- Understanding of the specific mechanism of bilirubin absorption in the intestine and the chemical composition of the component(s) in human milk that enhance bilirubin absorption
- Identification of interventions for breastfed infants with hyperbilirubinemia that would allow uninterrupted breastfeeding while reducing serum bilirubin concentrations to safe levels

(continued on next page)

Table 1
(continued)

Protocol[a]	Levels of Evidence					Research Gaps[b]
	I	II-1	II-2	II-3	III	
23. Nonpharmacologic Management of Procedure-Related Pain in the Breastfeeding Infant (2009)						• Most effective nonpharmacologic analgesic modalities for preterm infants and infants beyond newborn age
Total Annotated	28	0	0	0	2	• Effectiveness of BF and human milk for analgesia should be established in preterm infants, older infants, and in newborns undergoing multiple procedures, as should different combinations of nonpharmacologic modalities
Breastfeeding as analgesia	10	0	0	0	0	
Alternative to BF: sucrose taste	10	0	0	0	0	
Alternative to BF: Non-nutritive suckling	1	0	0	0	2	• Effectiveness of increasing concentrations of sweet taste should be studied in older infants and toddlers (and beyond)
Alternative to BF: skin-to-skin contact	3	0	0	0	0	
Comparison studies	4	0	0	0	0	
24. Allergic Proctocolitis in the Exclusively Breastfed Infant (2010)						• Incidence of allergic colitis in exclusively breastfed infants with attention to trend and familial patterns
Total Annotated	2	0	24	0	28	• Contribution of maternal immune factors transmitted to progeny during prenatal and/or postnatal life on the development of allergic responses in the neonate
Clinical course, laboratory and pathologic findings	2	0	16	0	26	• Define the immunologic mechanisms involved in the context of specific genetic, developmental, and environmental factors in mothers and infants
Maternal factors (prenatal or postnatal) that contribute to pathogenesis	0	0	8	0	2	• Investigation of the safety and efficacy of maternal pancreatic enzyme use in treating infant allergic colitis (current data are case reports/anecdotal)
						• Risk of developing major food allergies in infants who develop allergic proctocolitis
						• Should infants with a history of allergic proctocolitis delay or avoid exposure to other food allergens?
						• Determine additional laboratory tests for the diagnosis of allergic proctocolitis

25. "NPO" Guidelines (2010)					
Total Annotated	11	4	0	2	8
Pacifier	5	0	0	0	0
Gastric emptying	4	4	0	0	1
Lung injury	2	0	0	0	0
Aspiration	0	0	0	1	1
Review	0	0	0	1	3
Guidelines	0	0	0	0	1
Practice survey	0	0	0	0	2

- Variability of gastric emptying with variation in content of human milk (eg, increased fat in hindmilk)
- If comorbidities increase gastric acidity, volume, or emptying such that fasting requirements might differ
- Effect on gastric contents of non-nutritive sucking on a pacifier

Total annotated may not be sum of subtopics, as some studies address multiple areas.

a Year in table is year in which annotated bibliography was completed; in some cases the protocol was completed/revised in a subsequent year.

b Research gaps primarily identified at time of literature review and specified in annotated bibliography; in some cases these have been expanded by authors of this review (C.J.C., C.R.H.).

Abbreviations: BF, breastfeeding; NAS, neonatal abstinence syndrome; NICU, neonatal intensive care unit; NPO, nothing by mouth; RCT, randomized controlled trial; SIDS, sudden infant death syndrome; WIC, Special Supplemental Nutrition Program for Women, Infants, and Children.

From WHO/UNICEF. Protecting, Promoting and Supporting Breastfeeding: The Special Role of Maternity Services, a joint WHO/UNICEF statement published by the World Health Organization. Available at: http://whqlibdoc.who.int/publications/9241561300.pdf.

relevance, and rigor of ABM protocols, including translation into more languages. ABM's current process for protocol development is depicted in **Fig. 1**, and includes systematic assessment of the literature (**Table 2**). Development of these evidence-based guidelines is challenging on a number of levels, perhaps most notably because the evidence base itself is lacking. Research in this field is beginning to burgeon, yet remains challenged by lack of funding and ethical issues pertaining to randomization, among others. Developing protocols with global relevance is further made formidable by the wide diversity of health care settings in which they may be used.

ABM distributes its guidelines as widely as possible through its Website (www. bfmed.org), the National Guideline Clearinghouse (NGC; www.guideline.gov) and the journal *Breastfeeding Medicine* to promote evidence-based practice of breast-feeding medicine. The protocols most accessed electronically are shown in **Table 3**. Briefly, the ABM Web site protocol page is viewed on average more than

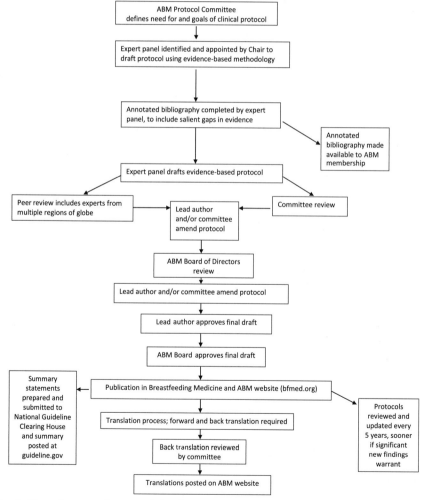

Fig. 1. Flow diagram of protocol development process used by Academy of Breastfeeding Medicine (ABM).

Table 2
US Preventive Services Task Force "quality of evidence" ranking used to assess the evidence base for Academy of Breastfeeding Medicine protocols

Level of Evidence	Explanation
I	Evidence obtained from at least one properly randomized controlled trial.
II-1	Evidence obtained from well-designed controlled trials without randomization.
II-2	Evidence obtained from well-designed cohort or case-control analytic studies, preferably from more than one center or research group.
II-3	Evidence obtained from multiple time series with or without the intervention. Dramatic results in uncontrolled experiments (such as the results of the introduction of penicillin treatment in the 1940s) could also be regarded as this type of evidence.
III	Opinions of respected authorities, based on clinical experience descriptive studies and case reports or reports of expert committees.

From Guide to Clinical Preventive Services. Report of the US Preventive Services Task Force. US Preventive Services Task Force. 2nd edition. Washington, DC: US Department of Health and Human Services; 1996.

6000 times monthly by more than 3000 viewers, whereas the protocols are accessed via the NGC Web site nearly 11,000 times monthly, suggesting that hundreds of providers are accessing these protocols daily. In addition to individual clinicians' use, they are used as teaching tools in conferences and by institutions as references for policies and practices; the extent of the latter uses is unknown.

To our knowledge, only one study has evaluated the effectiveness of protocol implementation using an ABM protocol. Using the "Breastfeeding-Friendly Office Protocol," Corriveau and colleagues[11] in Virginia documented an increase in exclusive breastfeeding rates through 6 months of age in a pediatric practice after protocol implementation. More such implementation analyses are needed.

ABM's 25 clinical protocols collectively address routine prenatal, peripartum, and postpartum (inpatient and outpatient) breastfeeding management, including supplementation, jaundice, human milk storage, cosleeping, procedural pain in the infant, and analgesia and anesthesia for the breastfeeding mother. These protocols also detail prevention and management of complications, such as hypoglycemia in the newborn and engorgement and mastitis in the mother. Guidelines detail management of breastfeeding for a variety of high-risk infants, including the late-preterm, and other special maternal and infant conditions. The brief review of each protocol that follows is intended to provide the reader with highlights; current protocols are available on-line in complete form. A clinical scenario illustrating the application of several protocols is provided (**Box 2**). ABM notes, however, that "these protocols serve only as guidelines for the care of breastfeeding mothers and infants and do not delineate an exclusive course of treatment or serve as standards of medical care. Variations in treatment may be appropriate according to the needs of an individual patient."

PROTOCOL SUMMARIES
ABM Clinical Protocol #1. Guidelines for Glucose Monitoring and Treatment of Hypoglycemia in Breastfed Neonates, Revised 2006 (Under Revision 2012)

Purpose
The purposes of the "hypoglycemia" protocol[12] for breastfed newborns are to provide health care professionals with evidence-based strategies to monitor blood glucose in

Table 3
Sample Internet usage of most accessed and translated protocols

Protocol	National Guideline Clearinghouse[a]	ABM Web Site[b]	Available Languages
	Monthly Views		
Analgesia and anesthesia for the breastfeeding mother[c]	2092		English, Korean, Chinese
Breastfeeding the late preterm infant ($34^{0/7}$ to $36^{6/7}$ wk gestation)	1277		English, Korean, Japanese, Spanish, Polish
Model breastfeeding Policy	1083		English, Chinese, Korean, Spanish
Guidelines for glucose monitoring and treatment of hypoglycemia in breastfed neonates[c]	1082	239	English, Spanish, Japanese, Korean, German, Chinese
Allergic proctocolitis in the exclusively breastfed infant	955		English, Spanish, Korean
Human milk storage information for home use for full-term infants	838	238	English, German, Spanish, Chinese, Korean
Use of galactogogues in initiating or augmenting the rate of maternal milk secretion	810	252	English, Korean, Spanish
Nonpharmacologic management of procedure-related pain in the breastfeeding infant	739		English, Spanish
Breastfeeding friendly physician's office, part 1: optimizing care for infants and children[c]	650		Expired
Contraception during breastfeeding[c]	572		Expired
Mastitis	515	233	English, Korean, Spanish, Chinese, Japanese, German
Hospital guidelines for the use of supplementary feedings in the healthy term breastfed neonate, revised 2009	411	349	English, Spanish, Japanese, Korean, Chinese

Includes 10 most accessed protocols via National Guideline Clearinghouse and 5 most accessed protocols via Academy of Breastfeeding Medicine (ABM) Web site.
[a] Average monthly page views between 8/1/11 and 8/1/12.
[b] During 7/12.
[c] Removed due to expiration 12/2/11.

at-risk late preterm and term infants, as well as to prevent and manage hypoglycemia, including establishing and/or preserving maternal milk supply when supplementation is necessary.

Overview
The protocol reviews newborn glucose physiology, outcomes in symptomatic and asymptomatic infants, suggested definitions of hypoglycemia (and rationale), risk factors, conditions in which monitoring is recommended, potential clinical manifestations, and general management recommendations, including treatment of documented hypoglycemia in both symptomatic and asymptomatic infants.

Box 2
Clinical scenario

E.M. is a 16-year-old single, primiparous mother of a newborn term healthy male infant. After delivery, her baby boy was placed skin to skin with mom and was breastfed for the first time within 45 minutes of birth (peripartum care protocol #5, hospital policy #7). He has breastfed 6 times thus far and mom states it is going well; he has had 2 urinations and 1 stool thus far. She says the nurses have been helping her get the baby positioned for breastfeeding and she will see the lactation consultant later today (peripartum care #5).

E.M. received her prenatal care at the hospital's obstetric clinic and learned about the breast-feeding from her nurse midwife and the nurses in the clinic; she planned to take a breastfeed-ing class offered by the hospital but wasn't able to get transportation to the class (prenatal care #19). E.M.'s prenatal history and labs are all unremarkable and her only medications during pregnancy were prenatal vitamins. She plans to bring her baby boy to the pediatric clinic at the hospital.

E.M. grew up locally but her nuclear family recently moved out of state. The father of the baby is in the military and is currently stationed overseas. E.M. has been living with her aunt and she plans to return there for the first few weeks postpartum. When the baby is several weeks old she plans to return to her parents' home out of state. She has supplies for the baby but no crib or bassinet and has been sleeping on a fold-out couch at her aunt's home. She heard that sleeping with your baby makes breastfeeding easier and plans for the infant to sleep with her.

Your examination conducted in the mother's room reveals a healthy, AGA term male infant. You congratulate the mother on her healthy son and encourage her to breastfeed exclusively for 6 months.

Hearing that she planned for baby to sleep with her on a couch you counsel her about safe sleep for the baby. You talk about the infant's need for a separate sleep space in the same room but not in the same bed and keeping loose bedding, stuffed animals, pillows, and so forth out of the space. She has a playpen for the baby that converts to a small potentially safe sleep space and you encourage her to use that as a bed for the baby for the first few months. You tell her she is correct that being close to the baby encourages frequent breastfeed-ing but that couches are particularly dangerous sleep surfaces for infants. Furthermore, you identify that the aunt is a smoker and you talk with E.M. about environmental smoke exposure for the baby and potential risks including SIDS and increased ear and respiratory infections. You also tell her that breastfeeding substantially lessens the risk of SIDS in her baby. She tells you she heard that a pacifier at bedtime also makes SIDS less likely. You tell her that she is correct but that breastfed babies feed more frequently than bottle-fed babies and that breast-feeding is very protective against SIDS and offers other long-term health advantages for her baby (co-sleeping #6). You recommend that until her milk supply is well established that she avoid using a pacifier and suggest that when the baby is about a month old would be a good time to start using one. You make a referral to the local WIC breastfeeding peer coun-selor and schedule her to see you in the office in 2 days where she can also follow-up with the lactation consultant (going home #2). You tell her you will see her and the baby in the morning for before she is discharged from the hospital and complete today's visit with anticipatory guid-ance about the remainder of testing and care that she can expect her baby to receive at the hospital (hearing screening, state metabolic testing, jaundice and cyanotic heart disease screening).

Routine screening of term, breastfed infants without additional risk factors is not recommended, as healthy, full-term infants do not develop symptomatic hypogly-cemia as a result of underfeeding. Further, ketogenesis occurs when there are pro-longed periods between feeding and the newborn brain is able to use ketone bodies as an energy substrate, thereby protecting neurologic function. When infants do develop documented asymptomatic hypoglycemia, breastfeeding every 1 to 2 hours or provision of 3 to 10 mL/kg of breastmilk or substitute nutrition should be accompanied with rechecking blood glucose before subsequent feeds to confirm acceptable and stable values. Intravenous glucose therapy should be instituted if glucose remains low despite feedings, or if hypoglycemia is symptomatic or severe.

A sample flow diagram for monitoring and treatment of hypoglycemia in breastfed newborns that is consistent with this ABM clinical protocol (but not part of the protocol per se) is shown in **Fig. 2**.

Evidence level and research gaps

The literature was most recently summarized for this protocol in 2006 and is summarized in **Table 1**. The only level I evidence is a randomized trial in rats demonstrating neuroprotective effects of fasting-induced hypoglycemia and ketonemia compared with both control animals and those with insulin-induced hypoglycemia during hypoxic-ischemic brain damage. Approximately half of the available publications were expert opinion with the other half divided between level II-2 and II-3.

ABM Clinical Protocol #2: Guidelines for Hospital Discharge of the Breastfeeding Term Newborn and Mother: "the Going Home Protocol," Revised 2007

Purpose

The purposes of the "Going Home Protocol"[13] are to provide guidelines that address the breastfeeding education and care management of the healthy mother and her term healthy baby around the time of peripartum hospital discharge.

Overview

The protocol recognizes that anticipatory attention to maternal and infant needs at the time of hospital discharge is critical to the successful establishment of breastfeeding and ultimately affects exclusive breastfeeding and breastfeeding duration.

A number of critical issues are addressed in this protocol, including documentation of infant feeding assessments, infant and maternal risk factors for breastfeeding problems/failure, educational needs of breastfeeding women (eg, hand expression/breast pump use, pacifier use, duration of breastfeeding, engorgement), appropriate sources of educational materials for use with breastfeeding dyads, arrangement of follow-up and referral to support organizations, and recommendations if mother and baby are not discharged together.

This protocol is consistent with the Ten Steps (see **Table 2**) and with existing statements of the AAP and ACOG around perinatal care of the breastfeeding dyad.

Evidence level and research gaps

Level I evidence is heavily weighted to the negative effects of commercial formula advertising products (eg, discharge bags) and the benefits of peer counselor support on breastfeeding duration (see **Table 1**). Many organizations have released statements about this topic and it is widely discussed by expert investigators; thus, approximately half of the cited publications are expert opinion with the other half divided between level II-2 and II-3.

ABM Clinical Protocol #3: Hospital Guidelines for the Use of Supplementary Feedings in the Healthy Term Breastfed Neonate, Revised 2009

Purpose

The purposes of the "supplementation" protocol[14] are to assist health care professionals caring for breastfed dyads during the birth hospitalization to minimize the number and volume of formula supplements given to breastfed infants based on evidence of what is medically appropriate and awareness of the adverse outcomes that may result from formula supplementation and the use of artificial nipples.

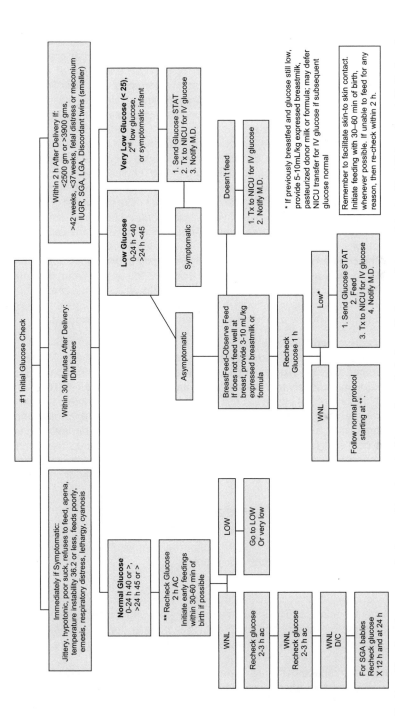

Fig. 2. Algorithm for glucose monitoring and treatment of hypoglycemia in breastfed neonates, consistent with ABM protocol. Units for glucose are mg/dL; AC, preprandial; DC, discontinue; IDM, infant of a diabetic mother; IUGR, intrauterine growth retardation; IV, intravenous; LGA, large for gestational age; NICU, neonatal intensive care unit; SGA, small for gestational age; Tx, transfer; WNL, within normal limits; **Indicates where protocol resumes after correction of hypoglycemia in asymptomatic infant.

Overview

Normal physiology of the breastfed newborn is reviewed, including weight loss, time to regain birth weight, and average reported colostrum intakes per feed over the first few days. Key early management strategies of the breastfeeding dyad are briefly discussed, including recommendations for hospitals to consider requiring physician's orders to dispense formula and documentation of provider education of mothers requesting nonmedically indicated supplementation. Common situations in which supplementation is often provided *inappropriately* are reviewed, along with associated risks of providing supplementation. Situation-specific responses that may preserve exclusive breastfeeding are provided.

Absolute and relative ("possible") medical indications for supplementation of healthy, term infants are outlined. *Choice of supplemental feedings* is discussed, with emphasis that expressed human milk is the first choice. Recognizing that adequate colostrum may not be available to some in the first few days, techniques with which to increase milk supply are reviewed, as are the risks and benefits of other supplemental feedings, including protein hydrolysate, standard, and soy formulas.

Suggested ranges of *volumes of supplemental feedings* at different ages are based on limited research on normal amounts of available colostrum and size of the infant's stomach and the age and size of the infant. Finally, *methods of providing supplementary feeds* are reviewed, along with the available evidence to support safety and efficacy of alternative feeding methods (supplemental nursing device at the breast, cup feeding, spoon or dropper feeding, finger-feeding, syringe feeding). Criteria to assist clinician's and families choose a method of supplementation are considered.

Evidence level and research gaps

The literature was most recently summarized for this protocol in 2008 (see **Table 1**). There are a number of well-designed studies documenting newborn transitional physiology and risks of unnecessary formula supplementation (II-1, II-2, and II-3). Randomized studies (I) document: (1) increased risk of cow's milk allergy in infants requiring supplements and receiving standard cow's milk formula versus whey-hydrolysate or pasteurized human milk, and (2) hydrolyzed formulas may reduce bilirubin levels faster than standard cow's milk formula. A level I study documents that cup feeds may preserve breastfeeding better for infants requiring multiple supplements and those born by cesarean deliveries, and other level I studies document safety of cup feeds in term and preterm infants.

ABM Clinical Protocol #4: Mastitis, Revised 2008

Purpose

The purpose of the mastitis protocol[15] is to optimize the prevention, diagnosis, and management of mastitis in the breastfeeding mother.

Overview

This brief protocol reviews the clinical definition of mastitis, recognizing the continuum from engorgement, noninfective mastitis, infective mastitis, and abscess. The protocol also summarizes the prevalence and predisposing factors as described in the literature and outlines indications and procedures for bacterial culture and sensitivity of the breastmilk, as recommended by WHO.

Key aspects of management are detailed, including effective milk removal, supportive measures, and pharmacologic management, including both analgesia and antibiotic treatment (when indicated, appropriate agents and length of treatment). Follow-up diagnosis and management for resistant cases is outlined. Potential complications of mastitis are discussed, including breastfeeding cessation and abscess formation, and management strategies for the latter. The potential diagnosis of candidal mastitis is discussed including the evolving evidence around this diagnostic dilemma. Finally, preventive strategies are reviewed.

Evidence level and research gaps
The literature was most recently summarized for this protocol in 2007 (see **Table 1**). There are several randomized trials that evaluate prevention of mastitis, and one that studied acupuncture for treatment. The vast majority of available evidence on prevalence, causes, treatment, and complications are from case-control or cohort studies (II-2). There is little high-quality evidence evaluating effect of antibiotic treatment, with only 2 randomized or quasi-randomized studies, one of which was very small.

ABM Clinical Protocol #5: Peripartum Breastfeeding Management for the Healthy Mother and Infant at Term, Revised 2008

Purpose
The purposes of the "peripartum care" protocol[16] are to provide guidelines that address the breastfeeding education and care of the healthy mother and her term healthy baby during prenatal care and the intrapartum and postpartum hospital time periods.

Overview
The protocol recognizes that hospital care of the breastfeeding couplet strongly influences the successful establishment of breastfeeding. Additionally, it addresses the prenatal time period and the education and evaluation of expectant women around breastfeeding.

Guidance is provided about prenatal care and evaluation of the expectant woman around breastfeeding. Issues include assessment of medical and physical conditions that affect mothers' ability to breastfeed, informed consent around infant feeding, effects of labor medications on breastfeeding, sources of patient education materials, and referral to antenatal support organizations. With regard to hospital care. the intrapartum, immediate postpartum, and ensuing hospital stays are addressed. This protocol is consistent with the WHO/UNICEF Ten Steps (as are all ABM protocols [see **Table 2**]) and with existing statements of the AAP and ACOG around perinatal care of the breastfeeding dyad. The protocol addresses details of incorporating the Ten Steps into maternal and infant peripartum care. Couplets at risk for breastfeeding problems that may benefit from lactation consultation are discussed, as is early discharge and maternal infant separation for medical indications.

Evidence level and research gaps
The literature was most recently summarized for this protocol in 2008 (see **Table 1**). The effectiveness of the Ten Steps is well supported in the literature and is supported by level 1 evidence for many recommendations in this protocol. Additionally, many guidelines, and statements from large professional organizations are cited in support of these recommendations.

ABM Clinical Protocol #6: Guideline on Cosleeping and Breastfeeding, Revised 2008

Purpose
The purpose of the "cosleeping" protocol[17] is to provide guidance about safe and unsafe infant sleep locations and practices. It specifically addresses the issues of cosleeping or bed sharing, parenting practices that may have significant positive impact on breastfeeding. Recommendations guide informed education of the breastfeeding mother/family that wishes to cosleep with an infant.

Overview

The practice of cosleeping is common in many areas of the world and is known to enhance breastfeeding frequency and duration. In recent years, the practices of bed sharing and cosleeping have received significant negative comment in developed countries. Some infant safe sleep guidelines (eg, United States) warn against cosleeping. Concerns center around mechanical suffocation and sudden infant death syndrome (SIDS) risks.

The protocol reviews the existing literature regarding cosleeping and asphyxiation risk, SIDS prevention and risk, with attention to ethnic diversity, and parental factors. It additionally reviews the effects of cosleeping on breastfeeding, which are positive. Of note, the document states that "there is not currently enough evidence to support routine recommendations against cosleeping." Most importantly, guidelines are provided in educating parents who wish to cosleep with their infant about the risks and benefits of cosleeping and unsafe cosleeping practices so that they may make an informed decision. To assist practitioners in counseling parents, attention is given to known unsafe practices related to cosleeping and the immediate sleep environment.

Evidence level and research gaps

The literature was most recently updated for this protocol in 2008 and will be again updated in 2013 (see **Table 1**). Owing to the relatively low incidence of infant death from either cosleeping or SIDS the empiric evidence around these topics is largely limited to epidemiologic studies (II-2) and meta-analyses and organizational statements (level III). It should be noted that the 2007 Agency for Healthcare Quality Research literature review on the effects of breastfeeding supports a 40% reduction in the risks of SIDS attributable to breastfeeding.[18]

ABM Clinical Protocol #7: Model Breastfeeding Policy, Revised 2010

Purpose

Recognizing that writing a breastfeeding policy in compliance with WHO/UNICEF Ten Steps requires hospitals to expend significant time and resources, ABM prepared this "hospital-policy" protocol[19] to reduce the burden of work for hospitals wishing to improve their maternity care practices around breastfeeding.

The purpose is to promote a philosophy and practice of maternal-infant care that advocates breastfeeding and to provide a model breastfeeding policy that incorporates the UNICEF/WHO evidence-based Ten Steps to Successful Breastfeeding (see **Table 2**) and make it readily available and adaptable to the needs of hospitals and birth centers worldwide.

Overview

The policy is written as a template, allowing hospitals to insert their institutional specifics and easily attain the basic form of a Ten Steps–compliant hospital policy on breastfeeding. It is based on recommendations from the most recent policy statements from the Office on Women's Health, US Department of Health and Human Services, AAP, ACOG, AAFP, WHO, ABM, and the UNICEF/WHO evidence-based Ten Steps to Successful Breastfeeding (see **Table 2**).

It has been adopted by New York State Health Department for use in their effort to change maternity care practices statewide and is additionally being used in the United States by The Joint Commission as a model for hospital use. Internationally, use of the protocol is more difficult to discern but it has been translated into many languages and republished broadly.

The protocol takes the mother/infant dyad through the entire peripartum stay, addressing all issues of care and delineating specific policies to ensure an optimal experience for the breastfeeding dyad.

Evidence level and research gaps

The policy and literature was most recently updated for this protocol in 2010 (see **Table 1**). As with ABM protocols #5 (Peripartum Care) and #3 (Going Home) the evidence is largely around incorporation of various aspects of the Ten Steps individually and in aggregate. Level 1 evidence is available for the Ten Steps and several epidemiologic studies indicate that breastfeeding improves incrementally as more steps are incorporated. Statements from maternal and child health agencies and health care organizations comprise most level III evidence.

ABM Clinical Protocol #8: Human Milk Storage Information for Home Use for Full-term Infants, Revised 2010

Purpose

The purpose of the "milk-storage" protocol[20] is to provide evidence-based guidelines for safe human milk handling and storage for home use for full-term infants with which health care providers can inform families.

Overview

The protocol systematically addresses recommendations for hand-washing, milk expression, containers of different materials, washing of containers, and washing of breasts and nipples.

Existing evidence is briefly reviewed regarding recommendations for length of storage at various 'room', 'cooler', refrigerator, and freezer temperatures. Studies at all temperatures have generally evaluated bacterial growth. Additionally, refrigerated and frozen samples have been evaluated by measuring decline in bactericidal capacity as a marker for milk quality and safety. The impact of freezing on specific nutrients is also discussed, as are alterations in smell and taste, which can occur with storage.

Finally, recommendations for use of stored milk are provided in terms of appropriate defrosting, temperature for drinking, shelf-life after thawing, and so forth.

Evidence level and research gaps

The literature for this protocol was last reviewed in 2010 (see **Table 1**). The vast majority of the work is level II-1 laboratory studies evaluating the effect of storage times, temperatures, and containers on human milk's bacterial growth, nutrient content (eg, vitamins, minerals, protein) and quality (eg, immunoglobulins, bactericidal capacity, cell count, antioxidants, enzymes). The level I study in this bibliography actually compared prestorage bacterial content of manually expressed versus pumped milk in mothers of very low birth weight infants.

ABM Clinical Protocol #9: Use of Galactagogues in Initiating or Augmenting the Rate of Maternal Milk Secretion, Revised 2011

Purpose

The purposes of the "galactagogue" protocol[21] are to assist health care providers who are caring for mothers with inadequate milk production to optimize their milk secretion by nonpharmacologic measures and understand the potential indications, risks, and benefits for specific galactagogues as documented by current evidence.

Overview

The protocol reviews the physiology of milk production with initial endocrine control of secretory activation (lactogenesis II) and subsequent autocrine control of the rate of milk synthesis. Potential indications for galactagogues are discussed, including "pump-dependent" women in whom milk supply often declines after a few weeks, other situations of faltering milk production, relactation, or adoption.

Available evidence for efficacy of specific pharmaceutical galactagogues is reviewed, with primary emphasis on domperidone and metoclopramide. At the time of protocol revision, there were several small randomized controlled trials in domperidone that suggested short-term efficacy, but otherwise scant evidence to support efficacy of either agent.

Evidence for use of herbals, foods, and beverages as galactagogues is also reviewed in an appendix, with the cautionary note that additional concerns for herbal preparations include lack of standardized dosing, possible contaminants, allergic potential, and drug interactions.

Recommendations for practice for women experiencing difficulties with low milk production are reviewed, with both term and preterm infants. This includes optimizing milk removal (through breastfeeding frequency and duration and/or milk expression); evaluation of medical causes of hypogalactia; weighing potential risks and benefits of specific galactagogues and informing the mother; use of pharmacologic agents for the shortest period of time and lowest possible dose; and consideration of dose-tapering.

Overall, in light of limited evidence for efficacy and potential for significant side effects of these drugs, this protocol recommends careful consideration before prescribing galactagogues in individual cases.

Evidence level and research gaps
The literature was most recently summarized for this protocol in 2009 (see **Table 1**). There are a number of RCTs of various pharmacologic agents, including metoclopramide and domperidone. Those with metoclopramide, however, are generally of low quality, small sample size, and with mixed results. Multiple small cohort studies II-1, II-3, and case reports document increase in milk supply with metoclopramide use. Several small blinded randomized controlled trials (RCTs) in domperidone suggest efficacy. A population-based study in the Netherlands (II-2) documented increased risk of sudden death with noncardiac QTc prolonging drugs, eg, domperidone. There are no placebo-controlled studies in herbals, only one RCT comparing fenugreek to torbangun (level I).

ABM Clinical Protocol #10: Breastfeeding the Late Preterm Infant (34^0–$36^{6/7}$ Weeks Gestation), Revised 2011

Purpose
The purposes of this "late-preterm" protocol[22] are to allow for as much breastfeeding and breastmilk feeding as possible in late preterms; heighten awareness of difficulties they may experience with breastfeeding; offer strategies to anticipate, promptly identify, and manage these problems so as to prevent medical complications; and finally, to maintain awareness of maternal needs, understanding of feeding plans, and coping ability.

Overview
This protocol reviews definitions of late preterm infants, noting applicability to some infants born at $37^{0/7}$ to $37^{6/7}$ weeks' gestation and reviews the reasons for and complication of the greater incidence of breastfeeding difficulties in these infants.

Principles of care are outlined and include optimizing communication (eg, inpatient and outpatient feeding plans among staff, family, and outpatient providers), clinical assessment, lactation support, minimal maternal-infant separation, prevention of complications, education (eg, family and staff in both inpatient and outpatient settings), discharge planning, close-follow-up, and monitoring care through quality improvement projects.

Specific recommendations for implementing these principles of care are then systematically provided for both inpatient and outpatient settings. These are chronologically divided into the inpatient (initial care, ongoing care, and discharge planning) and outpatient settings and incorporate the Ten Steps. Examples of late preterm-specific modifications include having a late preterm order set that can be easily modified, showing the mother techniques to facilitate effective latch with careful attention to adequate support of the jaw and head, early consideration of using an ultrathin silicone nipple shield for ineffective milk transfer, consideration of prefeeding and postfeeding weights, written discharge feeding plan that is communicated to the primary care provider, and so forth.

In the outpatient setting, emphasis is placed on late preterm–specific strategies for poor weight gain. Appropriate weight gain and frequency of outpatient weight checks are reviewed. Vitamin D and iron supplementation is addressed, as are screening recommendations for iron deficiency.

Evidence level and research gaps
The literature was most recently summarized for this protocol in 2010 (see **Table 1**). Overall, there are very few high level studies on breastfeeding assessment and management specifically in preterm infants. Many level II studies define physiologic vulnerability, normal maturation of feeding (suck/swallow/coordinated suck-swallow-breathe), increased morbidity (including readmissions) and mortality, and other outcomes. Studies on breastfeeding assessment are primarily level II-3, but none specifically were in preterm infants. Level I studies do exist on methods of feeding (cup, bottle, nasogastric feeds), with mixed results on short-term and long-term outcomes. A level II-2 study of nipple shields in premature infants documented increased milk transfer.

ABM Clinical Protocol #11: Guidelines for the Evaluation and Management of Neonatal Ankyloglossia and Its Complications in the Breastfeeding Dyad (Under Revision 2012)

Purpose
The purpose of the "tongue-tie" protocol[23] is to provide health care professionals with evidence-based guidelines to assess and treat ankyloglossia with associated breastfeeding problems and to further define areas of needed research.

Overview
The expired protocol reviews the definition, incidence and complications of ankyloglossia and recommendations for assessment of breastfeeding difficulties and severity of ankyloglossia. The frenulotomy procedure is described in detail. Recommendations for management of maternal complications of nipple pain, trauma, and suppressed lactation are provided.

Evidence level and research gaps
The literature was reviewed in 2012 for the protocol revision (see **Table 1**). Most of the evidence is level II-3, describing prevalence, associated breastfeeding difficulties, assessment, and outcomes with frenulotomy. There are 2 level I studies that randomize frenulotomy (versus sham or deferred procedure) and document greater improvement with frenulotomy (defined as maternal pain in one study, not defined in the other).

ABM Clinical Protocol #12: Transitioning the Breastfeeding/Breastmilk-fed Premature Infant from the Neonatal Intensive Care Unit to Home (Under Revision 2012)

Purpose
The purpose of this expired "Neonatal intensive care unit grad" protocol[24] is to assist health care providers monitor and optimize nutritional support for breastfed or

breastmilk-fed premature infants in anticipation of and following discharge from the hospital.

Overview

The expired protocol recommended careful review of nutritional status well before discharge, evaluating adequacy of both linear and ponderal growth and biochemical nutritional status, in conjunction with type, amount, and method of feeding. For those with optimal nutrition (defined in the protocol), a transition plan is described including recommendations for trialing human milk without fortifier or formula supplements in specific situations and guidelines for monitoring frequency of growth and biochemistry. Similarly, postdischarge assessments of growth and biochemistry are recommended, with corrective actions for those with inadequate growth or biochemical status, and content and frequency of subsequent evaluations.

The protocol includes detailed description of how to assess and optimize breastfeeding in premature infants, including assessment of latch, milk volume and transfer, frequency of feeds, maternal milk content, maternal satisfaction, and consideration of feeding devices and test weights.

Evidence level and research gaps

This protocol was originally approved in 2004, before ABM implemented the requirement that annotated bibliographies should be the initial step of protocol development (see **Table 1**). The protocol was acknowledged to be primarily expert opinion. Literature review for the revision is ongoing.

ABM Clinical Protocol #13: Contraception During Breastfeeding (Under Revision 2012)

Purpose

The purpose of the "contraception" protocol[25] is to identify contraceptive methods available for use during breastfeeding and provide additional information on the lactational amenorrhea method (LAM) and its use.

Overview

The protocol identifies relevant issues to be considered in the lactating woman when recommending a contraceptive method and cites effectiveness data for various methods, discusses advantages and disadvantages of methods, and the effect on lactation. Information about LAM, including the biologic basis, definition of the method, efficacy, considerations for physician counseling, management issues, and transitioning to other methods is discussed.

The update of the protocol is expected to address low-dose estrogen-containing contraceptives, the use of deproprovera in the immediate postpartum time period, and a number of new contraceptive methods, such as the vaginal ring and contraceptive patch.

Evidence level and research gaps

Literature cited in this protocol was last updated in 2005 and the protocol is currently being revised (see **Table 1**). Much of the evidence is dated, although it includes several RCTs and thus level 1 evidence. The information on LAM is well established and unlikely to be altered in the protocol update.

ABM Clinical Protocol #14: Breastfeeding-friendly Physician's Office, Part 1: Optimizing Care for Infants and Children (Under Revision 2012)

Purpose

The purpose of this protocol[26] is to describe the environment and practices of a physician's outpatient office that promotes, supports, and protects breastfeeding through a supportive office environment and education of health care professionals and families.

Overview

As with other ABM products, the recommendations made in this protocol are congruent with WHO/UNICEF Ten Steps (see **Table 2**) and provide detail about incorporation in a particular medical care setting. Based on strong empiric evidence that professional support of breastfeeding improves outcomes, the protocol provides recommendations to optimize support in the outpatient setting caring for children. The protocol draws on the fact that many aspects of the Ten Steps can be extended to outpatient settings and acknowledges that incremental changes to improve breastfeeding support are of value, as there is a dose-response relationship between the number of steps achieved and breastfeeding outcomes in inpatient settings.

The protocol provides guidance about incorporation of breastfeeding promotion, instruction, support, and clinical management into the routines of outpatient pediatric care.

Evidence level and research gaps

This protocol was first published in 2006 (see **Table 1**). ABM is currently reviewing the evidence around this topic in preparation for publication of an update. Previously cited evidence contained about 1/3 level I and II-2 evidence and 2/3 level III expert opinion or policy statements.

ABM Clinical Protocol #15: Analgesia and Anesthesia for the Breastfeeding Mother (Under Revision 2012)

Purpose

Recognizing that maternal anesthesia and analgesia may affect the neonate by passage into maternal breastmilk and that suboptimal choices may result in breastfeeding problems or unnecessary recommendations for breastfeeding cessation, the ABM published this "analgesia and anesthesia" protocol.[27] The protocol provides evidence around prudent practices with regard to labor and postpartum analgesia and anesthesia for the mother wishing to breastfeed.

Overview

The protocol summarizes evidence and recommendations for analgesia and anesthesia for labor, including pharmacologic and nonpharmacologic interventions, with attention to effects on breastfeeding. Uses of intravenous medications, epidural analgesia, and local anesthesia in vaginal and cesarean delivery are reviewed. Methods with the fewest effects on the neonate are identified and encouraged. Postpartum analgesia with nonopioid analgesics is encouraged to avoid maternal and infant sedation. Intravenous, oral and epidural/spinal methods are discussed. Surgical anesthesia for the lactating postpartum woman is reviewed, including specific guidance about infant age and when and if there is a need to interrupt breastfeeding. In a final section, specific medications are reviewed, including milk levels and infant effects.

Evidence level and research gaps

This protocol was last updated in 2006 and is undergoing revision (see **Table 1**). Randomized trials tracking breastfeeding outcomes in this area are rare, and subject to a great deal of crossover, which confounds results. Although significant controversy remains, new information has been published about maternal epidural anesthesia for labor and the effects on breastfeeding duration; information about this topic is expected to be expanded.

ABM Clinical Protocol #16: Breastfeeding the Hypotonic Infant, 2007

Purpose

The purpose of this "hypotonia" protocol[28] is to promote, support, and sustain breast-feeding in children with hypotonia.

Overview

The protocol begins with the definition of hypotonia, a list of common conditions in which hypotonia may occur or develop, and the reasons for which feeding problems often coexist. Down syndrome, as one of the more common and better studied causes of hypotonia, is used as an example. Other oral abnormalities typically coexist in Down syndrome and further complicate the feeding. Risks of formula feeding, which have not been specifically studied in Down syndrome or other hypotonic infants, are reviewed. Maternal experiences at diagnosis are briefly discussed, along with maternal reports of frustration and lack of support for breastfeeding.

A review of sucking behavior in Down syndrome details the multiple affected parameters, along with longitudinal changes in these parameters. For these infants specifically, feeding problems improve substantially by 3 to 4 months of age.

Recommendations address maternal education, measures to facilitate and assess feeding at the breast in the immediate postpartum period, preventive measures to preserve maternal milk supply, and recommendations for discharge and the remainder of the neonatal period. Many of the recommendations mirror the Ten Steps, with the recognition that these infants should be considered high risk.

Supporting the head and body is emphasized, with specific examples of how to do so (eg, the "Dancer" position). Other measures that may facilitate milk transfer include manual breast compression during breastfeeds and silicone nipple shields. Alternative feeding methods are discussed for infants unable to breastfeed or sustain suckling long enough to complete the feed, as are measures to protect the maternal milk supply for infants unable to fully breastfeed. Finally, infants with poor weight gain or coexisting cardiac, gastrointestinal, or renal anomalies may require additional calories; methods of enhancing the caloric density of breastmilk are discussed.

Evidence level and research gaps

The literature for this protocol was last reviewed in 2006 (see **Table 1**). Much of the evidence for these recommendations has been extrapolated from work in premature infants. There are level II-2 studies that evaluate the feeding decisions in mothers whose infants have Down syndrome, sucking behavior of infants with Down syndrome, and oxygen saturation during breast versus bottle feeds in infants with congenital heart disease. All other available evidence is of lower level (III) or extrapolated from premature infants or the general population.

ABM Clinical Protocol #17: Guidelines for Breastfeeding Infants with Cleft Lip, Cleft Palate, or Cleft Lip and Palate, 2007

Purpose

The purpose of the "cleft lip and palate" protocol[29] is to provide evidence-based guidelines with which to assist health care professionals optimize breastfeeding and/or provision of breastmilk for infants with cleft lip and/or cleft palate.

Overview

The background provides the definition and incidence of cleft lip and palate, separately and in combination. The anatomy and physiology of breastfeeding is briefly reviewed, with subsequent explanation of the impairment cleft lips and especially palates can cause for infants in generating suction and, for palates, also compression.

Practice recommendations include prenatal education whenever possible on the risks of formula feeding, as well as potential feeding difficulties and their management and referral for peer support. Mothers should be encouraged to provide as much breast-milk as possible.

Further recommendations are for individualized feeding assessment, provision of knowledgeable support, counseling about provision of breastmilk when direct breast-feeding is unlikely to be the sole source of nutrition (including assistance with hand expression and/or pumping beginning on day 1), delayed breastfeeding when the infant is unable to breastfeed directly, and monitoring of hydration and weight gain while feeding is established.

Specific modifications to breastfeeding via positioning are suggested, and are different for the infant with cleft lip versus cleft palate or cleft lip and palate. These should be individually evaluated for success. Parents should also be educated that orthopedic prostheses used for alignment preoperatively do not significantly increase feeding efficiency or effectiveness. Finally, guidelines for when infants can safely breastfeed postoperatively are provided. A list of frequently asked questions is provided as a protocol appendix.

Evidence level and research gaps

The literature for this protocol was last reviewed in 2007, and is limited, anecdotal, and includes studies with mixed results (see **Table 1**). Some of the reviews include level I studies, but were focused on all feeding interventions, not only breastfeeding. Many of the studies do not describe their populations in terms of size, location, and type of cleft, thus limiting utility of findings. There is level II-2 evidence that breastmilk provides extra benefits for infants with cleft lip and/or palate, beyond that expected in the normal population.

There is weak evidence that infants with cleft lip only are able to breastfeed and that infants with cleft palate have difficulty breastfeeding. Level III evidence guides management strategies and there is little evidence to guide assessment. There is level I evidence that obturators do not significantly facilitate feeding or weight gain and level II-1 evidence about when breastfeeding can occur postoperatively.

ABM Clinical Protocol #18: Use of Antidepressants in Nursing Mothers, 2008

Purpose

Recognizing that between 5% and 25% of women experience depression in the post-partum year, the ABM wrote the "antidepressant" protocol[30] to inform providers about treatment options and the risks and benefits to the breastfeeding woman and her infant. The protocol provides information on the risks of untreated depression, risks of medication to the infant and mother, and the benefits of treatment.

Overview

The protocol makes recommendations for active screening for and, when present, making the diagnosis of postpartum depression, and how treatment can be deter-mined. It specifically addresses the medications for which there is sufficient evidence to make recommendations and provides data (selective serotonin reuptake inhibitors [SSRIs] and tricyclic antidepressants [TCAs]/heterocyclic).

The protocol identifies appropriate validated tools and provides guidance about dis-tinguishing postpartum depression from the "baby blues" and about obtaining an appropriate history to illicit depressive symptoms.

Options for treatment are discussed. Psychotherapy is recommended as a first-line treatment for breastfeeding women with mild to moderate depression. The use of antidepressants is discussed when psychotherapy is not available or symptoms are severe. Guidance is provided about choice of antidepressant with specific detail about how to weigh risks and benefits in the individual lactating woman.

There is discussion of the pharmacokinetics of medication passage into breastmilk and infant factors that may affect the choice of medications and about specific classes of antidepressants, including SSRIs and TCAs/heterocyclic antidepressants, herbals including St John's wort and nutritional supplements, such as omega-3 fatty acids. The protocol does not supply a specific algorithm for treatment but recommendations address a number of important clinical considerations in diagnosis, selection of treatment options, and follow-up of women and their infants.

Evidence level and research gaps
This protocol was published in 2008 (see **Table 1**) and will undergo revision in 2013. There is a general lack of empiric evidence from which to make recommendations on this subject. Data on antidepressants to inform clinical decision making is largely from case reports or case series. There are very limited data on long-term effects on child development of antidepressant exposure via breastmilk.

ABM Clinical Protocol #19: Breastfeeding Promotion in the Prenatal Setting, 2009

Purpose
The ABM recognizes that a significant proportion of women make infant feeding decisions during the prenatal time period and that optimal support may influence a woman's choice of infant feeding method. The purpose of the "prenatal" protocol[31] is to provide guidelines for policies and practices that promote breastfeeding initiation and duration during outpatient prenatal care of the expectant woman.

Overview
As with ABM protocol #14 (outpatient pediatrics), guidance in this protocol extends breastfeeding supportive practices from the WHO/UNICEF Ten Steps (see **Table 2**) to the prenatal care setting. Issues addressed include the creation of a breastfeeding-friendly prenatal environment with guidance about staff education, appropriate patient education materials (free of commercial formula bias), and documentation in medical record. Specifics of an appropriate breastfeeding history are discussed including past experiences, plans for this child, and identification of potential complications or contraindications. Family traditions, expectations and support, and important elements of a woman's support system are recognized to have a significant influence on maternal success at breastfeeding. It is suggested that the initial physical examination is a good time to introduce the topic of infant feeding, reassure mother about her ability to breastfeed, and further identify any medical contraindications/ conditions that might affect breastfeeding success. Finally, recommendations are made for each trimester of prenatal care to help practitioners integrate breastfeeding support into the routines of office practice.

Evidence level and research gaps
This protocol was last updated in 2009. The literature in this area is relatively sparse (see **Table 1**). About one-third of the literature cited comes from RCTs, whereas most is observational (level II-2, III-3).

ABM Clinical Protocol #20: Engorgement, 2009

Purpose
The purpose of this "engorgement" protocol[32] is to provide evidence-based recommendations to prevent, recognize, and manage breast engorgement to facilitate successful breastfeeding.

Overview

The background of this brief protocol reviews the definition, proposed pathophysiology, and epidemiology of breast engorgement. It is acknowledged that there is a spectrum from expected, mild, physiologic engorgement during lactogenesis to severely symptomatic engorgement and, further, that there are no clinically useful tools for assessing engorgement. A differential diagnosis is provided.

Research on prevention, other than medical therapies to suppress lactation, is minimal. The currently recommended breastfeeding technique of emptying one breast at each feeding and alternating which breast is offered first is associated with less engorgement. Limited evidence suggests breast massage after feeds for the first 4 days postpartum may reduce engorgement.

Effective management strategies are reviewed, because prolonged symptomatic engorgement can negatively impact milk supply. There are 2 enzymatic preparations that have been shown to be more effective than placebo (one with anti-inflammatory properties and another in combination with an anti-inflammatory agent). Reverse pressure softening near the areola improves the infant's latch during engorgement. If the infant cannot nurse, manual expression or pumping should be performed either to soften the area to allow for latch, or for milk extraction to feed the infant.

A list of commonly recommended management strategies that have been shown to have no benefit (eg, cabbage leaves or extract and cold packs) is provided. Herbal treatments have not been studied.

Finally, recommendations for anticipatory guidance regarding engorgement to be provided before hospital discharge are summarized, including pain control, contact information for breastfeeding support, and advice and instructions on manual breast-milk expression. Providers seeing newborns or mothers after discharge should routinely inquire about engorgement.

Evidence level and research gaps

The literature for this protocol was last reviewed in 2006 and high-quality evidence is limited in lactating women (see **Table 1**). There are a number of older studies done in nonlactating women. There are several level I, II-1, and level II-2 studies supporting efficacy or nonefficacy of the treatments discussed previously. Eight randomized or quasi-randomized trials were considered high enough quality to include in a Cochrane review in 2001. Data supporting massage and reverse pressure softening are weak.

ABM Clinical Protocol #21: Guidelines for Breastfeeding and the Drug-dependent Woman, 2009

Purpose

The evaluation and management of the drug-dependent woman who wishes to breastfeed her infant unfortunately is an increasingly common concern for pediatric providers. The ABM wrote this protocol[33] to provide an evidence-based guideline for the evaluation and management of the drug-dependent woman choosing to breastfeed.

Overview

A background section addresses incidence and prevalence of drug use among women of childbearing age, issues of poly-substance use, other associated medical, mental health, social, and support concerns that are often associated with substance use and affect the risk-benefit assessment of breastfeeding in a particular mother baby couplet.

Further, the protocol discusses the limited information available about drugs of abuse and transfer into breastmilk; more information is available about methadone, and its use in breastfeeding is presented. Recommendations are made regarding prenatal education, evaluation, and preparation of the drug-dependent mother for breastfeeding her infant. Criteria are presented for selection of women who should be supported or discouraged in their decision to breastfeed. Recommendations for ongoing monitoring of the lactating woman with a history of substance use and the management of women who relapse are discussed.

Evidence level and research gaps

This protocol was last updated in 2009 (see **Table 1**). The literature in this area is sparse in total with most emphasis on methadone and lactation. The large majority of literature in this area constitutes primarily case reports. There are 4 reviews of general drug dependence and breastfeeding, and only case reports for illicit drug use (PCP, cocaine, marijuana) and breastfeeding; most conclude that illicit drug use and breastfeeding are incompatible. Few studies are level II, all regarding methadone use in lactation and only one case controlled study. Three small studies address buprenorphine and breastfeeding with conflicting results. All suffer from small numbers.

ABM Clinical Protocol #22: Guidelines for Management of Jaundice in the Breastfeeding Infant Equal to or Greater than 35 Weeks' Gestation, 2010

Purpose

Hyperbilirubinemia is a common neonatal problem often associated with breastfeeding problems with poor infant intake and dehydration. The purposes of this "jaundice" protocol[34] are to provide guidance about: (1) distinguishing causes of jaundice/hyperbilirubinemia in the newborn that are directly related to breastfeeding from those that are not; (2) monitoring and managing hyperbilirubinemia while preserving breastfeeding and protecting the infant from the potential toxicity risks of hyperbilirubinemia; and (3) hospital and office procedures for optimal management of jaundice and hyperbilirubinemia in the breastfed newborn and young infant.

Overview

All recommendations made in the protocol are consistent with the AAP Clinical Practice Guideline on Management of Hyperbilirubinemia in the Newborn Infant 35 or More Weeks of Gestation and the 2009 update to the guideline with additional information offered to provide specifics about breastfeeding concerns and management.[35,36]

The protocol begins with a discussion of the prevalence and etiology of neonatal hyperbilirubinemia delineating the normal rise in bilirubin that occurs in the healthy infant during the first week of life commonly termed "physiologic jaundice of the neonate."

In subsequent sections, important entities such as "breastmilk jaundice" and "starvation jaundice" and potential interactions between them are discussed. Understanding these concepts is central to appropriate management of hyperbilirubinemia in the breastfed infant. Problematic feeding is a significant contributor to neonatal hyperbilirubinemia and may be associated with neonatal weight loss and dehydration and, if not appropriately treated, bilirubin encephalopathy.

In the management of jaundice section, guidelines are made about monitoring and management of jaundice with attention to preservation of exclusive breastfeeding whenever possible. Breastfeeding practices that enhance success are encouraged, including early and frequent feeding, instruction of parents about feeding cues, and identification of infants at risk for hyperbilirubinemia because of poor breastfeeding and early lactation consultation in these cases.

Treatment guidelines use graphics for risk assessment and intervention from the AAP Guideline and are completely consistent with that publication.[35,37] Focus is placed on practices that allow for safe and effective treatment of hyperbilirubinemia with continued breastfeeding and minimal disruption of the process. Topics discussed include in-hospital administration of usual treatments with attention to breastfeeding supportive practices (eg, enhancing maternal milk supply, phototherapy in mother's room). Additionally, appropriate indications for alternative interventions, such as temporary breastfeeding cessation or formula supplementation, are discussed.

Evidence level and research gaps
The literature review focuses on basic and clinical research and on clinical guidance published between 1980 and 2005 relating directly to the relationship between neonatal jaundice and breastfeeding. Significant papers published before that period were also included (see **Table 1**). Broader issues of neonatal jaundice unrelated to breastfeeding, bilirubin metabolism, and sequelae of hyperbilirubinemia were not reviewed and readers are referred to the AAP guidelines[35] and the technical report by Ip and colleagues.[38] A total of 34 references were reviewed, of which 8 are level I and 22 are level II-1 or II-2 indicating that most research supporting this protocol is moderately strong epidemiologic evidence.

ABM Clinical Protocol #23: Nonpharmacologic Management of Procedure-related Pain in the Breastfeeding Infant, 2010

Purpose
The "pain" protocol[39] educates health care professionals on use of nonpharmacologic and behavioral interventions to relieve procedure-induced pain in breastfed infants with the overall goals of avoiding untreated pain and its sequelae while promoting breastfeeding.

Overview
The protocol background provides the rationale for treating pain in this population by summarizing the potential detrimental consequences of untreated pain, such as greater pain sensitivity in later childhood, parental distress, and so forth. The protocol then reviews evidence-based techniques for treating procedure-related pain in term newborns, premature newborns, and older infants (1 month–1 year of age), with emphasis that combining techniques may be more effective (eg, taste, sucking, skin-to-skin contact).

For term newborns, breastfeeding is the preferred choice, and itself is a multicomponent approach. For situations when breastfeeding is unavailable, the protocol methodically details the evidence for and practical aspects of using breastmilk, skin-to-skin contact, sucrose (with dosing recommendations), sucking, and combinations of these modalities.

There is less research in preterm infants, where medical and developmental status of the infant may preclude breastfeeding and even suck and swallow. There are concerns about prolonged sucrose exposure; one study documents lower motor scores and attention at term associated with receipt of more sucrose doses. Recommendations discuss the evidence for and practical aspects of providing relief via skin-to-skin contact, a pacifier dipped in sucrose, sucrose alone (doses provided), breastfeeding, and combinations of these modalities.

Evidence for and practical aspects of providing these measures for infants up to a year of age are also discussed.

Evidence level and research gaps
The evidence base for this protocol was reviewed in 2009 and overall there is a high level of evidence to support the recommendations (see **Table 1**). There are a relatively

large number of randomized, controlled studies evaluating breastfeeding, breastmilk, sucrose, and skin-to-skin contact as analgesics in term newborns.

ABM Clinical Protocol #24: Allergic Proctocolitis in the Exclusively Breastfed Infant, 2011

Purpose

The "allergic proctocolitis" protocol[40] explores the scientific basis, pathologic aspects, and clinical management of allergic proctocolitis in the breastfed infant and defines future research needs.

Overview

The protocol specifically addresses a clinical entity similarly known as allergic colitis, benign dietary protein proctitis, eosinophilic proctitis, or breast milk-induced proctocolitis. In a background section of this protocol, the definitions, incidence, clinical presentation, and pathophysiology of allergic proctocolitis are reviewed.

Maternal elimination diet is recommended as the first line of treatment, avoiding food containing the most likely allergen, cow's milk protein followed by other common food allergens (eg, soy, citrus fruits, eggs, nuts, peanuts, wheat, corn, strawberries, and chocolate). Geographic food differences are discussed with attention to common food allergens in different parts of the world. For more difficult cases, recommendations are made about the risk-benefit analysis weighing maternal concerns (restricted diet, nutritional needs, ability to comply) versus infant symptom resolution and benefits from breastfeeding. Treatment options are discussed should maternal elimination diet fail to resolve clinical symptoms. The addition of pancreatic enzymes in difficult cases is reviewed, including maternal dosing and available enzyme preparations.

An evaluation and management section includes recommendations about relevant history, breastfeeding assessment, evaluation of other allergic symptoms (eczema), assessment of infant growth, and laboratory evaluation. Clinical recommendations end with an algorithm of evaluation and treatment based on severity of clinical symptoms at presentation.

The protocol ends with a long section of research needs discussing a variety of poorly understood aspects of allergic proteolysis in the breastfed infant.

Evidence level and research gaps

This protocol was first published in 2011 (see **Table 1**). The literature review encompasses articles written in English and published between 1980 and 2010; a total of 54 papers were identified. A large proportion of the empiric evidence is level II-2. Very few RCTs have been conducted with regard to this entity with the exception of 2 trials, one of probiotics in addition to the elimination diet and one of maternal elimination diet alone. Most studies are observational in nature and center around clinical course, laboratory findings, and pathologic findings of allergic proctocolitis. A number of articles were identified about maternal prenatal and postnatal characteristics contributing to the development of allergic proctocolitis in the infant; most of these are prospective and observational in nature.

ABM Clinical Protocol #25 Recommendations for Pre-procedural Fasting for the Breastfed Infant: "NPO" Guidelines, 2012

Purpose

The "NPO" protocol[41] assists health care providers by defining minimum pre-procedural fasting requirements for breastfed infants with the overall goal of preventing pulmonary aspiration, hypoglycemia, and volume depletion, while also minimizing stress and anxiety in fasting infants and supporting optimal breastfeeding before and after procedures.

Overview

This protocol addresses procedures which require anything on the continuum between moderate sedation and general anesthesia, first reviewing the mechanism, incidence and sequelae of the potential consequence of inadequate fasting, ie, pulmonary aspiration. Evidence from animal studies and gastric-emptying times with different fluids, including human milk, and solids is reviewed.

Recommendations are provided for minor procedures not requiring sedation and diagnostic examinations requiring pharmacologic immobilization or sedation. Detailed recommendations are provided to maximize comfort of the infant with emphasis on not fasting longer than recommended, eg, to wake the infant to breastfeed so the last feed is completed 4 hours pre-anesthesia, continue clear liquids until 2 hours prior, offer a pacifier during fasting, and breastfeed as soon as the infant is awake if the type of surgery does not preclude oral intake.

Other important considerations that are discussed include having the mother express or pump milk during the fasting and operative periods so as not to interfere with ongoing milk production, when to administer versus hold medications and fasting requirements for other types of fluids and solids.

Evidence level and research gaps

The literature for this protocol was last reviewed in 2010 (see **Table 1**). There are several high-level studies evaluating gastric emptying that support clear liquids up to 2 hours presedation/anesthetic, and others document lung injury in animal models is similar between breastmilk and formula. Level I and II-1 studies have documented that breastmilk empties from the stomach faster than formula, and that breastmilk fortification does not alter emptying times. The overall evidence relating to preoperative intake of breastmilk, however, remains sparse.

SUMMARY

Clinical breastfeeding guidelines have been developed by many organizations to assist health care professionals provide evidence-based care for breastfeeding dyads. This article details the process and content for the Academy of Breastfeeding Medicine's clinical protocols, which are written for use by physicians globally. All ABM protocols are consistent with the Ten Steps to Successful Breastfeeding, and many are focused on their application in different settings and specific populations. The evidence base for these protocols ranged from strong to modest. There are wide research gaps in many of the protocols; the most salient of these are detailed.

ACKNOWLEDGMENTS

We acknowledge the Academy of Breastfeeding Medicine Protocol Committee for their tremendous amount of expertise and effort developing these protocols: Co-Chairs Kathleen Marinelli, MD, and Maya Bunik, MD, MSPH; Translations Chair Larry Noble, MD; and committee members Nancy Brent, MD, Alison Holmes, MD, MPH, Ruth Lawrence, MD, Nancy Powers, MD, Tomoko Seo, MD, and Julie Scott Taylor, MD, MSc. We also acknowledge the lead contributors of each protocol for their expertise and effort, the volunteer translators and back translators, and the Maternal and Child Health Bureau for partial support for protocol development.

REFERENCES

1. Field MJ, Lohr KN, editors. Clinical practice guidelines: directions for a new program, Institute of Medicine. Washington, DC: National Academy Press; 1990. p. 38.

2. American Academy of Pediatrics Section on Breastfeeding. Breastfeeding and the use of human milk. Pediatrics 2012;129(3):e827–41.

3. Family Physicians Supporting Breastfeeding, AAFP Breastfeeding Position Paper. Available at: http://www.aafp.org/online/en/home/policy/policies/b/breastfeeding positionpaper.html. Accessed September 14, 2012.

4. American College of Obstetricians and Gynecologists. Breastfeeding: maternal and infant aspects. Special report from ACOG. ACOG Clin Rev 2007;12(Suppl): 1S–16S.

5. WHO/UNAIDS/UNICEF infant feeding guidelines. Available at: http://www.unicef.org/programme/breastfeeding/feeding.htm. Accessed September 14, 2012.

6. International Lactation Consultant Association. Clinical Guidelines for the Establishment of Exclusive Breastfeeding. Available at: http://www.ilca.org/files/resources/ilca_publications/ClinicalGuidelines2005.pdf. Accessed September 30, 2012.

7. Registered Nurses Association of Ontario (RNAO). Breastfeeding best practice guidelines for nurses: supplement. Toronto: Registered Nurses Association of Ontario (RNAO); 2007. Available at: http://www.guideline.gov/content.aspx?id=11506. Accessed September 14, 2012.

8. World Health Organization. Guidelines on HIV and Infant Feeding. Principles and recommendations for infant feeding in the context of HIV and a summary of evidence. 2010. Available at: http://whqlibdoc.who.int/publications/2010/9789241599535_eng.pdf. Accessed September 14, 2012.

9. World Health Organization. Acceptable medical reasons for the use of breast-milk substitutes. Geneva (Switzerland): World Health Organization; 2009. Available at: http://whqlibdoc.who.int/hq/2009/WHO_FCH_CAH_09.01_eng.pdf. Accessed September 14, 2012.

10. World Health Organization. Mastitis, causes and management. Geneva (Switzerland): World Health Organization; 2000. Available at: http://whqlibdoc.who.int/publications/2003/9241562218.pdf. Accessed September 14, 2012.

11. Corriveau S, Drake E, Kellams A, et al. Evaluation of a clinical protocol in the primary care setting to increase the exclusivity and duration of breastfeeding. Poster presented at 17th Annual Academy of Breastfeeding Medicine Conference; Chicago, IL; October 11–12, 2012.

12. Wight N, Marinelli KA, Academy of Breastfeeding Medicine Protocol Committee. ABM clinical protocol #1: guidelines for glucose monitoring and treatment of hypoglycemia in breastfed neonates. Breastfeed Med 2006;1(3):178–84. Available at: http://www.bfmed.org/Media/Files/Protocols/hypoglycemia.pdf. Accessed September 12, 2012.

13. Academy of Breastfeeding Medicine Clinical Protocol Committee. ABM clinical protocol #2: guidelines for hospital discharge of the breastfeeding term newborn and mother: "the going home protocol." Breastfeed Med 2007;2(3):158–65. Available at: http://www.bfmed.org/Media/Files/Protocols/protocol_2goinghome_revised07.pdf. Accessed September 14, 2012.

14. Academy of Breastfeeding Medicine Clinical Protocol Committee. ABM clinical protocol #3: hospital guidelines for the use of supplementary feedings in the healthy term breastfed neonate. Breastfeed Med 2009;4(3):175–82. Available at: http://www.bfmed.org/Media/Files/Protocols/Protocol%203%20English%20Supplementation.pdf. Accessed September 12, 2012.

15. Academy of Breastfeeding Medicine Clinical Protocol Committee. ABM clinical protocol #4: mastitis. Breastfeed Med 2008;3(3):177–80. Available at: http://www.bfmed.org/Media/Files/Protocols/protocol_4mastitis.pdf. Accessed September 14, 2012.

16. Academy of Breastfeeding Medicine Clinical Protocol Committee. ABM clinical protocol #5: peripartum breastfeeding management for the health mother and infant at term. Breastfeed Med 2008;3(2):129–32. Available at: http://www.bfmed.org/Media/Files/Protocols/Protocol_5.pdf. Accessed September 14, 2012.
17. Academy of Breastfeeding Medicine Clinical Protocol Committee. ABM clinical protocol #6: guideline on co-sleeping and breastfeeding. Breastfeed Med 2008;3(1):38–43. Available at: http://www.bfmed.org/Media/Files/Protocols/Protocol_6.pdf. Accessed September 14, 2012.
18. Ip S, Chung M, Raman G, et al. A summary of the Agency for Healthcare Research and Quality's evidence report on breastfeeding in developed countries. Breastfeed Med 2009;4(Suppl 1):S17–30.
19. Academy of Breastfeeding Medicine Clinical Protocol Committee. ABM clinical protocol #7: model breastfeeding policy. Breastfeed Med 2010;5(4):173–7. Available at: http://www.bfmed.org/Media/Files/Protocols/English%20Protocol%207%20Model%20Hospital%20Policy.pdf. Accessed September 14, 2012.
20. Academy of Breastfeeding Medicine Clinical Protocol Committee. ABM clinical protocol #8: human milk storage information for home use for full-term infants. Breastfeed Med 2010;5(3):127–30. Available at: http://www.bfmed.org/Media/Files/Protocols/Protocol%208%20-%20English%20revised%202010.pdf. Accessed September 14, 2012.
21. Academy of Breastfeeding Medicine Clinical Protocol Committee. ABM clinical protocol #9: use of galactogogues in initiating or augmenting the rate of maternal milk secretion. Breastfeed Med 2011;6(1):41–9. Available at: http://www.bfmed.org/Media/Files/Protocols/Protocol%209%20-%20English%201st%20Rev.%20Jan%202011.pdf. Accessed September 14, 2012.
22. Academy of Breastfeeding Medicine Clinical Protocol Committee. ABM clinical protocol #10: breastfeeding the late preterm infant (34 0/7 to 36 6/7 weeks gestation). Breastfeed Med 2011;6(1):151–6. Available at: http://www.bfmed.org/Media/Files/Protocols/Protocol%2010%20Revised%20English%206.11.pdf. Accessed September 14, 2012.
23. Academy of Breastfeeding Medicine Clinical Protocol Committee. ABM clinical protocol #11: guidelines for the evaluation and management of neonatal ankyloglossia and its complications in the breastfeeding dyad. 2004. Published online. No longer accessible due to expiration. Available at: http://www.bfmed.org/Media/Files/Protocols/ankyloglossia.pdf. Accessed September 14, 2012.
24. Academy of Breastfeeding Medicine Clinical Protocol Committee. ABM clinical protocol #12: transitioning the breastfeeding/breastmilk-fed premature infant from the neonatal intensive care unit to home. Available at: http://www.bfmed.org/Media/Files/Protocols/Protocol_12.pdf. Accessed September 14, 2012.
25. Academy of Breastfeeding Medicine Clinical Protocol Committee. ABM clinical protocol #13: contraception during breastfeeding. Breastfeed Med 2006;1(1):43–51. Available at: http://www.bfmed.org/Media/Files/Protocols/Protocol_13.pdf. Accessed September 14, 2012.
26. Academy of Breastfeeding Medicine Clinical Protocol Committee. ABM clinical protocol #14: breastfeeding-friendly physician's office, part 1: optimizing care for infants and children. Breastfeed Med 2006;1(2):115–9. Available at: http://www.bfmed.org/Media/Files/Protocols/Protocol_14.pdf. Accessed September 14, 2012.
27. Montgomery A, Hale TW, Academy of Breastfeeding Medicine Clinical Protocol Committee. ABM clinical protocol #15: analgesia and anesthesia for the breastfeeding mother. Breastfeed Med 2006;1(4):271–7. Available at: http://www.bfmed.org/Media/Files/Protocols/Protocol_15.pdf. Accessed September 14, 12.

28. Thomas J, Marinelli KA, Hennessy M, Academy of Breastfeeding Medicine Clinical Protocol Committee. ABM clinical protocol #16: breastfeeding the hypotonic infant. Breastfeed Med 2007;2(2):112–8. Available at: http://www.bfmed.org/Media/Files/Protocols/Protocol_16.pdf. Accessed September 14, 2012.

29. Reilly S, Reid J, Skeat J, Academy of Breastfeeding Medicine Clinical Protocol Committee. ABM clinical protocol #17: breastfeeding infants with cleft lip, cleft palate or cleft lip and palate. Breastfeed Med 2007;2(4):243–50. Available at: http://www.bfmed.org/Media/Files/Protocols/Protocol_17.pdf. Accessed September 14, 2012.

30. Academy of Breastfeeding Medicine Clinical Protocol Committee. ABM clinical protocol #18: use of antidepressants in nursing mothers. Breastfeed Med 2008; 3(1):44–52. Available at: http://www.bfmed.org/Media/Files/Protocols/Protocol_18.pdf. Accessed September 14, 2012.

31. Academy of Breastfeeding Medicine Clinical Protocol Committee. ABM clinical protocol #19: breastfeeding promotion in the prenatal setting. Breastfeed Med 2009;4(1):43–5. Available at: http://www.bfmed.org/Media/Files/Protocols/Protocol%2019%20-%20Breastfeeding%20Promotion%20in%20the%20Prenatal%20Setting.pdf. Accessed September 14, 2012.

32. Academy of Breastfeeding Medicine Clinical Protocol Committee. ABM clinical protocol #20: engorgement. Breastfeed Med 2009;4(2):111–3. Available at: http://www.bfmed.org/Media/Files/Protocols/Protocol%2020%20-%20Engorgement%206-2009.pdf. Accessed September 14, 2012.

33. Academy of Breastfeeding Medicine Clinical Protocol Committee. ABM clinical protocol #21: guideline for breastfeeding and the drug-dependent women. Breastfeed Med 2009;4(4):225–8. Available at: http://www.bfmed.org/Media/Files/Protocols/Protocol%2021%20English.pdf. Accessed September 14, 2012.

34. Academy of Breastfeeding Medicine Clinical Protocol Committee. ABM clinical protocol #22: guidelines for management of jaundice in the breastfeeding infant equal to or greater than 35 weeks' gestation. Breastfeed Med 2010;5(2):87–93. Available at: http://www.bfmed.org/Media/Files/Protocols/Protocol%2022%20Jaundice.pdf. Accessed September 14, 2012.

35. AAP Subcommittee on Hyperbilirubinemia. Management of hyperbilirubinemia in the newborn infant of 35 or more weeks of gestation. Pediatrics 2004;114: 297–316.

36. Maisels MJ, Bhutani VK, Bogen D, et al. Hyperbilirubinemia in the newborn infant > or =35 weeks' gestation: an update with clarifications. Pediatrics 2009; 124:1193–8.

37. Screening of infants for hyperbilirubinemia to prevent chronic bilirubin encephalopathy: US Preventive Services Task Force recommendation statement. Pediatrics 2009;124:1172–7.

38. Ip S, Chung M, Kulig J, et al. An evidence-based review of important issues concerning neonatal hyperbilirubinemia. Pediatrics 2004;114:e130–53.

39. Academy of Breastfeeding Medicine Clinical Protocol Committee. ABM clinical protocol #23: non-pharmacologic management of procedure-related pain in the breastfeeding infant. Breastfeed Med 2010;5(6):315–9. Available at: http://www.bfmed.org/Media/Files/Protocols/Protocol%2023%20-%20Non-Pharmacologic%20Management%20of%20Procedure-Related%20Pain.pdf. Accessed September 14, 2012.

40. Academy of Breastfeeding Medicine Clinical Protocol Committee. ABM clinical protocol #24: allergic proctocolitis in the exclusively breastfed infant. Breastfeed Med 2011;6(6):435–40. Available at: http://www.bfmed.org/Media/Files/Protocols/Protocol24_English_120211.pdf. Accessed September 14, 2012.

41. Academy of Breastfeeding Medicine Clinical Protocol Committee. ABM clinical protocol #25: recommendations for preprocedural fasting for the breastfed infant: "NPO" guidelines. Breastfeed Med 2012;7(3):197–202. Available at: http://www.bfmed.org/Media/Files/Protocols/Protocol25_English_080312.pdf.   Accessed September 14, 2012.

Overcoming Clinical Barriers to Exclusive Breastfeeding

Marianne Neifert, MD, MTS[a,b], Maya Bunik, MD, MSPH[c],*

KEYWORDS

- Exclusive • Breastfeeding • Perceived insufficient milk (PIM)
- Breastfeeding support • Combination feeding

KEY POINTS

- Barriers to exclusive breastfeeding include lack of prenatal education, comfort and ease with formula feeding, perception of insufficient milk, misinterpretation/understanding of normal infant crying, inadequate support, maternal employment, and early introduction of solids.
- Despite the brevity of the postbirth hospitalization, the provision of supportive maternity care practices, especially exclusive breast milk feeding, represents an evidence-based intervention to increase exclusive and extended breastfeeding.
- When supplementation is required for a breastfed newborn, using mother's own expressed milk provides the health benefits of exclusive breast milk feeding and helps ensure an abundant milk supply.
- Potential sources of essential support to help mothers increase breastfeeding exclusivity in the first 6 months postpartum include the federal WIC program, Nurse-Family Partnership (NFP), families, mother-peers, health care professionals, and employers.
- A newborn follow-up visit at 3 to 5 days and a second ambulatory visit at 2 weeks are critical to evaluate the onset of breastfeeding, monitor infant weight gain, discuss infant feeding cues, and provide ongoing support to the mother.

THE CASE FOR EXCLUSIVE BREASTFEEDING

In their most recent breastfeeding policy statement, the American Academy of Pediatrics (AAP) reaffirmed their long-standing recommendation of exclusive breastfeeding for about the first 6 months of life, with continued breastfeeding through 12 months and beyond, as appropriate complementary foods are introduced.[1] The World Health Organization (WHO) similarly recommends that infants worldwide be

[a] Department of Pediatrics, Children's Hospital Colorado, University of Colorado Denver, 13123 East 16th Avenue, B065, Aurora, CO 80045, USA; [b] Dr. Mom® Presentations LLC, PO Box 880, Parker, CO 80134, USA; [c] Children's Outcomes Research, Department of Pediatrics, Children's Hospital Colorado, University of Colorado Denver, 13123 East 16th Avenue, B032, Aurora, CO 80045, USA
* Corresponding author.
E-mail address: maya.bunik@childrenscolorado.org

Pediatr Clin N Am 60 (2013) 115–145
http://dx.doi.org/10.1016/j.pcl.2012.10.001
0031-3955/13/$ – see front matter © 2013 Elsevier Inc. All rights reserved.

pediatric.theclinics.com

exclusively breastfed for the first 6 months, with breastfeeding continuing for up to 2 years or beyond, as safe and nutritionally adequate complementary foods are added.[2]

Exclusive breastfeeding is defined as an infant receiving only breast milk and no other liquids or solids except for drops or syrups consisting of vitamins, minerals, or medicines.[3] Although being ever breastfed, compared with never breastfed, is linked with numerous improved infant and maternal health outcomes, mounting research evidence confirms that the health benefits of breastfeeding are dose-related, with exclusive breastfeeding conferring the maximum health benefits for infants and mothers.[1,4] The promotion of breastfeeding is a recognized public health strategy for preventing childhood obesity,[5,6] based on the documented dose-related, protective effect of breastfeeding in reducing childhood overweight.[7]

Whereas some infant feeding experts have argued that solid foods can be introduced safely after 4 months of exclusive breastfeeding,[8] the AAP recommends exclusive breastfeeding for about 6 months rather than 4 months because the longer recommendation extends the period of lactational amenorrhea and provides greater infant protection against lower respiratory tract illnesses, otitis media, and diarrheal disease.[1,9] Not only does exclusive breastfeeding for about 6 months provide ideal infant nutrition and the maximum short- and long-term health benefits for infants and mothers, it has long been observed that shortened exclusive breastfeeding owing to supplementation with infant formula is linked with a shortened duration of breastfeeding.[10–14] As soon as regular formula feedings are started, breastfeeding frequency and suckling duration decrease sharply.[13] Thus, the younger infants are when regular formula feeds are introduced, the younger they are at cessation of breastfeeding.

EXCLUSIVE BREASTFEEDING RATES IN THE UNITED STATES

Fortunately, decades of ongoing breastfeeding promotion efforts have been successful in steadily raising national breastfeeding rates. Among 2009 US births, breastfeeding initiation has risen to 76.9%,[15] achieving the Healthy People 2010 (HP2010) national objective of 75% and representing the highest initiation rate in nearly 7 decades.[16] In 2007, following the HP2010 midcourse review, target goals for exclusive breastfeeding at 3 and 6 months were added to the HP2010 objectives for breastfeeding initiation and duration.[17] The new HP2020 objectives reflect even higher targets for all breastfeeding outcome measures (**Table 1**).

Although more than three-quarters of US mothers begin breastfeeding, the current low rates of breastfeeding continuation and exclusivity indicate that most US infants and mothers are not receiving the maximum health benefits associated with full and

Table 1
U.S. National breastfeeding rates compared to HP breastfeeding objectives

	Ever Breastfed, %	Breastfeeding at 6 mo, %	Breastfeeding at 12 mo, %	Exclusively Breastfeeding at 3 mo, %	Exclusively Breastfeeding at 6 mo, %
2009[a] US	76.9	47.2	25.5	36.0	16.3
HP2010 objectives	75.0	50.0	25.0	40.0	17.0
HP2020 objectives	81.9	60.6	34.1	46.2	25.5

Abbreviation: HP, Healthy People.
    [a] Centers for Disease Control and Prevention National Immunization Survey, Provisional Data, 2009 births.

extended breastfeeding. In addition, the substantial racial and economic differences in breastfeeding contribute to infant and maternal health disparities. Similar to the socio-demographic disparities in breastfeeding initiation and duration, for children born in 2007, rates of exclusive breastfeeding through 3 and 6 months were lowest among black infants and infants of mothers who were young, unmarried, had lower incomes, were less educated, or who were living in rural areas.[17] Raising exclusive breastfeeding rates remains a critical public health strategy to improve infant and maternal health, especially among populations at risk.

BARRIERS TO EXCLUSIVE BREASTFEEDING

More than 85% of expectant mothers recruited for the national 2005–2007 Infant Feeding Practices Study II[18] (IFPS II) intended to exclusively breastfeed for 3 months or longer[19]; yet, only 32% of mothers achieved their intended exclusive breastfeeding goal.[19] Although the study mothers, who were drawn from a nationally distributed, self-selected consumer opinion panel, were not nationally representative, they characterized the population of US women most likely to succeed with breastfeeding,[18] thus underscoring the need for effective strategies to enable more women to reach their exclusive breastfeeding goals.

The *2011 Surgeon General's Call to Action to Support Breastfeeding* identifies diverse personal and societal barriers to breastfeeding, including lack of knowledge, embarrassment, widespread exposure to infant formula, inappropriate maternity care practices, lactation difficulties and concerns about insufficient milk, employment and child care, insufficient family and social support, and inadequate physician knowledge and support.[20] The *Call to Action* appropriately shifts the emphasis in breastfeeding promotion from an individual woman's personal choice to the essential need to make society-wide institutional changes that reduce women's barriers to successful breastfeeding.[20] The numerous and varied factors that create barriers to exclusive breastfeeding (**Box 1**) call for multifaceted, society-wide approaches, involving families, communities, clinicians, hospitals and health care systems, employers, and others, to ensure that expectant and new mothers receive the necessary information, clinical services, and ongoing support to achieve exclusive and sustained breastfeeding.

PRENATAL PREPARATION FOR EXCLUSIVE BREASTFEEDING

Prenatal breastfeeding education is critically important to inform pregnant women about the infant and maternal health benefits of breastfeeding, strengthen their intention to breastfeed, elicit and address perceived barriers, and identify key sources of support. Although most expectant mothers are aware that breastfeeding trumps infant formula in nutritional quality and immune benefits, few know that the health benefits are dose-related or that the small quantities of colostrum available in the first day or two after birth are sufficient to meet the needs of term, healthy newborns. A 2005 Cochrane review of intervention trials to promote the initiation of breastfeeding found that health education, especially needs-based, informal, repeat sessions, and peer support interventions, significantly increase breastfeeding initiation rates among US economically disadvantaged mothers.[21]

Relevant topics to be addressed in prenatal breastfeeding education include the nutritional superiority of human milk; why exclusive breastfeeding is recommended; how to get an optimal start breastfeeding in the hospital; reasons to avoid formula supplementation; the importance of an early follow-up visit; practical aspects of breastfeeding, including strategies for combining breastfeeding and employment; sources of support and clinical lactation services; and the timing of the introduction

---

Box 1
Personal and societal barriers to exclusive breastfeeding

Lack of information

Low attendance at prenatal breastfeeding classes

Ambivalence

Embarrassment

Breastfeeding myths

Inappropriate maternity care practices

Lack of timely follow-up after hospital discharge

Maternal employment and child care practices

Early introduction of complementary foods

Misinterpretation of normal infant behaviors

Inadequate family and social support

Lack of breastfeeding role models

Real and perceived insufficient milk

Comfort level with formula feeding

WIC formula availability

Inappropriate formula marketing practices

Inadequate availability of banked donor human milk

Lack of access to and availability of clinical breastfeeding services

Delayed intervention for breastfeeding difficulties

Inadequate clinician knowledge and support

---

of complementary foods. Because relatively few expectant mothers currently attend a prenatal breastfeeding class, breastfeeding information needs to be integrated into childbirth education curricula and reinforced by prenatal providers. The recent addition of 8 categories of women's preventive services, mandated without cost sharing under The Patient Protection and Affordable Care Act, includes comprehensive lactation support and counseling from trained providers, as well as breastfeeding equipment.[22] These new lactation benefits may help reduce breastfeeding disparities by improving socially and economically disadvantaged women's access to prenatal breastfeeding classes, breast pumps, and counseling.

Unfortunately, many of the infant-feeding messages that pregnant women receive come from formula company promotional materials that target expectant and new mothers though prenatal offices, the Internet, and parenting magazines.[23,24] Pregnant women often receive unsolicited "gifts" from formula manufacturers through the mail or at their physician's office, which implies a medical endorsement. These new mother, infant-feeding kits include powdered formula samples and formula coupons, which encourage the early supplementation of breastfeeding. Handouts and market materials that begin with "for breastfeeding and supplementing moms"[25] or "whether you decide to breastfeed, supplement, or formula feed"[26] serve to undermine exclusive breastfeeding and normalize the use of formula in infant feeding. Prenatal and pediatric providers should decline to partner with infant formula manufacturers under the guise of providing "gifts" for their patients.

Preparing Expectant Mothers for an Optimal Hospital Breastfeeding Experience

Pediatricians, obstetric care providers, staff from the Special Supplemental Nutrition Program for Women, Infants, and Children (WIC), public health nurses, childbirth educators, doulas, and others who interact with expectant mothers should help prepare families for an optimal hospital breastfeeding experience. Even when hospitals offer supportive maternity practices, staff often find it difficult to implement optimal breastfeeding policies, such as mother-infant skin-to-skin contact immediately after birth or round-the-clock rooming-in, when ideal practices conflict with parental expectations of allowing eager family members to hold the newborn immediately after birth or having the baby cared for in the nursery at night. Lack of preparation for what the early postpartum period will be like, including unrealistic expectations about newborn crying, waking, and feeding behaviors and mothers' own need for rest, has been identified as a key trigger for low-income breastfeeding mothers' in-hospital use of supplemental formula.[27] The Joint Commission national public education Speak Up campaign[28] includes free breastfeeding educational materials in English and Spanish, endorsed by the AAP and other organizations, to prepare expectant and new mothers for the successful initiation of breastfeeding, including exclusive breastfeeding in the hospital.[29]

PROMOTING EXCLUSIVE BREASTFEEDING IN THE HOSPITAL

Despite the brevity of the postbirth hospitalization, the maternity care experience is recognized as a critical period in the establishment of breastfeeding. The provision of supportive maternity care practices, especially exclusive breast milk feeding, represents an important evidence-based intervention to increase exclusive and extended breastfeeding.

The Baby-Friendly Hospital Initiative

In 1991, the United Nations International Children's Emergency Fund (UNICEF) and WHO jointly launched the global Baby-Friendly Hospital Initiative (BFHI), to promote, protect, and support breastfeeding by recognizing hospitals and birthing centers that implement the evidence-based, ideal practice standards, known as the Ten Steps to Successful Breastfeeding (**Box 2**).[30] Baby-Friendly designated hospitals, compared with non–Baby-Friendly facilities, consistently have been linked with increases in breastfeeding initiation, duration, and exclusivity.[31–33] Despite the evidence that supportive breastfeeding maternity practices affect breastfeeding outcomes well beyond the hospital stay, only a small percentage of US maternity hospitals and birthing centers have pursued the Baby-Friendly designation.[34] Results of the Centers for Disease Control and Prevention's (CDC's) biennial National Survey of Maternity Practices in Infant Nutrition and Care (mPINC) survey show that few US hospitals have implemented policies that fully support and encourage mothers to breastfeed.[35]

Although implementing all Ten Steps represents the gold standard for breastfeeding support in maternity facilities, making incremental changes in Baby-Friendly practices has been linked with significant improvements in breastfeeding outcomes.[11,12,36] In a large, nationally representative survey of new mothers, primiparas who delivered in hospitals that practiced 6 or 7 of the Ten Steps were 6 times more likely to be exclusively breastfeeding at 1 week, as intended, compared with those in hospitals that practiced none or 1.[36] A large, population-based study in Colorado found that 5 of the Ten Steps were linked with a longer duration of breastfeeding: breastfeeding within the first hour, breast milk only, infant rooming-in, no pacifier use, and receipt of a telephone number for postdischarge help.[12] The combined effect of the 5 practices had

---

Box 2
WHO/UNICEF Ten Steps to Successful Breastfeeding

1. Have a written breastfeeding policy that is routinely communicated to all health care staff.
2. Train all health care staff in skills necessary to implement this policy.
3. Inform all pregnant women about the benefits and management of breastfeeding.
4. Help mothers initiate breastfeeding within one hour of birth.
5. Show mothers how to breastfeed and how to maintain lactation even if they are separated from their infants.
6. Give newborn infants no food or drink other than breast milk, unless medically indicated.
7. Practice rooming-in (allow mothers and infants to remain together) 24 hours a day.
8. Encourage breastfeeding on demand.
9. Give no artificial nipples or pacifiers to breastfeeding infants.
10. Foster the establishment of breastfeeding support groups and refer mothers to them on discharge from the hospital or clinic.

From World Health Organization. Evidence for the ten steps to successful breastfeeding. Available at: http://whqlibdoc.who.int/publications/2004/9241591544_eng.pdf. Accessed August 31, 2012.

---

the strongest impact, with breastfeeding duration being significantly longer among mothers, independent of socioeconomic status, who reported all 5 successful maternity practices compared with those who did not.

Reducing In-Hospital Formula Supplementation of Breastfed Infants

Numerous studies have found a significant link between exclusive breastfeeding during the postbirth hospitalization and subsequent breastfeeding duration and exclusivity,[11,12,19,37] including the likelihood of achieving mothers' exclusive breastfeeding intention.[19,36] Giving formula supplements to breastfed newborns in the hospital has been linked with a decreased likelihood of full breastfeeding at 6 months of age.[10,19,37] Yet, results of the 2009 national mPINC survey show that 24.6% of US hospitals routinely supplement healthy breastfed newborns with formula.[35]

Optimal maternity practices require that formula supplementation of breastfed infants be used only for a valid medical indication (or on specific maternal request after appropriate education).[1,30,35,38,39] Nevertheless, much of the in-hospital use of formula supplements for breastfed newborns is by maternal request, particularly among low-income mothers who have not attended a prenatal breastfeeding class.[27] A recent survey of low-income, African American mothers found that 60% initiated breastfeeding, and 78% of the breastfed newborns received formula supplementation in the hospital, predominantly because of maternal request.[40] Although nurses recognize that formula use should be rare, knowledge deficits and lack of teaching time, maternal complaints of fatigue, insufficient colostrum or sore nipples, and infant challenges, such as fussiness, sleepiness, or latch difficulties, contribute to frequent formula use on the part of nursing staff.[27,41–43] Because mothers tend to continue at home the infant care practices begun in the hospital, those using in-hospital formula supplements require close follow-up and monitoring to transition to full breastfeeding as quickly as possible.

To improve maternity care practices, optimize breastfeeding initiation, and highlight the health benefits of exclusive breastfeeding, the Joint Commission recently added measurement of exclusive breast milk feeding among term newborns during the birth hospitalization as a Core Quality Measure of a hospital's performance.[38,44,45] This step has helped to change the long-standing paradigm among clinicians that supplementing a breastfed baby necessarily means using infant formula. More clinicians now appreciate the feasibility and desirability of using mother's own breast milk, whether expressed by hand or with a pump, to supplement an infant who is unable to obtain sufficient milk by direct breastfeeding. Alternatively, screened, processed donor milk may be prescribed, if available.[1,38,44] Expressing mother's own milk when an infant is unable to obtain sufficient quantities by nursing ensures that the mother establishes an abundant milk supply and the infant accrues all the health benefits of exclusive breast milk feeding. In addition, the preferential use of mother's own milk conveys a powerful message that human milk represents ideal infant nutrition and is highly valued.

Immediate skin-to-skin contact has been shown to facilitate the early initiation of exclusive breastfeeding and extend breastfeeding duration.[46,47] A recent, large, prospective study of the duration of skin-to-skin mother-infant contact during the first 3 hours following birth demonstrated a dose-response relationship between early skin-to-skin contact and exclusive breastfeeding during the maternity hospital stay.[46] Instituting extended, uninterrupted skin-to-skin contact during the early postpartum period should be a key strategy in promoting exclusive breastfeeding behaviors.

Continuous, round-the-clock rooming-in of mother and infant potentially creates a private, intimate atmosphere that supports the new mother in learning to recognize and respond to her infant's feeding cues, continue skin-to-skin contact, become comfortable latching her baby and breastfeeding, and gain confidence in her ability to care for her infant. However, these would-be benefits of rooming-in can be undermined when frequent, erratic, and lengthy interruptions by visitors and diverse hospital personnel take precedence over breastfeeding and essential self-care. A study of healthy mother-infant dyads recorded a mean of 54 interruptions (people entering the mother's room or phone calls), averaging 17 minutes each, between 8 AM and 8 PM on postpartum day 1.[48]

A steady stream of visitors may interfere with skin-to-skin contact and cue-based breastfeeding, promote the use of a pacifier to appease a hungry baby while guests are present, prevent the lactation consultant from offering one-on-one instruction, or so deplete a new mother that she asks to have her baby cared for in the nursery at night, increasing the risk of formula supplementation. Many hospitals have implemented a designated afternoon "quiet time" or "nap time" to give new mothers more time alone with their newborns and the opportunity to rest and renew.[48] Counseling expectant parents to limit the number of postpartum visitors and their length of stay may be a simple strategy to help promote early exclusive breastfeeding.

Being given a phone number to call for help with breastfeeding after discharge is another Baby-Friendly practice that helps promote exclusive breastfeeding. Thirty-four percent of breastfeeding mothers in a prospective study reported having 1 or more problems with breastfeeding in the first 4 weeks.[49] Women who experienced early breastfeeding difficulties were significantly more likely to discontinue full breastfeeding before 6 months and to have a shorter duration of any breastfeeding. In a retrospective, cohort study of infant-feeding practices at 6 months of age, infants of mothers who were given a telephone number for breastfeeding help, compared to infants whose mothers were not, had 6 times the odds of being almost exclusively breastfed at 6 months (some infants were infrequently fed water, juice, or solid food).[37]

For decades, maternity hospitals routinely have distributed formula company discharge bags to new mothers, unwittingly implying their endorsement of the products and indirectly serving as marketing agents for formula manufacturers. Multiple studies show that receiving a commercial discharge pack containing formula samples and promotional materials reduces the duration of exclusive breastfeeding.[50,51] This long-standing and seemingly innocuous practice is in violation of the WHO International Code of Marketing of Breastmilk Substitutes and undermines a hospital's mission to promote optimal health.[52] As hospitals reevaluate the ethics of their relationships with industry, more than a third nationwide, including all maternity hospitals in Rhode Island and Massachusetts, have discontinued the practice of distributing formula gift bags, and this trend is gaining momentum.[53,54]

NEWBORNS AT-RISK FOR INEFFECTIVE BREASTFEEDING

Many infant biologic variables, including birth weight, gestational age, labor medications, oral anatomic variables, neurologic status, and medical conditions, can influence an infant's ability to latch on to the breast, suckle effectively, extract milk, and promote ongoing milk production.[55,56] Late-preterm infants, born at $34^{0/7}$ through $36^{6/7}$ weeks' gestation, represent the largest subgroup of at-risk newborns managed in level 1 (basic) nurseries. In 2010, the proportion of all US births that were late preterm was 8.49%, representing nearly 340,000 infants.[57] Late-preterm infants are physiologically and metabolically immature and are at increased risk, compared with term infants, for infant mortality, morbidity during the birth hospitalization, and hospital readmission, most commonly for jaundice, suspected sepsis, and feeding difficulties.[58]

Breastfeeding may initially appear successful during the birth hospitalization, but not be sustained after discharge when the mother's milk comes in. Many factors contribute to the late-preterm infant's impaired ability to extract milk from the breast, including fewer awake-alert periods, immature oromotor skills, weak intraoral suction pressures, difficulty attaching to the breast effectively, and immature suck-swallow-breathe cycles.[59] Although the use of an ultrathin silicone nipple shield may enable late-preterm infants to transfer milk more effectively, most will temporarily require supplemental feedings with expressed breast milk in addition to direct breastfeeding.

If the late-preterm infant does not nurse actively for at least 15 minutes 8 to 10 times in 24 hours, the mother should begin prevention pumping with a hospital-grade breast pump to ensure regular, effective breast stimulation and drainage.[59] As with other newborns at risk for inadequate breastfeeding (**Box 3**), the primary goals during the critical first 2 weeks after birth are to ensure that the mother establishes an abundant milk supply and that the infant is adequately nourished, ideally with exclusive breast milk feedings.[56,59] This triple-feeding regimen (breastfeeding 5–10 minutes per side, supplementing the infant with ad libitum expressed milk, pumping residual milk until the breasts are well drained) is continued as the infant matures and progressively takes more milk with direct breastfeeding. The mother can discontinue pumping when the infant consistently gains appropriate weight with exclusive breastfeeding. Periodically weighing the identically clothed infant before and after feeding ("test weighing" procedure) can help document the infant's ability to transfer milk with direct breastfeeding (**Fig. 1**).[56,59,60]

Alternative feeding methods, such as a plastic spoon or medicine cup, can be used in the hospital to offer small quantities of expressed colostrum/breast milk or donor milk (or formula, if required), and avoid the use of a bottle and nipple while the infant learns to latch and nurse effectively.[60] Once the infant is discharged, however, the most expedient method of "triple feeding" typically involves using a bottle. With ongoing skin-to-skin contact, frequent opportunities to latch on to the breast, and an abundant maternal milk supply, chances are good that the infant will successfully transition to full breastfeeding.

Box 3
Examples of potential newborn risk factors for ineffective breastfeeding

1. Preterm, late-preterm, or early term ($37^{0/7}$ to $38^{6/7}$ weeks of gestation)

2. Birth weight less than 6 pounds

3. Multiple birth

4. Oral anatomic variations (eg, ankyloglossia, micrognathia, cleft defects)

5. Jaundice

6. Systemic illness, such as oxygen requirement, cardiac defect, or infection

7. Neuromotor abnormality, such as Down syndrome or impaired sucking ability

8. Difficulty latching correctly or using a nipple shield

9. Weight loss >7% or continued weight loss after "milk comes in"

10. Maternal risk factors for delayed lactogenesis or lactation failure (such as diabetes mellitus, obesity, perinatal stress, older maternal age, postpartum hemorrhage, breast variations, or breast surgery)

Clinicians need to identify other newborns at risk for ineffective breastfeeding (see **Box 3**), so that an appropriate feeding plan can be tailored prior to discharge and close follow-up ensured. Whenever a breastfed infant is unable to extract milk effectively, the mother's milk supply will down regulate within a few days unless regular milk removal is accomplished. When recognized early, potential problems in the initiation of lactation can be addressed in a way that supports exclusive and extended breastfeeding.

ESTABLISHING AN ABUNDANT MILK SUPPLY

Because insufficient milk is a chief reason that breastfeeding women begin supplementing with formula or wean early,[13,61,62] helping women establish an abundant milk supply is a critical strategy in promoting exclusive and extended breastfeeding. In a study comparing milk output among mothers of preterm and term infants, mean milk output at days 6 and 7 was highly associated with week 2 milk output and moderately associated with week 6 output for both gestation groups.[63] For both mothers of

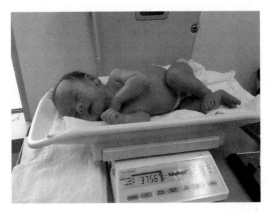

Fig. 1. Infant on scale, accurate to 2 grams, for prefeeding and postfeeding test weights. (*Courtesy of* M. Bunik, MD, Aurora, CO.)

term and preterm infants, mean milk volumes produced by day 6 and 7 predicted whether the mother would achieve adequate milk production at week 6 postpartum. These data emphasize the importance of the first 1 to 2 weeks postpartum in establishing a plentiful milk supply that will facilitate exclusive breastfeeding.

Endocrine and Autocrine Control of Lactation

Prolactin, secreted by the anterior pituitary gland, is the key lactogenic hormone necessary for the establishment and maintenance of lactation.[64] Prolactin secretion is promoted by infant suckling and regular milk removal. Blood levels are highest in early lactation, with basal levels declining and postfeeding spikes continuing as lactation progresses.[65] Oxytocin is the essential hormone involved in the milk ejection reflex, which is critical to successful lactation.[66] Infant suckling triggers oxytocin release from the posterior pituitary, causing contraction of myoepithelial cells surrounding the mammary alveoli and ducts. This squeezing action expels stored milk into the collecting ducts and propels it toward the nipple, where it is removed by the suckling infant. Noxious stimuli, including pain, stress, or embarrassment, can partially inhibit the milk ejection reflex, reducing the volume of milk transferred to the infant.[66]

Hormones alone do not fully explain how milk synthesis is regulated in the breastfeeding woman or account for the variability in milk production in each breast. Lactating mothers regulate milk secretion independently in each breast, according to the proportion of stored milk that the infant removes at a feeding.[67,68] This regulatory mechanism is believed to involve a chemical inhibitor of milk secretion that increases in concentration as milk accumulates in the breast and decreases as milk is removed. Frequent, effective breastfeeding stimulates milk secretion by limiting the accumulation of inhibitory protein, whereas infrequent, or ineffective, breastfeeding decreases milk production, as the concentration of the inhibitor rises in stored milk. This locally regulated negative feedback mechanism is known as autocrine control of lactation.[65] After a mother's milk "comes in" (lactogenesis II), the frequency and efficacy of milk removal appears to be the most powerful determinant of the milk volume produced in each breast.[67]

Lactogenesis II

The onset of copious milk production (lactogenesis II or secretory activation), typically occurring between day 2 and 3 postpartum, is a critical stage of lactation, during which the concentration of milk components changes rapidly as milk volume dramatically increases.[64,65] Mothers perceive their "milk coming in" as breast enlargement, fullness, firmness, and the leakage of colostrum/breast milk. Milk volumes consumed by term infants rapidly increase from 36 to 96 hours postpartum, after which infant milk intake tends to plateau at an average volume of 750 to 800 mL per 24 hours by 1 month postpartum.[65,69] Clinicians need to screen and intervene for early breastfeeding problems that limit milk removal, such as infants who breastfeed ineffectively, severe maternal nipple pain that impairs milk let-down, or long intervals without breastfeeding or expressing milk, to prevent a significant decrease in mother's milk supply once lactogenesis II has occurred.

Risk factors associated with delayed lactogenesis II include primiparity, urgent cesarean delivery, prolonged stage 2 labor, maternal diabetes, maternal obesity, older maternal age, and an infant who is not breastfeeding well.[70–73] Among mothers who intend to breastfeed for at least 6 months, delayed onset of lactation beyond 72 hours postpartum is linked with a shorter duration of breastfeeding, compared with women who report an earlier onset of lactation.[74] With frequent breast stimulation and milk removal, mothers with delayed lactogenesis may be able to produce an adequate milk supply by 7 to 10 days postpartum. However, such women require ongoing support and close monitoring of infant weight gain until full breastfeeding is established.

Women's breasts vary widely in their capacity to store milk that is available to the infant.[67] Once breastfeeding is well established, a mother with a larger breast storage capacity has greater flexibility in breastfeeding patterns compared with a mother with a smaller breast storage capacity, who will need to breastfeed or express milk more often. The longest interval between breastfeeds or milk expression may be a more important determinant of milk production than the total number of times milk is removed from the breasts daily.[67]

DECREASING COMMON BARRIERS TO EXCLUSIVE BREASTFEEDING

Despite high breastfeeding initiation rates, the vast majority of US infants also are fed formula during their first year. Among breastfeeding mothers in the IFPS II, 42% were supplementing with formula at 1 month.[75] Formula feeding is highly visible in US society, and comfort with formula feeding is widespread among expectant first-time mothers, who often have no knowledge of the practical aspects of breastfeeding.[76] Formula is widely viewed by mothers and practitioners alike as the solution to breastfeeding problems rather than a cause or contributor to breastfeeding problems.[77] Among low-income breastfeeding mothers, formula use is not typically considered detrimental nor associated with regret.[78]

Perceived Insufficient Milk

Although breastfeeding mothers supplement their babies with formula for many reasons (convenience, mother-baby separations, breastfeeding challenges, the father's desire to feed, or the choice to begin weaning) the belief that her milk is insufficient for her infant's needs is the major reason mothers start regular formula feeds.[13] Respondents in the IFPS II cited "I didn't have enough milk" as 1 of the top 3 reasons in their decision to stop breastfeeding through 8 months, and "breast milk alone did not satisfy my infant" was consistently ranked among the top 3 reasons why mothers discontinued breastfeeding regardless of weaning age.[62] Perceived insufficient milk (PIM) is well documented as one of the most common and influential deterrents to breastfeeding duration and exclusivity.[61,62,79]

Potential strategies to prevent PIM include reinforcing appropriate early infant feeding routines and closely monitoring breastfeeding dyads during the first postpartum weeks to ensure that breastfeeding is well established. Frequent infant weight checks and periodic test weighing (prenursing weight compared with a postnursing weight) can provide concrete evidence for breastfeeding mothers concerned about the adequacy of their milk supply.[80] Education about normal infant feeding volumes also can reassure mothers of thriving infants who lack confidence about their milk production.

To help lactating mothers maintain an abundant milk supply, clinicians should counsel breastfeeding women to avoid allowing their breasts to remain overly full.[67] If an infant begins sleeping through the night, the mother can express milk before she retires to shorten the nighttime interval that her breasts go without being drained. Similarly, if both breasts have not softened after the morning feeding, she can remove extra milk to help keep her supply plentiful. Because a large majority of breastfeeding mothers in the United States use a breast pump, expressing and storing surplus milk can ensure that a mother continues to produce a plentiful supply, and the frozen reserves can serve as a visual reminder that she has more than enough milk.

Combination Breast and Formula Feeding

Combination breast and formula feeding (CBFF) is defined as breastfeeding and offering daily supplemental formula from the first week of life.[81] CBFF, also known as "los dos," is a common cultural practice among Latinas. This practice is also prevalent among African American mothers and WIC enrollees.[81] In a national representative sample, CBFF was found to be associated with a significantly shorter duration of breastfeeding.[81] Among the study children, CBFF and formula feeding, when compared with 4 months of exclusive breastfeeding, were associated with an increased risk for overweight/obesity between ages 2 and 6 years.[81]

A recent randomized controlled trial investigated the impact of daily telephone education and support on the use of elective supplementation in the first 2 weeks postpartum among low-income primiparous, primarily Latina breastfeeding women.[78] None of the 300 Latina subjects breastfed exclusively, and few study mothers received any prenatal breastfeeding education. Mothers with a prior intent to "only breastfeed" were more likely to be in the "predominant breastfeeding" category, feeding less than 4 ounces of formula per day, underscoring the importance of prenatal education, especially for low-income mothers, to strengthen women's breastfeeding knowledge and intent.[78]

A qualitative study among low-income Latina women and their families found that Latina mothers assumed they could have "the best of both worlds" by combination feeding, even if they knew that breastfeeding was healthier and more convenient.[82] Universal exposure to formula feeding in the United States and strategic advertising of new formula additives to expectant and new mothers have a powerful influence, particularly among Latinas, who desire to provide both the benefits of breastfeeding and the highly touted "innovations" in infant formula. Believing that any breastfeeding confers all the health advantages, formula use is seen as enhancing breastfeeding, rather than diminishing the health benefits of exclusive breastfeeding.

In another qualitative study using structured interviews with expectant and new Latina mothers, the investigators explored beliefs surrounding "las dos cosas."[83] None of the women interviewed expressed familiarity with medical recommendations around breastfeeding exclusivity or duration,[83] thus highlighting the need to educate expectant and new mothers about the dose-related health benefits of breastfeeding and the negative dose-response effect of formula use on breastfeeding benefits and duration.[82,83]

Parents' Misinterpretation of Infant Crying

Many common infant health and behavior symptoms are mistakenly attributed to breastfeeding, both by parents and providers. Breastfeeding often gets the blame for infant spitting, frequent feeding, gassiness, and especially unexplained fussiness and crying. Low-income breastfeeding mothers with fussy infants often introduce solids or formula in an attempt to calm their baby or increase sleep duration.[84] Breastfeeding mothers also may restrict their own diets, try to manipulate the balance of fore milk and hind milk, or offer a specialty formula that claims to ease infant fussiness and gas. Infant crying is a common concern raised at pediatric medical visits, and the complaint often gets "medicalized" with diagnostic labels, such as colic or gastroesophageal reflux.

Mothers of breastfed infants report more challenging temperaments at 3 months of age compared with mothers of formula-fed infants.[85] It is possible that breastfeeding mothers are more attuned to their infants' behaviors owing to the intimacy of the nursing relationship. Although the perception of infant distress can be taxing and unsettling for parents, irritability among offspring of a variety of bird and mammalian species is a normal component of signaling to parents that helps ensure the nutritional needs of the young are met.[85] Yet, excessive or unexplained infant crying can undermine a breastfeeding mother's confidence and lead her to believe that there is something wrong with her milk or her baby, or that breastfeeding alone does not satisfy her infant. Pediatric providers can help mothers of fussy babies maintain exclusive breastfeeding by providing empathic support, educating parents concerning normal crying patterns in early infancy, offering effective coping strategies, and reassuring mothers that the period of increased crying will come to an end. Helpful national resources include The Period of PURPLE Crying, www.purplecrying.info/, and The Fussy Baby Network, www.fussybabynetwork.com.

The common misinterpretation of infant behaviors among WIC staff and clients contributes to low exclusive breastfeeding rates among WIC enrollees, but may be a modifiable factor. The widespread perception that crying, night-waking, and other normal infant behaviors are a result of hunger contributes to the early introduction of solids and formula. The FitWIC Baby Behavior Study investigated whether randomly training WIC staff and participants to better understand normal infant behavior and promote positive caregiver-infant interactions would affect infant feeding practices and the distribution of the exclusive breastfeeding food package.[86] The study found that providing education about normal infant behavior improved compliance with infant-feeding recommendations. Combination feeding in the first 4 months postpartum decreased among WIC participants at intervention sites, compared with those in the control group, and significantly fewer infants in the intervention group were above the 95th percentile for weight-for-age at the end of the study.[86]

Early Introduction of Complementary Foods

Many breastfeeding mothers introduce solid foods to their infants before 6 months based on cultural practices and the advice of female relatives, the belief that cereal will help an infant sleep longer at night or reduce spitting up, or the conviction that eating solids represents an important developmental milestone.[87] Among respondents in the national IFPS II, 41% reported that their infants were consuming solid foods at 4 months.[88] Mothers who began feeding their infants solids by 4 months, compared with those who did not, were more likely to have discontinued breastfeeding at 6 months.[88] Clinicians may help achieve greater compliance with delaying the introduction of complementary foods until about 6 months by providing ongoing consistent messaging, including an explanation of the scientific basis for exclusive breastfeeding recommendations, and helping mothers sort through conflicting infant feeding advice.

Maternal Employment

More than half of all new mothers become employed during their infant's first year.[89] Although more mothers today continue to breastfeed after returning to work than a decade ago, duration of breastfeeding is significantly shorter for employed mothers, and simply anticipating returning to work or school may prompt mothers to begin supplementing with formula.[90,91] A longer maternity leave increases breastfeeding duration and exclusivity.[90–93] In a large, longitudinal, nationally representative sample, women returning to work at 13 or more weeks had the highest proportion of predominant breastfeeding beyond 3 months, whereas those returning within 1 to 6 weeks had the lowest proportion.[90] Regularly pumping the breasts during the work day is associated with longer breastfeeding duration and intensity than not removing milk during working hours.[94] Working part time versus full time and having a flexible work schedule also are linked with a longer duration of breastfeeding.[91,95] Breastfeeding mothers who return to work full time are most likely to wean between the month before and 2 months after they become employed.[91] To promote exclusive breastfeeding, providers can encourage expectant and new mothers to delay their return to work as long as possible, and, if feasible, work part time before resuming full-time employment. Affirming and encouraging employed breastfeeding mothers at each well-baby visit may help women persevere in their efforts.

Diminished milk production is a major obstacle among employed breastfeeding women and often leads to breast refusal by the infant and the need for formula supplementation. Suggested strategies to help employed mothers maintain an abundant milk supply and breastfeed exclusively include (1) early initiation of milk expression, ideally within the first 2 weeks postpartum, after 1 or 2 morning feedings to establish a generous milk supply and accumulate frozen stores of expressed milk as a buffer against a dwindling supply,[96] and (2) using the "Magic Number" teaching tool to ensure that mothers maintain their daily frequency of draining their breasts after returning to work.[97] In addition, having opportunities during the work day to breastfeed directly (for example, by telecommuting, using onsite child care, or having a child care provider or family member bring the infant to the mother to nurse) has been shown to maintain breastfeeding "intensity" and increase breastfeeding duration.[94]

Child care providers often offer a breastfed infant larger volumes of milk by bottle than the infant would receive when nursing directly at the breast. This practice may cause the infant to lose interest in nursing and the mother to perceive that her milk supply is inadequate.[98] Communicating with the child care provider about typical feeding volumes for breastfed infants, how to read infant satiety cues, use of a slow flow nipple, and the acceptability of discarding unused expressed milk at the end of a feeding can create a collaborative partnership that promotes exclusive breastfeeding.

The Business Care for Breastfeeding is a comprehensive, national, government-sponsored initiative designed to educate employers about the economic benefits of supporting breastfeeding employees in the workplace and offer toolkits for the creation of workplace lactation programs.[99] The 2010 workplace breastfeeding support provision in the Patient Protection and Affordable Care Act grants new rights to lactating mothers in the workplace by amending the Fair Labor Standards Act. Under the new provision, employers are required to provide reasonable, unpaid break time and a private location (other than a bathroom) for an employee to express breast milk for her nursing child as often as needed for 1 year after the child's birth.[100] Both of these strategies provide hope for changing the workplace culture to better support breastfeeding employees to maintain exclusive breastfeeding.[99,100] A mother should meet with her employer, preferably during pregnancy or before returning to work, to clarify the location of the lactation space and anticipated break times. Expedient milk expression is best accomplished using an automatic-cycling electrical pump with a double collection system every 3 to 4 hours while mother is separated from her infant, depending on the infant's age and the mother's breast storage capacity.[96,101] The use of a hands-free pumping bra allows the mother to multitask during milk expression.

SOURCES OF SUPPORT AND CONFIDENCE FOR BREASTFEEDING MOTHERS

A 2012 Cochrane Review of the effectiveness of support for breastfeeding mothers found that all forms of extra support, including lay and professional, analyzed together, show an increase in breastfeeding duration and exclusivity.[102] The most effective support is provided in person and on a recurring basis at regular scheduled visits.

The Special Supplemental Nutrition Program for Women, Infants and Children

Over half of all newborns in the United States are enrolled in WIC, which represents a major source of support and practical assistance for the nation's most vulnerable population of breastfeeding mothers.[103] WIC promotes breastfeeding as the optimal source of nutrition for infants and offers many incentives for breastfeeding mothers, who receive a greater amount and variety of foods than those who feed only formula, with fully breastfeeding mothers receiving the most substantial food package. Breastfeeding mothers are eligible to participate in WIC longer than nonbreastfeeding mothers, and they may receive follow-up support through peer counselors, in addition to breast pumps and other aides to help support the initiation and continuation of breastfeeding. As of August 2009, WIC promotes exclusive breastfeeding by no longer routinely issuing infant formula in the first month to breastfeeding mothers to support the establishment of successful breastfeeding. Moreover, compelling evidence shows that WIC Breastfeeding Peer Counselors effectively improve rates of breastfeeding initiation, duration, and exclusivity.[104]

However, individual WIC agencies differ widely in their breastfeeding services, as well as in staff knowledge and attitudes concerning breastfeeding.[105] Although breastfeeding rates among WIC mothers have steadily increased, breastfeeding initiation, duration, and exclusivity among WIC participants remain significantly lower than non-WIC mothers.[106] Counseling challenges for WIC staff and nutritionists include the contradiction of WIC as both supporting breastfeeding and providing free formula, clients' perception that free formula is more valuable than the exclusive breastfeeding food package, and the belief in having a critical reserve of formula "just in case."[107] Encouraging WIC clients to accumulate frozen stores of their own milk by expressing milk remaining after breastfeeding (particularly in the morning when milk production is higher) may increase mothers' confidence about the adequacy of their milk supply and reduce requests for "just in case" formula. The trend toward including international board-certified lactation consultants (IBCLC) as part of WIC staffing shows promise in raising exclusive breastfeeding rates by providing timely intervention for clinical lactation challenges.[108]

The Baby's Father

Fathers should be considered vital members of a mother's "breastfeeding team," providing essential physical help and emotional support.[109] Qualitative data from mothers and fathers with breastfeeding infants confirm that a father's support makes a big difference, and fathers want to be empowered to fulfill this support role.[110] A controlled clinical intervention trial found that teaching new fathers about managing common breastfeeding difficulties, including fear of insufficient milk, significantly increased full breastfeeding at 6 months and reduced PIM.[111] In a study exploring maternal and paternal attitudes toward breastfeeding, fathers planning exclusive breastfeeding described breastfeeding as more natural and responded more strongly that breastfeeding helped mothers feel closer to their infants, compared with peers planning mixed feeding.[112] Health professionals should educate fathers about ways to help their breastfeeding partners and promote frank discussion among partners to strengthen their exclusive breastfeeding intention.

Mother-to-Mother Support

The importance of mother-to-mother support is reflected in the CDC's ongoing monitoring of the number of La Leche League Leaders per 1000 live births as a measure of comprehensive breastfeeding support included in each state's annual Breastfeeding

Report Card.[15] Established in 1956, at the height of the US formula-feeding era, La Leche League International provides mother-to-mother support, empowering information, and modeling of breastfeeding norms through group meetings, telephone counseling, publications, and the Internet.[113]

Today, many additional sources of mother-to-mother support are available through WIC Breastfeeding Peer Counselors, the growing number of hospital-based follow-up support groups, breastfeeding boutiques, postnatal yoga studios, and, more recently, Breastfeeding Cafés (**Fig. 2**).[114] Internet breastfeeding support groups, Mommy Blogs, and other social media communities now overcome problems of geographic isolation for new mothers. The emergence of breastfeeding support groups specifically targeting black mothers represents a promising grass-roots movement to raise African American breastfeeding rates by providing community breastfeeding role models and culturally competent information to help women of color begin and sustain breastfeeding.[115–118] Similar to undertaking other life challenges, when new mothers share their insecurities and learn that others feel the same way, they gain confidence in taking on the difficult challenge of breastfeeding. Task mastery and mutual empowerment are at the center of the mother-to mother support and confidence-building movement.[119]

Nurse-Family Partnership

The Nurse-Family Partnership (NFP) is a long-standing, evidence-based, nurse-home visitation program for low-income, first-time mothers, with proven long-term positive health and psychosocial outcomes for both the mother and child.[120,121] This federally funded, national program currently provides services in 41 states. Bi-weekly home visits by specially trained public health nurses begin during the mother's pregnancy and continue until her child is 2, creating a strong therapeutic relationship with the registered nurse that fosters maternal self-efficacy. Although the goals of NFP are to improve pregnancy outcome, child health and development, and the economic self-sufficiency of the family, a recent study found breastfeeding rates were higher for at-risk NFP clients than for similar WIC enrolled and eligible counterparts.[122] With more frequent home visits during the early postpartum period and ongoing regular contacts throughout infancy, NFP nurses are in a unique position to offer

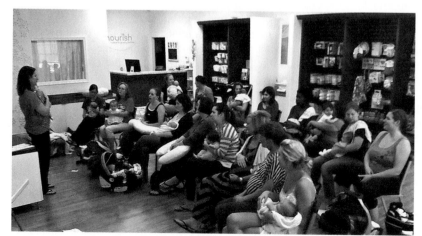

Fig. 2. Community-based breastfeeding support group. (*Courtesy of* M. Neifert, MD, Aurora, CO.)

strategic assessment, education, and support to help at-risk mothers successfully establish and maintain exclusive breastfeeding. Evaluation of the NFP's role in positively affecting breastfeeding outcomes among low-income, at-risk mothers warrants further investigation as a key strategy to improve infant health and development and increase child spacing.

THE ROLE OF THE PRIMARY CARE PROVIDER IN PROMOTING EXCLUSIVE AND EXTENDED BREASTFEEDING

Pediatricians and other pediatric care providers have a key role to play in the promotion of exclusive breastfeeding, ideally beginning in the prenatal period.[123,124] Taking advantage of training opportunities to improve breastfeeding knowledge, problem solving, and counseling can increase clinicians' effectiveness and comfort in providing breastfeeding management and support.[125] A targeted breastfeeding curriculum for residents in pediatrics, family medicine, and obstetrics and gynecology was effective in increasing physician knowledge, confidence, and practices and significantly increased exclusive breastfeeding at 6 months.[124]

Pediatricians can work with their local hospitals to promote breastfeeding-friendly maternity practices,[1] and consider taking the lead in their hospital's pursuit of the Baby-Friendly designation.[34] Pediatricians and their team should screen newborns for breastfeeding risk factors, and tailor an initial feeding plan that ensures that an at-risk infant is adequately nourished and the mother establishes an abundant milk supply.

The AAP recommends that newborn postdischarge visits be scheduled at 3 to 5 days (within 48–72 hours of hospital discharge).[1] The provider or lactation-trained office staff should observe and evaluate the onset of breastfeeding (ie, lactogenesis II has occurred, latch is effective and comfortable, infant's weight and elimination patterns are appropriate).[1] Recognizing that problems in the initiation of breastfeeding often lead to insufficient milk and excessive infant weight loss, pediatricians need to identify and ensure timely intervention for early breastfeeding complaints that impair milk transfer, such as latch-on difficulties, marked postpartum breast engorgement, or severe nipple soreness, to ensure the establishment of an abundant milk supply in the critical first weeks after birth (**Figs. 3** and **4**).[56,63] Yet, compliance with AAP recommendations for early follow-up after birth hospitalization remains inconsistent, and delayed follow-up of newborns commonly occurs.[126,127] Encouraging new mothers to complete a daily infant feeding and elimination log during the postbirth hospitalization and the first weeks at home helps facilitate the physician's assessment of breastfeeding. In addition, completing a breastfeeding log for at least 3 weeks has been linked with an increased likelihood of full breastfeeding at 6 months.[128]

A second, early follow-up ambulatory visit at 2 weeks is recommended to monitor infant weight gain and provide ongoing support to the mother during the challenging first weeks of breastfeeding and new parenthood.[129] In a prospective, randomized trial, mothers whose infants received a routine, preventive, outpatient visit between 4 days and 2 weeks in the office of a primary care physician trained to support breastfeeding were significantly more likely to report exclusive breastfeeding at 4 weeks and a longer duration of breastfeeding, when compared with mothers whose infants received usual care at 1 month with an untrained physician.[125]

Because the busy office practice cannot realistically address all breastfeeding challenges,[130] physicians should know their local IBCLCs or breastfeeding counselors and communicate closely with these individuals when referring clients for help.[131] They should keep informed about and refer mothers to available community breastfeeding resources, including hospital outpatient lactation services and WIC breastfeeding

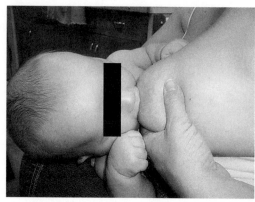

Fig. 3. Using breast compressions while breastfeeding to deliver a spray of milk and entice a sleepy baby to resume nursing effectively. (*Courtesy of* M. Neifert, MD, Aurora, CO.)

support. This role is facilitated when local WIC agencies, hospitals, and/or breastfeeding coalitions take on the task of compiling and making available to practitioners a current resource list for local breastfeeding clinical services and support.

Breastfeeding mothers commonly report that a health care professional recommended formula supplement for their infant in response to maternal complaints, such as breast and nipple pain, fatigue, apparent infant hunger, and problems with infant latching-on.[77,130] With appropriate clinical management and extra counseling, however, such common breastfeeding concerns usually can be resolved while maintaining exclusive breast milk feeding. Pediatricians also should ensure that breastfeeding continues in the context of diagnoses such as hyperbilirubinemia, gastroesophageal reflux, allergic colitis, transient gassiness with certain maternally ingested foods or overactive let-down of milk that temporarily causes infant distress during feeding.[132] The Academy of Breastfeeding Medicine has developed numerous peer-reviewed, evidence-based clinical protocols that can guide the practitioner in the management of various breastfeeding problems and medical issues affected by breastfeeding.[133]

Physicians often underestimate the power of their words to promote breastfeeding by enthusiastically affirming, informing, and encouraging breastfeeding mothers at each office visit. In a large prospective cohort study, mothers who reported receiving

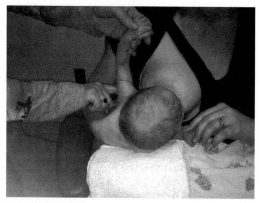

Fig. 4. Using tactile stimulation to keep a sleepy infant awake and actively breastfeeding. (*Courtesy of* M. Bunik, MD, Aurora, CO.)

clinician support were about half as likely to discontinue breastfeeding by 12 weeks as those who did not.[123] Physicians can help strengthen mothers' commitment to breast-feeding by regularly complimenting them on continuing to nurse their baby, and increase mothers' confidence in the adequacy of their milk supply by reassuring them about their infant's well-being and rate of weight gain. Primary care providers should repeatedly remind breastfeeding mothers to schedule an infant weight check between visits whenever they are concerned about their milk supply or are considering starting supplemental formula.

Additional strategies to promote exclusive breastfeeding in the pediatric office include reinforcing the value of exclusive breastfeeding at well-baby visits and routinely inquiring about the introduction of supplemental formula or solids (**Box 4**). Pediatric providers should incorporate age-related breastfeeding anticipatory guidance at each visit, including information about normal infant crying, expressing and storing breast milk, infant appetite spurts, maternal employment, infant teething, and delaying solid foods (**Table 2**).[134]

Box 4
Evidence-based strategies to promote exclusive breastfeeding

1. Strengthen health professionals' commitment to promote and support breastfeeding.

2. Educate expectant mothers about breastfeeding, including the nutritional superiority of human milk, why exclusive breastfeeding is recommended, how to get an optimal breastfeeding start in the hospital, reasons to avoid formula supplementation, sources of support and clinical lactation services, strategies for combining breastfeeding and employment, and the timing of the introduction of complementary foods.

3. Widely implement supportive maternity care practices, including immediate skin-to-skin mother-baby contact; continuous rooming-in of mother and infant; unrestricted, cue-based breastfeeding; avoidance of formula supplementation of breastfed newborns; avoidance of routine pacifier use; and postdischarge access to support and professional services to overcome breastfeeding challenges.

4. Change the traditional paradigm that supplementation of breastfed infants requires the use of formula; instead, begin milk expression and preferentially supplement with mother's own milk when a medical indication exists.

5. Help breastfeeding mothers establish and maintain an abundant milk supply in the critical first postpartum weeks.

6. Identify infants at risk for ineffective breastfeeding, and begin "prevention pumping" to ensure that the mother establishes an abundant milk supply and the infant is adequately nourished with exclusive breast milk feedings.

7. Restrict formula distribution in hospitals and ambulatory facilities.

8. Ensure timely follow-up and evaluation of breastfeeding dyads within 48 hours of hospital discharge and again at 2 weeks postpartum by knowledgeable and supportive providers.

9. Provide ongoing breastfeeding anticipatory guidance and support from pediatricians and other health professionals.

10. Know about and refer nursing mothers to local breastfeeding resources, and promote collaboration and communication among primary care providers, hospital and community-based lactation consultants, and WIC and public health staff.

11. Promote maternal self-efficacy through broad social support systems, including WIC Breastfeeding Peer Counselors, NFP nurses, hospital-based and community breastfeeding support groups, and family and partner support.

12. Encourage adequate maternity leave and workplace lactation programs.

Table 2
Breastfeeding touchpoints for overcoming obstacles to exclusivity

Breastfeeding Touchpoint	Parental Concern	Main Obstacles	Provider Advice
Prenatal	"I want to breastfeed, but since I am going to work, I need to be able to give formula too."	• Lack of information about combining breastfeeding and working • Lack of information about milk expression and access to pumps	• Strongly encourage attendance at a prenatal breastfeeding class (deserves equal time to birthing class education). • Consider a longer maternity leave, if possible. • Prepare to simplify life during the transition to parenting.
	"My husband and other family members will want to help feed the baby. Won't they feel excluded if I only breastfeed?"	• Family members wanting to feed the baby	• Enlist father's help in supporting his nursing partner. Fathers can interact with their infant by holding baby skin-to-skin or taking baby out while mother sleeps. • After breastfeeding is well established, others can feed expressed milk by bottle.
	"I want to do combination feeding, or Los Dos."	• Desire for "the best of both worlds" by combination feeding • Lack of knowledge about the importance of frequent and exclusive breastfeeding during the early postpartum weeks for establishing mother's milk supply	• "Puro pecho," or only mother's own milk, provides greater health benefits and helps maintain an abundant milk supply. • If eligible, enrollment in WIC offers breastfeeding mothers a substantial food package, counseling, breast pumps, and peer counselors.
Birth	"My friend says it is a good idea to ask the nurses to care for my baby at night, so I can get some sleep."	• Unrealistic expectations for the postbirth hospital stay • Lack of prenatal education • Frequent interruptions and excessive visitors deplete new mothers. • Increased risk of formula supplements for nighttime births from 9 PM to 6 AM	• Promote immediate skin-to-skin contact after birth to facilitate initiation of breastfeeding within the first hour. • Teach mother to interpret her infant's feeding cues and breastfeed as often as baby wants. Advocate for no routine formula use in the system of care. • Advise mother to request help in the hospital with breastfeeding to promote task mastery. • Encourage continuous rooming-in, where mother can practice being with her baby in a controlled setting and learn to latch baby comfortably and effectively.
	"The yellow milk does not look like much. A little formula won't hurt, will it?"	• Belief that the small amount of colostrum is insufficient until "milk comes in"	• Explain the potency and adequacy of colostrum and the rapid increase in milk production from 36 to 96 h.

3–5 d	"Now that we are home, the baby seems to be feeding every hour. She or he doesn't seem satisfied."	• Lack of knowledge about normal frequency of feedings for breastfed newborns • Infants typically begin feeding more frequently the second night after birth, when baby is at home. • Concern about whether the infant is getting enough milk, due to mother's inability to see what the infant takes at the breast • Sleepy infant	• Explain that 8–12 feedings in 24 h are typical and necessary to establish an abundant milk supply. • Provide a hand-pump, or teach hand expression, so mother can see that she has milk. • Explain normal infant elimination patterns once mother's milk comes in (3–5 voids and 3–4 stools per day by 3–5 d; onset of yellow, seedy milk stools by 4–5 d). • Perform infant test weights (before and after feeding) to reassure mother about baby's milk intake at a feeding. • Teach mother the difference between infant "flutter sucking" or "nibbling" that results in only a trickle of milk at breast versus "drinking" milk, with active sucking and regular swallowing. • Tickling under axilla or holding hand can help keep baby on task at breast. Or, compressing the breast when the baby stops slow, deep sucking can deliver a spray of milk to entice him or her to start drinking again (see **Figs. 3** and **4**). • Anticipate infant appetite spurt at about 10–14 d of age.
	"My nipples are sore and cracked. Can I take a break and give my baby a little formula?"	• Sore nipples usually are attributable to incorrect latch-on technique and are a common reason that mothers discontinue breastfeeding early or start supplements.	• Observe a nursing session to evaluate latch. Consider referring mother to a lactation consultant for one-on-one assistance with latch.
2 wk	"My breasts do not feel very full anymore. I'm afraid my milk went away."	• As postpartum breast engorgement resolves, and the breasts adjust to making and releasing milk, mothers may perceive they have insufficient milk.	• Expect infant to be above birth weight by 10–14 d, and reassure mother about infant's rate of weight gain since the 3–5-d visit. • Although mother's breasts are less swollen than during postpartum engorgement, they should feel fuller before feedings and softer afterward.
	"How can I know my baby is getting enough?"	• The 10–14-d appetite spurt can cause mother to doubt the adequacy of her milk supply.	• Consider performing test weights (before and after feeding) to reassure mother about her infant's intake. • Anticipate another appetite spurt at about 3 wk of age.

(continued on next page)

Table 2
(continued)

Breastfeeding Touchpoint	Parental Concern	Main Obstacles	Provider Advice
1 mo	"My baby is crying a lot, and I am tired and need sleep."	• Normal infant crying peaks at about 6 wk (3–5 h in 24 h). • Mother may attribute infant crying to hunger or an adverse reaction to her milk.	• Congratulate mother on a full month of breastfeeding! • If infant has gained weight appropriately, reassure mother about the adequacy of her milk supply. • Offer coping strategies for infant crying, including holding baby skin-to-skin; 5 Ss (however, swaddling with hands up near head to help assess feeding cues); use of infant carrier; stroller or car ride; Period of PURPLE Crying.
	"Nothing seems to calm her/him except the bottle."	• If infant drinks milk from a bottle that is offered, mother may assume infant is not satisfied by breastfeeding.	• Explain that infant sucking is reflexive, and drinking from an offered bottle doesn't always mean that the baby was hungry. Baby "can't scream and suck at the same time," so the bottle may appear to calm baby, just as a pacifier might. • If mom desires to offer a bottle, use expressed milk as the supplement. • Forewarn mother about cluster feeds (late afternoon/evening) and upcoming appetite spurts, occurring about 6 wk and 3 mo.
2 mo	"My mother said that, if I give rice cereal in a bottle before bedtime, the baby may sleep longer at night."	• Parental sleep deprivation • Mother may already have returned to work, which often increases fatigue and leads to a decrease in milk supply.	• Explain the lack of evidence that rice cereal or other solid foods increase infant sleep. • Remind mother that adding complementary foods is a project and increases workload for parents. • Reinforce the benefits of exclusive breastfeeding for maternal-infant health and mother's milk supply.
	"I am going back to work, and am worried that I do not have enough frozen stores of milk. Are there any herbs I can take to keep my milk supply strong?"	• Lack of knowledge about the principles of milk production and unrealistic beliefs about the efficacy of galactogogues	• Enlist help from others, including support for returning to work. • Explain that there is no "magic pill" or special tea to increase mother's milk supply. The key to ongoing milk production is frequent, effective milk removal (every 3–4 h). • Caution mother to avoid going long intervals without draining her breasts.

Age			
4 mo	"My baby seems to only eat for a few minutes, and when I try to put her/him back to the breast, she/he refuses."	• Misinterpretation of infant's efficiency in nursing causes concern about infant milk intake.	• Explain that infants become more efficient at breastfeeding, and by 3 mo, they may drain the breast in 4–7 min. • Reinforce continuing to delay the introduction of solid foods.
	"My baby seems more interested in everything around him/her than in nursing at the breast."	• Normal infant distractibility causes mother to believe her infant is self-weaning.	• Explain that distractibility is a normal developmental behavior at this age, and that short, efficient feeds are common. • Nurse in a quiet, darkened room.
6 mo	"My baby is drooling and rubbing on her/his gums all the time. I do not think that I can continue to breastfeed because my baby might bite me."	• Common myth that a mother needs to wean when her baby gets teeth to avoid being bitten while breastfeeding	• Congratulate mother on 6 mo of exclusive breastfeeding! • Explain that infants cannot bite and actively breastfeed at the same time. Biting tends to occur if the breast is offered when the infant is not interested or at the end of the feeding. • If the infant bites, say "No biting," touch the infant's lips, set the baby down, and briefly leave the room.
	"My baby has refused to breastfeed for almost a whole day now. Is she/he ready to wean?"	• Misinterpretation of sudden breastfeeding refusal ("Nursing Strike") to mean that a baby is self-weaning.	• Explain that some babies may suddenly refuse the breast between 4 and 7 mo of age for no apparent reason. Common causes include an upper respiratory infection, ear infection, teething, regular exposure to bottle-feeding, use of a new soap/perfume, maternal stress, or a decrease in milk supply. • Because many babies will nurse while asleep, try offering the breast when the baby is drowsy or asleep. • Regularly express milk if the baby won't nurse, and feed the pumped milk until the infant resumes breastfeeding.

Courtesy of M. Bunik, MD, Aurora, CO.

SUMMARY

Most US infants and mothers are not receiving the maximum, short-term and long-term health benefits associated with exclusive breastfeeding, and substantial racial and economic differences in breastfeeding contribute to infant and maternal health disparities. Women's personal and societal barriers to exclusive breastfeeding include lack of prenatal education, inappropriate maternity practices, being comfortable with formula feeding, perception of insufficient milk, misinterpretation of normal infant crying, early introduction of complementary foods, maternal employment, inadequate support, and lack of access to clinical breastfeeding services. Despite the brevity of the postbirth hospitalization, substantial evidence confirms the role of supportive maternity care practices in increasing breastfeeding duration and exclusivity. Because perceived insufficient milk is a chief reason that breastfeeding mothers begin supplementing with formula or wean early, helping women establish and maintain an abundant milk supply, and feel confident that they have enough milk, is a critical strategy in promoting exclusive and extended breastfeeding. A newborn postdischarge visit at 3 to 5 days of life and a second, early follow-up appointment at 2 weeks are essential to monitor infant weight and provide support and encouragement to the mother during the establishment of breastfeeding. Potential sources of essential support to help mothers increase breastfeeding duration and exclusivity include the federal WIC program, NFP nurses, families, mother-peers, health care professionals, and employers. All practitioners need to increase their own breastfeeding knowledge, problem solving, and counseling, as well as work closely with their hospital-based and community lactation consultants and WIC agencies to best support exclusive breastfeeding for the first 6 months.

REFERENCES

1. Eidelman AI, Schanler RJ. Breastfeeding and the use of human milk. Pediatrics 2012;129:e827–41 PM:22371471.
2. World Health Organization. Infant and child nutrition: global strategy on infant and young child feeding. Available at: http://apps.who.int/gb/archive/pdf_files/WHA55/ea5515.pdf. Accessed August 31, 2012.
3. World Health Organization. Indicators for assessing infant and young child feeding practices. Available at: http://www.ifpri.org/sites/default/files/publications/childfeeding.pdf. Accessed August 31, 2012.
4. Ip S, Chung M, Raman G, et al. Breastfeeding and maternal and infant health outcomes in developed countries. Evid Rep Technol Assess (Full Rep) 2007;(153):1–186 PM:17764214.
5. White House Task Force on Childhood Obesity. Solving the problem of childhood obesity within a generation. Available at: http://www.letsmove.gov/whitehouse-task-force-childhood-obesity-report-president. Accessed August 31, 2012.
6. Accelerating Progress in Obesity Web site. Available at: http://www.iom.edu/Reports/2012/Acclerating-Progress-in-Obesity-Prevention.aspx. Accessed September 19, 2012.
7. Harder T, Bergmann R, Kallischnigg G, et al. Duration of breastfeeding and risk of overweight: a meta-analysis. Am J Epidemiol 2005;162:397–403 PM:16076830.
8. Fewtrell M, Wilson DC, Booth I, et al. Six months of exclusive breast feeding: how good is the evidence? BMJ 2011;342:c5955 PM:21233152.
9. Kramer MS, Kakuma R. Optimal duration of exclusive breastfeeding. Cochrane Database Syst Rev 2012;(8):CD003517. PM:22895934.

10. Bolton TA, Chow T, Benton PA, et al. Characteristics associated with longer breastfeeding duration: an analysis of a peer counseling support program. J Hum Lact 2009;25:18–27 PM:18971503.
11. DiGirolamo AM, Grummer-Strawn LM, Fein SB. Effect of maternity-care practices on breastfeeding. Pediatrics 2008;122(Suppl 2):S43–9 PM:18829830.
12. Murray EK, Ricketts S, Dellaport J. Hospital practices that increase breastfeeding duration: results from a population-based study. Birth 2007;34:202–11 PM: 17718870.
13. Hornell A, Hofvander Y, Kylberg E. Solids and formula: association with pattern and duration of breastfeeding. Pediatrics 2001;107:E38 PM:11230619.
14. Feinstein JM, Berkelhamer JE, Gruszka ME, et al. Factors related to early termination of breast-feeding in an urban population. Pediatrics 1986;78:210–5.
15. Centers for Disease Control and Prevention. Breastfeeding report card—United States. 2012. Available at: http://www.cdc.gov/breastfeeding/pdf/2012BreastfeedingReportCard.pdf. Accessed August 31, 2012.
16. Bain K. The incidence of breast feeding in hospitals in the United States. Pediatrics 1948;2:313–20 PM:18880101.
17. Breastfeeding trends and updated national health objectives for exclusive breastfeeding—United States, birth years 2000-2004. Morb Mortal Wkly Rep 2007;56:760–3 PM:17673896.
18. Fein SB, Labiner-Wolfe J, Shealy KR, et al. Infant feeding practices study II: study methods. Pediatrics 2008;122(Suppl 2):S28–35 PM:18829828.
19. Perrine CG, Scanlon KS, Li R, et al. Baby-Friendly hospital practices and meeting exclusive breastfeeding intention. Pediatrics 2012;130:54–60 PM: 22665406.
20. Surgeon General's report: US Department of Health and Human Services. The Surgeon General's call to action to support breastfeeding. Washington, DC: US Department of Health and Human Services, Office of the Surgeon General; 2011.
21. Dyson L, McCormick F, Renfrew MJ. Interventions for promoting the initiation of breastfeeding. Cochrane Database Syst Rev 2005:CD001688. PM:15846621.
22. US Department of Health and Human Services. Women's preventive services: Required health plan coverage guidelines. Available at: http://www.hrsa.gov/womensguidelines/. Accessed August 31, 2012.
23. Dusdieker LB, Dungy CI, Losch ME. Prenatal office practices regarding infant feeding choices. Clin Pediatr (Phila) 2006;45:841–5 PM:17041172.
24. Wright CM, Waterston AJ. Relationships between paediatricians and infant formula milk companies. Arch Dis Child 2006;91:383–5 PM:16632663.
25. Enfamil. Certificate for Free Breastfeeding Kit. Available at: http://www.enfamil.com/app/iwp/enfamil/certificate.do?dm=enf&id=/Consumer_Home3/Offers/BreastfeedingKit&iwpst=B2C&ls=0&csred=1&r=3523980718. Accessed September 2, 2012.
26. Abbott Laboratories. Similac Homepage. Available at: https://similac.com/. Accessed September 2, 2012.
27. Damota K, Banuelos J, Goldbronn J, et al. Maternal request for in-hospital supplementation of healthy breastfed infants among low-income women. J Hum Lact 2012;28:476–82.
28. The Joint Commission. Speak up initiatives. Available at: http://www.jointcommission.org/speakup.aspx. Accessed August 31, 2012.
29. The Joint Commission. Speak Up: What you need to know about breastfeeding. Available at: http://www.jointcommission.org/speakup_breastfeeding/. Accessed August 31, 2012.

30. World Health Organization. Evidence for the ten steps to successful breastfeeding. Available at: http://whqlibdoc.who.int/publications/2004/9241591544_eng.pdf. Accessed August 31, 2012. 2012.

31. Braun ML, Giugliani ER, Soares ME, et al. Evaluation of the impact of the baby-friendly hospital initiative on rates of breastfeeding. Am J Public Health 2003;93:1277–9 PM:12893612.

32. Kramer MS, Chalmers B, Hodnett ED, et al. Promotion of Breastfeeding Intervention Trial (PROBIT): a randomized trial in the Republic of Belarus. JAMA 2001;285:413–20 PM:11242425.

33. Merewood A, Mehta SD, Chamberlain LB, et al. Breastfeeding rates in US Baby-Friendly hospitals: results of a national survey. Pediatrics 2005;116:628–34 PM:16140702.

34. Baby Friendly USA. Available at: http://www.babyfriendlyusa.org/eng/index.html. Accessed August 31, 2012.

35. Vital signs: hospital practices to support breastfeeding—United States, 2007 and 2009. Morb Mortal Wkly Rep 2011;60:1020–5 PM:21814166.

36. Declercq E, Labbok MH, Sakala C, et al. Hospital practices and women's likelihood of fulfilling their intention to exclusively breastfeed. Am J Public Health 2009;99:929–35 PM:19299680.

37. Dabritz HA, Hinton BG, Babb J. Maternal hospital experiences associated with breastfeeding at 6 months in a northern California county. J Hum Lact 2010;26:274–85 PM:20484659.

38. The Joint Commission. Perinatal care. Available at: http://www.jointcommission.org/perinatal_care/. Accessed August 31, 2012.

39. Philipp BL. ABM clinical protocol #7: model breastfeeding policy (revision 2010). Breastfeed Med 2010;5:173–7 PM:20590476.

40. Tender JA, Janakiram J, Arce E, et al. Reasons for in-hospital formula supplementation of breastfed infants from low-income families. J Hum Lact 2009;25:11–7 PM:18971505.

41. Gagnon AJ, Leduc G, Waghorn K, et al. In-hospital formula supplementation of healthy breastfeeding newborns. J Hum Lact 2005;21:397–405 PM:16280555.

42. Akuse RM, Obinya EA. Why healthcare workers give prelacteal feeds. Eur J Clin Nutr 2002;56:729–34 PM:12122548.

43. Reiff MI, Essock-Vitale SM. Hospital influences on early infant-feeding practices. Pediatrics 1985;76:872–9 PM:4069855.

44. United States Breastfeeding Committee. Implementing The Joint Commission perinatal care core measure on exclusive breast milk feeding. Available at: http://www.usbreastfeeding.org/Portals/0/Coalitions/2010-NCSBC/BTT-Handouts/BTT-29-Handout.pdf. Accessed August 31, 2012.

45. The Joint Commission. Specifications Manual for Joint Commission National Quality Measures (v2010B2): Perinatal Care. Available at: http://manual.jointcommission.org/releases/TJC2010B/MIF0170.html. Accessed September 2, 2012.

46. Bramson L, Lee JW, Moore E, et al. Effect of early skin-to-skin mother–infant contact during the first 3 hours following birth on exclusive breastfeeding during the maternity hospital stay. J Hum Lact 2010;26:130–7 PM:20110561.

47. Moore ER, Anderson GC, Bergman N, et al. Early skin-to-skin contact for mothers and their healthy newborn infants. Cochrane Database Syst Rev 2012;(5):CD003519. PM:22592691.

48. Morrison B, Ludington-Hoe S, Anderson GC. Interruptions to breastfeeding dyads on postpartum day 1 in a university hospital. J Obstet Gynecol Neonatal Nurs 2006;35:709–16 PM:17105635.

49. Scott JA, Binns CW, Oddy WH, et al. Predictors of breastfeeding duration: evidence from a cohort study. Pediatrics 2006;117:e646–55 PM:16585281.
50. Rosenberg KD, Eastham CA, Kasehagen LJ, et al. Marketing infant formula through hospitals: the impact of commercial hospital discharge packs on breastfeeding. Am J Public Health 2008;98:290–5 PM:18172152.
51. Snell BJ, Krantz M, Keeton R, et al. The association of formula samples given at hospital discharge with the early duration of breastfeeding. J Hum Lact 1992;8: 67–72 PM:1605843.
52. Merewood A, Grossman X, Cook J, et al. US hospitals violate WHO policy on the distribution of formula sample packs: results of a national survey. J Hum Lact 2010;26:363–7 PM:20871089.
53. Sadacharan R, Grossman X, Sanchez E, et al. Trends in US hospital distribution of industry-sponsored infant formula sample packs. Pediatrics 2011;128:702–5 PM:21949146.
54. Centers for Disease Control and Prevention. CDC National survey of maternity care practices in infant nutrition and care (mPINC). Available at: http://www.cdc.gov/breastfeeding/pdf/mpinc_overview.pdf. Accessed August 31, 2012.
55. Dewey KG. Maternal and fetal stress are associated with impaired lactogenesis in humans. J Nutr 2001;131:3012S–5S PM:11694638.
56. Neifert MR. Prevention of breastfeeding tragedies. Pediatr Clin North Am 2001; 48:273–97 PM:11339153.
57. Hamilton BA, Martin JA, Ventura SJ. Births: preliminary data for 2010. Natl Vital Stat Rep. 2011;60:1–26. Available at: http://www.cdc.gov/nchs/data/nvsr/nvsr60/nvsr60_02.pdf. Accessed August 31, 2012.
58. Engle WA, Tomashek KM, Wallman C. "Late-preterm" infants: a population at risk. Pediatrics 2007;120:1390–401 PM:18055691.
59. Meier PP, Furman LM, Degenhardt M. Increased lactation risk for late preterm infants and mothers: evidence and management strategies to protect breast-feeding. J Midwifery Womens Health 2007;52:579–87 PM:17983995.
60. ABM clinical protocol #10: breastfeeding the late preterm infant (34(0/7) to 36(6/7) weeks gestation). Breastfeed Med 2011;6:151–6 PM:21631254.
61. Gatti L. Maternal perceptions of insufficient milk supply in breastfeeding. J Nurs Scholarsh 2008;40:355–63 PM:19094151.
62. Li R, Fein SB, Chen J, et al. Why mothers stop breastfeeding: mothers' self-reported reasons for stopping during the first year. Pediatrics 2008; 122(Suppl 2):S69–76 PM:18829834.
63. Hill PD, Aldag JC, Chatterton RT, et al. Comparison of milk output between mothers of preterm and term infants: the first 6 weeks after birth. J Hum Lact 2005;21:22–30 PM:15681632.
64. Neville MC. Anatomy and physiology of lactation. Pediatr Clin North Am 2001; 48:13–34 PM:11236721.
65. Czank C, Henderson JJ, Kent JC, et al. Hormonal control of the lactation cycle. In: Hale TW, Hartmann PE, editors. Textbook of human lactation. 1st edition. Amarillo (TX): Hale Publishing, LP; 2007. p. 89–111.
66. Prime DK, Geddes DT, Hartmann PE. Oxytocin: milk ejection and maternal-infant well-being. In: Hale TW, Hartmann PE, editors. Textbook of human lactation. 1st edition. Amarillo (TX): Hale Publishing, LP; 2007. p. 141–55.
67. Daly SE, Hartmann PE. Infant demand and milk supply. Part 2: the short-term control of milk synthesis in lactating women. J Hum Lact 1995;11:27–37 PM:7718103.

68. Daly SE, Hartmann PE. Infant demand and milk supply. Part 1: infant demand and milk production in lactating women. J Hum Lact 1995;11:21–6 PM:7718102.

69. Neville MC, Allen JC, Archer PC, et al. Studies in human lactation: milk volume and nutrient composition during weaning and lactogenesis. Am J Clin Nutr 1991;54:81–92 PM:2058592.

70. Chapman DJ, Perez-Escamilla R. Identification of risk factors for delayed onset of lactation. J Am Diet Assoc 1999;99:450–4 PM:10207398.

71. Nommsen-Rivers LA, Chantry CJ, Peerson JM, et al. Delayed onset of lactogenesis among first-time mothers is related to maternal obesity and factors associated with ineffective breastfeeding. Am J Clin Nutr 2010;92:574–84 PM:20573792.

72. Dewey KG, Nommsen-Rivers LA, Heinig MJ, et al. Risk factors for suboptimal infant breastfeeding behavior, delayed onset of lactation, and excess neonatal weight loss. Pediatrics 2003;112:607–19 PM:12949292.

73. Hartmann PE, Cregan M. Lactogenesis and the effects of insulin-dependent diabetes mellitus and prematurity. J Nutr 2001;131:3016S–20S.

74. Chapman DJ, Perez-Escamilla R. Does delayed perception of the onset of lactation shorten breastfeeding duration? J Hum Lact 1999;15:107–11 PM:10578785.

75. Shealy KR, Scanlon KS, Labiner-Wolfe J, et al. Characteristics of breastfeeding practices among US mothers. Pediatrics 2008;122(Suppl 2):S50–5 PM:18829831.

76. Nommsen-Rivers LA, Chantry CJ, Cohen RJ, et al. Comfort with the idea of formula feeding helps explain ethnic disparity in breastfeeding intentions among expectant first-time mothers. Breastfeed Med 2010;5:25–33 PM:20043707.

77. Taveras EM, Li R, Grummer-Strawn L, et al. Mothers' and clinicians' perspectives on breastfeeding counseling during routine preventive visits. Pediatrics 2004;113:405–11 PMID:15121981.

78. Bunik M, Shobe P, O'Connor ME, et al. Are 2 weeks of daily breastfeeding support insufficient to overcome the influences of formula? Acad Pediatr 2010;10:21–8 PM:20129478.

79. Ahluwalia IB, Morrow B, Hsia J. Why do women stop breastfeeding? Findings from the Pregnancy Risk Assessment and Monitoring System. Pediatrics 2005;116:1408–12 PM:16322165.

80. Wilhelm S, Rodehorst-Weber TK, Flanders Stepans MB, et al. The relationship between breastfeeding test weights and postpartum breastfeeding rates. J Hum Lact 2010;26:168–74 PM:20015841.

81. Holmes AV, Auinger P, Howard CR. Combination feeding of breast milk and formula: evidence for shorter breast-feeding duration from the National Health and Nutrition Examination Survey. J Pediatr 2011;159:186–91 PM:21429512.

82. Bunik M, Clark L, Zimmer LM, et al. Early infant feeding decisions in low-income Latinas. Breastfeed Med 2006;1:225–35 PMID: 17661603.

83. Bartick M, Reyes C. Las dos cosas: an analysis of attitudes of Latina women on non-exclusive breastfeeding. Breastfeed Med 2012;7:19–24 PM:22007765.

84. Heinig MJ, Follett JR, Ishii KD, et al. Barriers to compliance with infant-feeding recommendations among low-income women. J Hum Lact 2006;22:27–38 PM:16467285.

85. Lauzon-Guillain B, Wijndaele K, Clark M, et al. Breastfeeding and infant temperament at age three months. PLoS One 2012;7:e29326 PM:22253712.

86. Heinig MJ, Banuelos J, Goldbronn J, et al. Fit WIC baby behavior study: Helping you understand your baby. Available at: http://www.nal.usda.gov/wicworks/Sharing_Center/spg/CA_report2006.pdf. Accessed August 31, 2012.

87. Olson BH, Horodynski MA, Brophy-Herb H, et al. Health professionals' perspectives on the infant feeding practices of low income mothers. Matern Child Health J 2010;14:75–85 PM:18982434.

88. Grummer-Strawn LM, Scanlon KS, Fein SB. Infant feeding and feeding transitions during the first year of life. Pediatrics 2008;122(Suppl 2):S36–42 PM:18829829.

89. Bureau of Labor Statistics, US Department of Labor. Employment characteristics of families–2011. Available at: http://www.bls.gov/news.release/pdf/famee.pdf. Accessed August 31, 2012.

90. Ogbuanu C, Glover S, Probst J, et al. The effect of maternity leave length and time of return to work on breastfeeding. Pediatrics 2011;127:e1414–27 PM:21624878.

91. Guendelman S, Kosa JL, Pearl M, et al. Juggling work and breastfeeding: effects of maternity leave and occupational characteristics. Pediatrics 2009;123:e38–46 PM:19117845.

92. Erkkola M, Salmenhaara M, Kronberg-Kippila C, et al. Determinants of breast-feeding in a Finnish birth cohort. Public Health Nutr 2010;13:504–13 PM:19825208.

93. Kristiansen AL, Lande B, Overby NC, et al. Factors associated with exclusive breast-feeding and breast-feeding in Norway. Public Health Nutr 2010;13:2087–96 PM:20707948.

94. Fein SB, Mandal B, Roe BE. Success of strategies for combining employment and breastfeeding. Pediatrics 2008;122(Suppl 2):S56–62 PM:18829832.

95. Mandal B, Roe BE, Fein SB. The differential effects of full-time and part-time work status on breastfeeding. Health Policy 2010;97:79–86 PM:20400199.

96. Neifert M. Great expectations: essential guide to breastfeeding. New York: Sterling Publishing; 2009.

97. Mohrbacher N. The magic number and long-term milk production. Clinical Lactation 2011;2:15–8.

98. Batan M, Li R, Scanlon K. Association of child care providers breastfeeding support with breastfeeding duration at 6 months. Matern Child Health J 2012 [Epub ahead of print]. PM:22706997.

99. womenshealth.gov. Breastfeeding. Available at: http://www.womenshealth.gov/breastfeeding/government-in-action/business-case-for-breastfeeding/. Accessed August 31, 2012.

100. The Patient Protection and Affordable Care Act. Available at: http://www.gpo.gov/fdsys/pkg/PLAW-111publ148/pdf/PLAW-111publ148.pdf. Accessed August 31, 2012.

101. Lawrence RA, Lawrence RM. Breastfeeding, a guide for the medical professional. 7th edition. Maryland Height (MO): Elsevier Mosby; 2011.

102. Renfrew MJ, McCormick FM, Wade A, et al. Support for healthy breastfeeding mothers with healthy term babies. Cochrane Database Syst Rev 2012;(5):CD001141. PM:22592675.

103. USDA Food and Nutrition Service. WIC at a glance. Available at: http://www.fns.usda.gov/wic/aboutwic/wicataglance.htm. Accessed August 31, 2012.

104. Chapman DJ, Morel K, Anderson AK, et al. Breastfeeding peer counseling: from efficacy through scale-up. J Hum Lact 2010;26:314–26 PM:20715336.

105. Suitor CW. Planning a WIC research agenda: workshop summary. Washington, DC: National Academy Press; 2011.

106. Centers for Disease Control and Prevention. Provisional breastfeeding rates by socio-demographic factors, among children born in 2007. Available at: http://www.cdc.gov/breastfeeding/data/NIS_data/2007/socio-demographic_any.htm. Accessed August 31, 2012.
107. Holmes AV, Chin NP, Kaczorowski J, et al. A barrier to exclusive breastfeeding for WIC enrollees: limited use of exclusive breastfeeding food package for mothers. Breastfeed Med 2009;4:25–30 PM:19196037.
108. Yun S, Liu Q, Mertzlufft K, et al. Evaluation of the Missouri WIC (Special Supplemental Nutrition Program for Women, Infants, and Children) breast-feeding peer counselling programme. Public Health Nutr 2010;13:229–37 PM: 19607746.
109. Rempel LA, Rempel JK. The breastfeeding team: the role of involved fathers in the breastfeeding family. J Hum Lact 2011;27:115–21 PM:21173422.
110. Tohotoa J, Maycock B, Hauck Y, et al. Supporting mothers to breastfeed: the development and process evaluation of a father inclusive perinatal educa-tion support program in Perth, Western Australia. Health Promot Int 2011;26: 351–61 PM:21156662.
111. Pisacane A, Continisio GI, Aldinucci M, et al. A controlled trial of the father's role in breastfeeding promotion. Pediatrics 2005;116:e494–8 PM:16199676.
112. Chezem JC. Breastfeeding attitudes among couples planning exclusive breast-feeding or mixed feeding. Breastfeed Med 2012;7:155–62 PM:22224507.
113. La Leche League International. Available at: http://www.llli.org/ab.html?m=1. Accessed August 31, 2012.
114. Parkes A. A breastfeeding cafe: could it work for you? Available at: www.llli.org/llleaderweb/lv/lvoctnov05p112.html. Accessed August 17, 2012.
115. Green K. 10 must-dos for successful breastfeeding support groups. Breastfeed Med 2012;7:346–7 PM:22857643.
116. Black Mothers' Breastfeeding Association. Available at: http://www.black mothersbreastfeeding.org/HOME.html. Accessed August 31, 2012.
117. US Department of Health and Human Services, Office on Women's Health. Your guide to breastfeeding for African American women. Available at: http://www.womenshealth.gov/publications/our-publications/breastfeeding-guide/breastfeedingguide-africanamerican-english.pdf. Accessed August 31, 2012.
118. Mattox KK. African American mothers: bringing the case for breastfeeding home. Breastfeed Med 2012;7:343–5 PM:22924942.
119. McQueen KA, Dennis CL, Stremler R, et al. A pilot randomized controlled trial of a breastfeeding self-efficacy intervention with primiparous mothers. J Obstet Gynecol Neonatal Nurs 2011;40:35–46 PM:21244493.
120. Olds DL, Robinson J, Pettitt L, et al. Effects of home visits by paraprofessionals and by nurses: age 4 follow-up results of a randomized trial. Pediatrics 2004; 114:1560–8 PM:15574615.
121. Nurse-Family Partnership. Available at: http://www.nursefamilypartnership.org/. Accessed August 31, 2012.
122. Bunik M, Krebs NF, Beaty B, et al. Breastfeeding and WIC enrollment in the Nurse Family Partnership Program. Breastfeed Med 2009;4:145–9 PM: 19243262.
123. Taveras EM, Capra AM, Braveman PA, et al. Clinician support and psychosocial risk factors associated with breastfeeding discontinuation. Pediatrics 2003;112: 108–15 PM:12837875.
124. Feldman-Winter L, Barone L, Milcarek B, et al. Residency curriculum improves breastfeeding care. Pediatrics 2010;126:289–97 PM:20603262.

125. Labarere J, Gelbert-Baudino N, Ayral AS, et al. Efficacy of breastfeeding support provided by trained clinicians during an early, routine, preventive visit: a prospective, randomized, open trial of 226 mother-infant pairs. Pediatrics 2005;115:e139–46 PM:15687421.

126. Profit J, Cambric-Hargrove AJ, Tittle KO, et al. Delayed pediatric office follow-up of newborns after birth hospitalization. Pediatrics 2009;124:548–54 PM:19651578.

127. Feldman-Winter LB, Schanler RJ, O'Connor KG, et al. Pediatricians and the promotion and support of breastfeeding. Arch Pediatr Adolesc Med 2008;162:1142–9 PM:19047541.

128. Pollard DL. Impact of a feeding log on breastfeeding duration and exclusivity. Matern Child Health J 2011;15:395–400 PM:20177755.

129. American Academy of Pediatrics. Bright Futures. Available at: http://brightfutures.aap.org. Accessed September 1, 2012.

130. Taveras EM, Li R, Grummer-Strawn L, et al. Opinions and practices of clinicians associated with continuation of exclusive breastfeeding. Pediatrics 2004;113:e283–90 PM:15060254.

131. International Lactation Consultant Association. Available at: http://www.ilca.org/i4a/pages/index.cfm?pageid=1. Accessed August 31, 2012.

132. Cloherty M, Alexander J, Holloway I. Supplementing breast-fed babies in the UK to protect their mothers from tiredness or distress. Midwifery 2004;20:194–204 PM:15177864.

133. Academy of Breastfeeding Medicine. Available at: http://www.bfmed.org/Resources/Protocols.aspx. Accessed August 31, 2012.

134. Brazelton TB. Touchpoints—birth to three. 2nd edition. Cambridge (MA): Pereus Book Group; 2006.

Establishing Successful Breastfeeding in the Newborn Period

Alison V. Holmes, MD, MPH, FABM

KEYWORDS

- Breastfeeding • Baby-friendly hospital initiative • Newborn nursery policy/protocol
- Breastfeeding initiation • Skin-to-skin

KEY POINTS

- Patient education and preparation for successful breastfeeding should occur before and during pregnancy.
- The immediate period after delivery is crucial for breastfeeding success. Time skin-to-skin and early, unrestricted breastfeeding should be strongly promoted.
- The Baby-Friendly Hospital Initiative's "Ten Steps" are evidence-based measures that birth facilities can employ to improve breastfeeding initiation, duration, and exclusivity.
- Breastfeeding can be supported and continued through common medical problems in the newborn period such as hypoglycemia and hyperbilirubinemia, and in the late preterm infant.

The health benefits of breastfeeding are so significant that stronger support of breast-feeding has become a public health priority. Target breastfeeding rates are ensconced in national and international health policies.[1-3] In the clinical realm, however, the start of the breastfeeding relationship in the first few days after birth can have a variety of individualized barriers that can be difficult to overcome. Some early barriers to breast-feeding are owing to unavoidable medical complications of the mother or infant, but other common challenges may be ameliorated by changes in hospital policies or via better training of medical, nursing, and other health care staff members in the medical management of breastfeeding.[4,5]

This review focuses on summarizing the best available evidence concerning the establishment of successful breastfeeding in the neonatal period. We begin by summa-rizing interventions from the prenatal period that positively affect immediate breast-feeding outcomes postnatally. Prenatal preparation also implies preparation for any anticipated medical complications; many of these can be met successfully with good planning. Second, we review the literature regarding immediate post-delivery

Division of Pediatric Hospital Medicine, The Geisel School of Medicine at Dartmouth, One Rope Ferry Road, Hanover, NH 03755, USA
E-mail address: Alison.v.holmes@hitchcock.org

Pediatr Clin N Am 60 (2013) 147–168
http://dx.doi.org/10.1016/j.pcl.2012.09.013   **pediatric.theclinics.com**

care of the mother–infant dyad, including the importance of time spent skin-to-skin, the delay of nonurgent procedures for the infant, and achieving an early and successful first breastfeed. Third, we analyze the most recent evidence regarding the World Health Organization's (WHO) Baby Friendly Hospital Initiative (BFHI) and its Ten Steps.[6] To conclude, we explore how to troubleshoot common newborn nursery issues such as hyperbilirubinemia, hypoglycemia, and the late preterm infant, while still optimizing the breastfeeding relationship.

PRENATAL PREPARATION FOR BREASTFEEDING
The Decision to Breastfeed

Women make the decision to breastfeed before becoming pregnant, or early in the first trimester—often before their first prenatal visit.[7,8] The influence of the primary care clinician on the decision to breastfeed is strong.[9–11] In a 2001 study of 1229 women, Lu and colleagues[10] found that prenatal encouragement to breastfeed was most influential for women from population groups that were least likely to breastfeed. Prenatal encouragement from a physician was associated with a more than 3-fold increase in breastfeeding initiation among low-income, young, and less educated women; with a 5-fold increase among black women, and by a nearly 11-fold increase among single women. Guise and colleagues[11] conducted a meta-analysis of 30 randomized, controlled trials and 5 systematic reviews, and found that prenatal education was among the most important potential interventions for increasing breastfeeding initiation and duration.

As discussed in greater detail later in this review, implementation of the BFHI Ten Steps can lead to much higher breastfeeding rates.[12,13] Step 3 of the BFHI states that all pregnant women should be informed of the benefits of breastfeeding.[6] A Cochrane review concluded that the most effective type of prenatal education is a repeated, needs-based, clinician and patient dyadic informal education that occurs as a part of routine care.[14] In a 2008 systematic review, Chung and colleagues[15] studied the outcomes of structured breastfeeding education, and concluded that for every 3 to 5 women who attend a prenatal education program, 1 more woman will initiate and continue breastfeeding for up to 3 months. A smaller, but very recent, study indicates that training women prenatally about normal infant feeding cues can increase breastfeeding duration.[16]

Many municipalities and some regions and nations have undertaken awareness and advertising campaigns such that women of childbearing age (and those who support them) are informed of the extensive health benefits of breastfeeding. **Fig. 1** shows some examples of print advertising from around the globe. The effectiveness of such campaigns has been mixed.[7,17,18] The extensive United States breastfeeding awareness campaign of 2005–2006 did seem to improve public sentiment about breastfeeding, but a causal link with improved breastfeeding rates cannot be determined from a mass intervention of this kind.[19]

The Prenatal Visit, Community Supports

Many pediatricians offer prenatal visits to prospective parents.[20] In addition to reviewing the workings of the office practice, this visit presents a great opportunity to provide anticipatory guidance about a choice that likely affects overall maternal and child health more than any of the other decisions that have to be made for the newborn around the time of delivery. Although pediatricians do not provide prenatal care, their influence may be able to work in a similar manner to the primary care counseling described if they encounter soon-to-be mothers during pregnancy.[10,11,14,15]

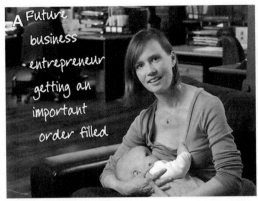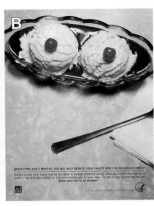

Fig. 1. Two breastfeeding promotion campaigns. *(A)* A New Zealand campaign aims to normalize out-of-the-house breastfeeding and links breastfeeding with positive futures for the infants pictured. *(B)* One of the images from the U.S. AdCouncil 2005–2006 campaign that emphasized the health risks of formula feeding—this one about the link between not breastfeeding and childhood obesity. ([A] Copyright © New Zealand Ministry of Health. Available at: www.breastfeeding.org.nz. [B] *From* US Department of Health and Human Services, National Breastfeeding Campaign. Available at: http://womenshealth.gov/breastfeeding/government-in-action/national-breastfeeding-campaign/.)

Unfortunately, the role of the pediatric prenatal visit specifically on breastfeeding initiation and duration has not been subject to study. Other prenatal preparation available to prospective breastfeeding women include informative books, classes, text messaging services (Text4Baby), lay support networks (La Leche League), and breastfeeding services provided by the Women, Infants and Children (WIC) program.[21]

Of the aforementioned breastfeeding support services, those provided by WIC have been subject to the most study.[22–24] Since 2008, WIC food packages have been changed such that women who are breastfeeding receive a substantially bigger and more nutritious food package. The first study of the impact of this food package change on breastfeeding outcomes was published in 2012, and found that more mothers are now receiving the full breastfeeding food package (without formula), but the overall breastfeeding initiation rate in the WIC population has not been impacted by the change.[25]

Anticipating Probable Perinatal Medical Issues

Although the BFHI Ten Steps address the care of the healthy term newborn, not every birth of a baby is low risk and after 38 completed weeks of gestation. Although some medical issues arise acutely at delivery, there are others that can be anticipated during pregnancy, and the detrimental effects of these medical issues on breastfeeding can be mitigated with good preparation. For a woman with a history of preterm birth and/or ongoing preterm labor, there can be some degree of planning for how to achieve successful breastfeeding in the preterm neonate. A full review of breastfeeding the preterm infant is beyond the scope of this article, but is discussed by Underwood and colleagues elsewhere in this issue. Families that are anticipating a possible preterm delivery, however, can become familiar with the lactation support services at the hospital with the newborn intensive care unit where the infant will likely be born. They can familiarize themselves with techniques and services helpful for supplying milk for preterm infants, including pasteurized donor human milk, pumping, and hand expression.[26]

Mothers with gestational or preexisting diabetes mellitus can anticipate a high likelihood of neonatal hypoglycemia after delivery. The first intervention for mild to moderate hypoglycemia in a newborn is often enteral supplementation with infant formula, often delivered via bottle and standard nipple; however, the breastfed infant with mild hypoglycemia can first be put directly to breast for a feed of colostrum. If there is an ineffective latch, the infant can be fed with colostrum that has been expressed by hand (**Fig. 2**).[27,28]

Avoiding formula supplementation preserves the health benefits of early, exclusive breastfeeding and may assist with better development of a full maternal milk supply.[29] Some advocate the use of pasteurized human donor milk for any supplementation of the breastfed newborn; this approach is controversial, because the supply of this expensive resource is quite limited, and may ethically need to be reserved for preterm neonates.[30]

AFTER DELIVERY
The Importance of Skin-to-Skin Contact

Immediately after delivery, the placement of the newborn skin-to-skin on his or her mother's chest has immense positive effects both on newborn physiologic parameters, and on numerous metrics of breastfeeding success (**Fig. 3**). In a 2012 systematic review, Moore and colleagues[31] demonstrated that skin-to-skin contact in the immediate post-delivery period improves physiologic transition in the newborn, increases the success of the first breastfeed, and leads to more effective breastfeeding. More babies that had been placed skin-to-skin continued to breastfeed through 1–4 months, compared with those receiving standard care.

Smaller studies of skin-to-skin contact have shown direct changes in infant behavior. Preterm infants exposed to their mother's milk odor—a natural byproduct of skin-to-skin care—suckle for longer periods of time at each feeding, and consume more milk at each feeding when they reach 35 weeks post-conceptional age.[32] In a study of 72 infants randomized to skin-to-skin contact versus isolation, the majority of those who were left in contact breastfed in the first hour. Whenever the first breastfeed occurred, 63% in the contact group had an effective sucking technique, whereas only 21% in the control group (left in isolation) demonstrated good breastfeeding skills at the first feed.[33]

The First Breastfeed

Once in skin-to-skin contact with their mother, many infants find their own way to the breast and begin to feed without significant assistance. A dramatic example of this can be seen in the WHO/United Nations Children's Fund (UNICEF)–sponsored video "The Breast Crawl," in which a newborn girl finds the breast and begins to suckle without any assistance from her mother or from other adult observers (**Fig. 4**, video link).[34] An early first breastfeed seems to help with increased milk supply in the first days of life, earlier passage of meconium, and a greater likelihood of continued breastfeeding. Conversely, delay in the first feed can lead to issues of poor milk supply and to greater odds of discontinuing breastfeeding.[35–37]

Newborn Procedures

To align hospital policies with the clear benefits of early skin-to-skin contact and early breastfeeding, nurseries may find they need to alter the timing of routine newborn procedures. Unless a newborn is of significantly low birth weight (<1800–2000 g), is born at less than 34 weeks gestational age, or has signs and symptoms of illness

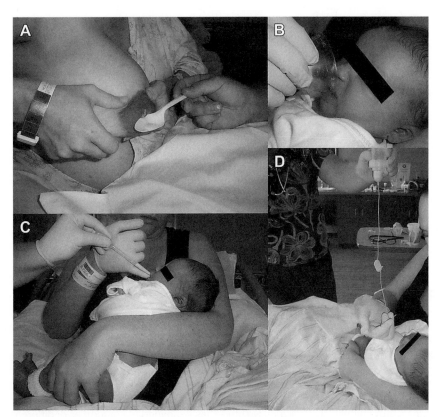

Fig. 2. Devices for medically necessary supplementation. (*A*) A spoon is very useful for colostrum, because it can be held under the breast by an assistant for hand expression. It is perfect for collecting 1 or 2 teaspoons—the typical amount of colostrum expressed in the first 48 hours. Expressed colostrum can be fed to the infant right from the spoon, without loss of milk in collecting materials. (*B*) Feeding cups are the most common method for supplemental feeds worldwide, and the only bottle alternative subject to rigorous research methods. (*C*) A dropper is most useful for smaller amounts of early milk. It can be inserted on the inside of the cheek and given slowly, shown here while the newborn sucks on the mother's finger. (*D*) Supplemental nursing system allows for supplementation either via finger, as pictured here, or directly at the breast. The small tube is taped to the areola, and the infant takes both tube and areola into his mouth simultaneously. The main advantage is continued stimulation of nipple and pituitary–mammary axis during supplementation. Disadvantages include expense, difficulty with cleaning in places where water is scarce, and lack of rigorous study of its efficacy. The mother in this picture had significant nipple erosions, and was therefore supplementing via fingerfeeding. Gloves are not necessary; they were used here owing to the mother's long fingernails. ([*B*] *Data from* Howard CR, Howard FM, Lanphear B, et al. Randomized clinical trial of pacifier use and bottle-feeding or cupfeeding and their effect on breastfeeding. Pediatrics 2003;111:511–8.)

requiring a transfer to a special care nursery, weighing of the infant can be deferred until after a few hours of skin-to-skin time. The only medically necessary reason to weigh a late preterm or term newborn immediately after delivery would be to administer correct dosages of weight-based medications or intravenous fluids—interventions that are not necessary for well-appearing neonates in this gestational age range.

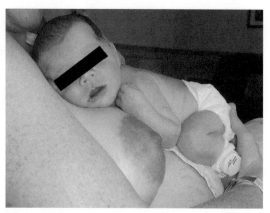

Fig. 3. The ideal place for a newborn—skin-to-skin with his mother.

The efficacy of the newborn dose of hepatitis B vaccine in preventing silent vertical hepatitis transmission is optimized when it is administered as close to delivery as possible. Parenteral vitamin K is the most effective form of phytonadione for preventing both early and late hemorrhagic disease of the newborn.[38] Both of these injections can be delivered while the newborn is skin-to-skin and/or breastfeeding, because both skin-to-skin contact and breastfeeding have been demonstrated to diminish pain responses in the newborn.[39–41] Newborns who require blood sampling for asymptomatic hypoglycemia may also have these heel lances done while they remain skin-to-skin.

Erythromycin eye ointment for prevention of opthalmia neonatorum need not be applied immediately after delivery. No study has examined the outcomes of differential timing of application, but waiting for an hour or 2 of skin-to-skin time before application should not have adverse effects from a microbiological perspective.[42]

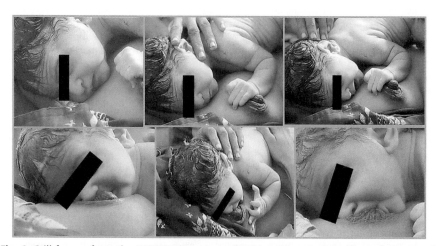

Fig. 4. Still frames from the UNICEF "Breast crawl" video. View at: http://www.breastcrawl. org/video.htm. (*Courtesy of* UNICEF India; with permission. Available at: http://breastcrawl. org/video.shtml.)

Normal Breastfeeding Patterns in the First Days

If new parents or extended family of the newborn, or the nursery medical, nursing, and other hospital staff are unfamiliar with normal breastfeeding patterns, this can be detrimental for the establishment of successful breastfeeding. The American Academy of Pediatrics (AAP), Academy of Breastfeeding Medicine (ABM), American Academy of Family Physicians, American College of Obstetricians and Gynecologists, WHO/UNICEF, and the U.S. Surgeon General all recommend 6 months of exclusive breastfeeding, because of the particular health benefits of breast milk as the only enteral intake (also discussed in detail by Dieterich and colleagues elsewhere in this issue).[1–4,43–46] Many new families, however, are more familiar with the patterns of formula-fed infants, who generally consume higher volumes with less frequency than is normative for breastfed infants. In addition, because milk consumption with breastfeeding is not "seen" and not easily "measured," many families worry that the "baby is not getting enough"; these families need particular reassurance from medical professionals.[23,47,48]

Normal breastfeeding patterns during the first week of life, including timing, volume, and related output, are summarized in **Table 1**. During the first 24 hours, a significant subset of newborns does not have a good latch. Most neonates have some effective latch and suckle by 48 hours of life, and supplementation for poor feeding not associated with significant illness in the mother or infant is not necessary in the first 2 days.[30,49] If there is poor feeding with weight loss of greater than 7%, supplementation can be considered. Weight loss of 7% alone, however, in the absence of poor feeding, is not an indication for supplementation.[30] We should take great care to reassure mothers that lack of effective feeding for the first day or so is quite normal, because medically unnecessary supplementation undermines maternal confidence in the ability to breastfeed and has an adverse effect on breastfeeding outcomes.[50,51]

The first day can be a slower day for feeding, with many newborns having a long period of sleep after the first hour or two after they are born.[52,53] Many infants only feed 4–6 feeds in the first 24 hours, although others will feed more frequently than this even during their first day. By day 2, feeding frequency typically increases to 8–12 times in each 24-hour period, but is generally not spaced at even intervals. Lower volumes of early milk (colostrum) then transition to mature milk (lactogenesis II), with higher volumes any time between 24 and 120 hours after delivery. Urine and stool output increase each day. A good rule of thumb for measuring sufficient intake in the first week is 1 urine and 1 stool for each day of life.[30,54–59]

Table 1					
Normal breastfeeding patterns, volumes, timing and output in the first week of life—term infant					
Day of Life	Number of Feeds in 24 h	Volume per Day (cc/kg/d)	Volume per Feed for 3 kg Baby (mL)	Number Urine Outputs	Number Stools
1	4–5	3–17	2–10	1	1
2	6–10	10–50	5–15	2	2
3	8–12	40–120	15–30	3	3
4	8–12	80–160	30–60	4–6	4–5
5	8–12	120–160	45–60	4–7	4–6
6	8–12	130–160	50–60	5–8	4–8
7	8–12	140–170	55–65	>6	>5

Data from Refs.[54–61]

Certain physiologic cues can be useful to reassure families and the care team that breastfeeding is going well. Normal patterns of intake and output are a first good measure. The sensation of uterine cramping during feeding can reassure that the hypothalamic–pituitary–mammary gland axis is intact and that oxytocin release during suckling are occurring. Strong, early cramping is more common in multiparous women than in primiparous women; many in the latter category do not feel significant cramping for the first few days. At the onset of lactogenesis II, many but not all lactating women feel a sense of fullness in their breasts that diminishes after an effective breastfeed. Many women experience the feeling of "let-down" at the beginning of a breastfeed. This tingling sensation of milk flowing forward is caused by oxytocin release, but it can be absent in the first few days after delivery.[54,60]

BABY-FRIENDLY HOSPITALS AND THE TEN STEPS

In 1991, the WHO and UNICEF sponsored the BFHI, based on the "Ten Steps to Successful Breastfeeding" as a global health initiative to protect, promote, and support breastfeeding. The BFHI uses evidence-based interventions to promote breastfeeding initiation, duration, and exclusivity by educating hospital staff, reviewing and changing hospital policies, and decreasing the influence of commercial formula in the hospital setting.[6]

More than 10,000 hospitals world-wide have achieved BFHI certification, with significant geographic variation. As of May 2012, 143 U.S. birth facilities are certified by Baby Friendly USA, accounting for only about 4% of all infants delivered.[4,61] In Canada, there were 18 Baby-Friendly Hospitals in 2008, and the provinces of New Brunswick and Quebec have efforts underway to have all of their hospitals certified.[62] In contrast, all 65 Swedish birth facilities were certified by the end of 1997.[63]

The next section of the article reviews the Ten Steps individually, because each has a significant basis in the scientific literature.

Step 1: Have a Written Breastfeeding Policy That Is Communicated to All Health Care Staff

There are models for ideal hospital breastfeeding policies from both the AAP and the ABM.[64,65] The goal of a written policy should be to have breastfeeding supportive procedures that are consistent with the Ten Steps of the BFHI. Policies provide a written resource available at all hours of the day and night for hospital staff; they can foster consistency in language and practice, and can help to set budgetary priorities. Written breastfeeding policies are associated with increases in breastfeeding initiation and higher rates of breastfeeding continuation at 2 weeks.[66,67] Better outcomes are seen at hospitals that have more comprehensive policies; the ABM and AAP model policies incorporate a sufficient level of detail.[64,65,67]

Step 2: Train All Health Care Staff in Skills Necessary to Implement This Policy

The BFHI requires that nursing staff members who care for the mother–newborn dyad complete 20 hours of formal breastfeeding training, 3 hours of which must be clinical. Any physicians caring for 1 or both members of the couplet must complete 3 hours of continuing medical education.[68] Resources for nurse and physician training are listed in **Boxes 1** and **2**. The prior requirement of 18 hours of nurse training had been shown to increase rates of exclusive breastfeeding, likely because the bedside caregivers obtained increased skills to help mothers, and are not as likely to resort to formula supplementation to solve breastfeeding problems.[69,70]

Box 1
The WHO/UNICEF BFHI Ten Steps to successful breastfeeding

1. Have a written breastfeeding policy that is routinely communicated to all health care staff.

2. Train all health care staff in skills necessary to implement this policy.

3. Inform all pregnant women about the benefits and management of breastfeeding.

4. Help mothers initiate breastfeeding within one half-hour of birth.

5. Show mothers how to breastfeed and maintain lactation, even if they should be separated from their infants.

6. Give newborn infants no food or drink other than breast milk, not even sips of water, unless medically indicated.

7. Practice rooming in—that is, allow mothers and infants to remain together 24 hours a day.

8. Encourage breastfeeding on demand.

9. Give no artificial teats or pacifiers (also called dummies or soothers) to breastfeeding infants.

10. Foster the establishment of breastfeeding support groups and refer mothers to them on discharge from the hospital or clinic.

From WHO/UNICEF. Protecting, Promoting and Supporting Breastfeeding: The Special Role of Maternity Services, a joint WHO/UNICEF statement published by the World Health Organization. Available at: http://whqlibdoc.who.int/publications/9241561300.pdf.

Historically, physicians received little training in breastfeeding.[71] Although the studies showing knowledge and skill deficits are 2 decades old, there have not been further studies to show that the situation has improved. A 2008 study by Feldman-Winter and colleagues[72] actually demonstrated a deterioration of practicing pediatricians' attitudes toward breastfeeding over a recent 10-year period. Fortunately, there is evidence to show that a breastfeeding training program for resident physicians in family medicine, obstetrics–gynecology, and pediatrics, not only improved knowledge and skills, but also led to an increase in breastfeeding rates in the 7 academic centers that participated in the curriculum.[73] The 3 hours of BFHI physician training have not been formally evaluated, but the influence of physician opinion and support on breastfeeding success is strong.[9–11,74,75]

Box 2
Options for physician and nurse breastfeeding training

Live meetings

ABM International Conference www.bfmed.org

International Lactation Consultant Association Conference http://www.ilca.org/i4a/pages/index.cfm?pageid=3305

Online or distance

Breastfeeding Continuing Education Program—18 hours, designed for nursing staff http://www.risingstareducation.net/default.asp?a=home

Wellstart International Self-Study Modules, 3rd edition, 2009 http://www.wellstart.org/

Breastfeeding Training—University of Virginia http://www.breastfeedingtraining.org/

Breastfeeding Basics http://www.breastfeedingbasics.org/

Step 3: Inform All Pregnant Women About the Benefits and Management of Breastfeeding

The importance of prenatal breastfeeding education and the influence of primary care and prenatal clinicians on breastfeeding outcomes are summarized early in this article in the section "Prenatal preparation for breastfeeding–The decision to breastfeed." Although more than half of women make their breastfeeding decision before they become pregnant, education during pregnancy is still crucial.[76] Prenatal providers should provide consistent and up-to-date breastfeeding information and should speak clearly to the superiority of breastfeeding over formula.[77]

Step 4: Help Mothers to Initiate Breastfeeding Within One Half-Hour of Birth

The evidence for early and prolonged skin-to-skin contact and breastfeeding within the first hour was reviewed earlier in this article in the sections: "After delivery: The importance of skin-to-skin" and "The first breastfeed." We note here that although step 4 says that breastfeeding should begin within the first one-half hour after birth, the U.S. rule for this part of BFHI has been extended to 1 hour after delivery.[68]

Step 5: Show Mothers How to Breastfeed/Maintain Lactation if Separated From the Infant

Breastfeeding is more likely to be successful if mothers and their infants have skilled help. Health care providers are responsible for teaching and assisting with proper breastfeeding techniques, and for providing counsel for how to maintain lactation if there is mother–infant separation. A full description of correct breastfeeding technique is beyond the scope of this article, but can be found elsewhere.[54] The basics of correct technique include an effective latch, good suck, proper positioning of the infant relative to the mother's body and breast, a satisfied infant, and a mother who does not experience excessive pain.

To begin a breastfeed, the infant should be positioned "belly to belly" with her or his mother. In any of the common positions for holding, including the cradle hold, across the chest, and sideling belly-to-belly, there should be an excellent positioning of abdomens flat to each other. For the football hold, the mother's and baby's bodies should lie in the same plane. The infant's mouth should open wide, to take in a 2- to 3-cm radius of areola into the mouth. When viewing a correctly latched infant in profile, his lips should be flanged outwards in any of the positions (see **Fig. 4**). Although there may be some pain during the latching on process in normal breastfeeding, breast pain or even significant discomfort should not persist during the feeding. Pain is indicative of improper latch.[54]

The importance of good breastfeeding technique to eventual breastfeeding outcomes is quite strong. Mothers and infants who either initially demonstrated a correct technique or who received help to correct poor technique experienced lower rates of low milk production, sore nipples, and engorgement, and had increased breastfeeding rates up to 4 months later.[76,77] Teaching mothers optimal latch and positioning significantly increased infant weight gain for those who had previously not been gaining ideally.[77] Conversely, incorrect technique can lead to sore nipples, decreased milk supply, engorgement, insufficient infant weight gain, and eventually to decreased breastfeeding duration and exclusivity.[37,38,76,78]

Mothers and infants do sometimes have to be separated for medical reasons. In these events, alternative methods of providing a mother's own milk to her newborn are preferred over artificial alternatives. Trained staff should teach mothers effective milk expression both via hand expression and with a hospital-grade double electric breast pump, because these are the most effective methods for milk removal. There is emerging evidence that hand expression may be most effective in the first day or two, after which use of an electric pump is superior for milk removal.[26,79,80] See the article by Flaherman elsewhere in this issue for further exploration of this topic. Families should also be instructed on the proper storage of expressed milk.[81]

Step 6: Give Newborn Infants No Food Other Than Breast Milk, Unless Medically Indicated

Given the strength of the emerging medical evidence about the particular importance of exclusive breastfeeding to maximize breastfeeding's health benefits, the 2-decade-old BFHI recommendation in step 6 to not supplement infants unless medically necessary has withstood the test of time.[29,46] The most recent data from the U.S. Centers for Disease Control and Prevention show that 42% of breastfed newborns in U.S. hospitals are given supplemental formula; clearly, not that many have medical conditions that call for supplementation.[82] In-hospital supplementation has been associated with fewer breastfeeds, low maternal milk supply, and earlier breastfeeding termination. No decrease in jaundice has been found for breastfed babies who were supplemented.[37,82–84]

Medical indications for recommending supplementation are outlined in **Table 2**; contraindications to breastfeeding are reviewed elsewhere in this issue. See the article by Lawrence in this issue for further exploration of this topic.[85] **Table 2** also reviews a few common scenarios where infants frequently are supplemented, but really do not require supplementation for medical reasons. Volumes to supplement should reflect the physiology of the normal breastfed newborn (see **Table 1**). The first choice for supplementation is the mother's own milk, followed by pasteurized human donor milk (where it is available, and the supply is sufficient to allow for use in the term newborn) and hydrolysate formula.[1,26,29,85] Protein hydrolysate formulas are preferable as supplements; they avoid exposure to full cow's milk proteins, reduce bilirubin levels more rapidly, and may better convey the message that the supplementation is a transient medical intervention.[29,85]

The most challenging aspect of Step 6 for many U.S. hospitals is that BFHI requires its certified hospitals to abide by the International Code of Breastmilk Substitutes, to pay fair market value for infant formula, and to not distribute any commercial materials from formula manufacturers. The majority of U.S. birth hospitals receive no-cost or heavily discounted infant formula directly from formula manufacturers. Birth hospitals also distribute formula promotion materials in the form of "diaper bag" gifts to new mothers, although this practice is decreasing.[86] These promotional materials have been shown to lead to lower rates of exclusive breastfeeding.[87,88] One important note for hospitals who seek BFHI status is that "fair market value" does not mean retail price. If the nursery purchases diapers, receiving blankets, and infant T-shirts at 75% discount over retail from suppliers, BFHI allows for the purchase of formula at a commensurate discount (Baby Friendly USA, personal communication, 2009).

Step 7: Practice Rooming In: Mothers and Infants Should Remain Together 24 Hours a Day

Newborns who room with their mothers have increased opportunities to suckle at the breast, leading to increased breastfeeding frequency and decreased need for supplementation. Their feeding cues are identified earlier, they cry less, and they weigh more by the end of the first week. Mothers who have their babies with them all day and night have increased milk volumes, increased bonding, and increased parenting confidence.[35,89,90] Infants who room-in have more quiet sleep than those who stay in

Table 2
Medical indications for supplementation of breastfeeding

Absolute Medical Indications to Supplement Breastfeeding	Relative Medical Indications to Supplement Breastfeeding	Not Reasons to Supplement Breastfeeding
Mother–infant separation	Asymptomatic hypoglycemia	A sleepy infant in the first 24–48 h with <7% weight loss
Severe maternal illness	Significant dehydration not improved with breastfeeding help	Bilirubin <18 after 72 h with <7% weight loss, with good feeding and stooling
Inborn error of metabolism[a]	Weight loss of 8%–10% with delay of lactogenesis II past 120 h	Infant fussy at night or who feeds for several hours
Infant unable to feed at breast owing to illness or malformation	Poor stool output at 120 h	Tired/sleeping mother
Rare maternal medications	Poor milk transfer	
	Jaundice owing to starvation, or breast milk jaundice with bilirubin >18	
	Macronutrient needs	
	Maternal history of breast surgery that would likely preclude full milk supply	
	Intolerable pain during feedings	

[a] Depending on the particular inborn error, human milk can sometimes be used to comprise a portion of the special metabolic formula. Consultation with a physician specialist in medical genetics, and a certified nutritionist with expertise in metabolic disorders would be required.

From The Academy of Breastfeeding Medicne Protocol Committee. Academy of Breastfeeding Medicine Clinical Protocol #3: hospital guidelines for the use of supplementary feedings in the healthy term breastfed neonate. Breastfeed Med 2009;4(3):175–82; with permission.

nurseries; mothers have the same amount of sleep whether their newborn is with them or in the nursery, but the rooming-in mothers have higher sleep quality scores.[90,91]

Step 8: Encourage Breastfeeding on Demand

BFHI permits no restrictions on the frequency or duration of breastfeeds, and acknowledges that breastfeeding does not occur at regular time intervals. Unrestricted feeding allows the newborn to indicate her or his own feeding readiness, and to self-regulate feedings. Frequent breastfeeding leads to earlier passage of meconium, higher day 3–4 weight nadir, less supplementation, increased breast milk intake volume on day 3, earlier lactogenesis, and decreased hyperbilirubinemia.[57] In addition, ad libitum feeding stabilizes neonatal glucose levels, increases the rate of infant weight gain, and prevents engorgement.[92–94]

Step 9: Give No Artificial Nipples or Pacifiers to Breastfeeding Infants

Step 9 has a weaker evidence base compared with the other 9 steps, with a number of prominent contradictory findings. BFHI certification does, however, require that breastfeeding infants not be offered any pacifiers unless they have certain medical conditions. A recent systematic review on pacifier use and breastfeeding found that the 5 included randomized, controlled trials had high degrees of crossover between the pacifier and non-pacifier arms, and that there were significant amounts of heterogeneity among the trials, making analysis difficult. The 20 observational studies were also challenging to interpret in that it is difficult to know whether pacifiers were being used because mothers desired to wean, or if the pacifiers cause earlier breastfeeding cessation. The conclusion of fairly comprehensive systematic review was that the current body of literature did not suggest any association between pacifier use and breastfeeding duration or exclusivity.[95]

In the highest quality individual randomized, controlled trials with the most subjects, best randomization schema, and lowest degree of crossover included in the above review, early (at 4 days of life) pacifier use was significantly associated with only a small reduction in the length of exclusive breastfeeding (28 vs. 21 days); overall breastfeeding duration was not affected.[96]

BFHI allows for the use of pacifiers where they are medically indicated (**Box 3**).

When the breastfed infant requires in-hospital supplementation for any of the indications in **Table 2**, BFHI requires use of a method other than a bottle with nipple. Some supplementation options include a cup, spoon, dropper, syringe, or supplemental feeding system (see **Fig. 2**). There is little literature supporting the use of 1 device over another in terms of breastfeeding outcomes. One large, randomized trial of more than 700 breastfed infants randomized the subgroup requiring supplements to either cup or bottle, and did not find breastfeeding outcome differences between the 2 groups overall. They did find that the subgroup that required 4 or more supplements had better breastfeeding outcomes if the supplements were fed via cup. The authors concluded that cups should be used preferentially, because providers do not know at the outset (for an individual baby) how many supplements might be required.[95]

Step 10: Foster Breastfeeding Support Groups and Refer Mothers to Them at Discharge

The tenth step of BFHI states that new mothers be referred to community-based breastfeeding support at the time of discharge. Data from the U.S. Centers for Disease

---

Box 3
Medical use of pacifiers

- Maternal–infant separation
- Infant too ill to feed (respiratory distress)
- Prematurity, for suck training during gavage feeds
- Painful procedures
- Neonatal abstinence syndrome
- After breastfeeding is well-established (reduction of sudden infant death syndrome risk)[a]

[a] This should not be an issue in the hospital after delivery because breastfeeding is not well established then. The AAP recommends pacifier use after 4 weeks of age (if breastfeeding is going well) for prevention of sudden infant death syndrome.

Data from American Academy of Pediatrics, Task Force on Sudden Infant Death Syndrome (SIDS). The changing concept of sudden infant death syndrome: diagnostic coding shifts, controversies regarding the sleeping environment, and new variables to consider in reducing risk. Pediatrics 2005;116(5):1245–55.

Control and Prevention National Survey of Maternity Practices in Infant Nutrition and Care finds that only 27% of U.S. birth hospitals provide adequate discharge support services.[97] Referrals to lay support groups such as La Leche League, governmental programs (WIC), postnatal education programs, home visitor programs, and telephone support have all been found to improve breastfeeding outcomes.[36,70,98–100]

Efficacy of the Ten Steps in Combination

Because the BFHI has been in existence for over 20 years, there is now a substantial body of literature that has evaluated the efficacy of 10 steps implementation in the United States and around the world. The achievement of BFHI certification leads to substantially improved breastfeeding outcomes, including increases in breastfeeding initiation, exclusivity, and duration.[12,13,101–103]

SUPPORTING BREASTFEEDING DURING MEDICAL PROBLEMS

Although the BFHI Ten Steps work well for term newborns without medical problems, there are common issues in the well nursery that can have detrimental effects on breastfeeding if they are addressed without concern for preserving an exclusive diet of human milk. Three of the most common are hyperbilirubinemia, hypoglycemia, and the late preterm infant.

Hyperbilirubinemia

The AAP recommends that all newborns 35 weeks gestation and older be monitored for jaundice, and that bilirubin levels should be managed per standardized nomograms.[104,105] In some cases, poor enteral intake plays a role in infant hyperbilirubinemia, but in many other instances, the cause is related to isoimmune reaction or a genetic factor, such as Gilbert disease. The first step for the clinician is to fully understand the individual infant's causal factors for jaundice, and to not advocate for any supplementation if the newborn's intake, output, and pattern of weight loss and gain are within normal limits:[106] If poor enteral intake is determined to be a factor in jaundice requiring phototherapy, the first (and many times the only needed) supplement should be the mother's own expressed milk, which should be provided via one of the methods pictured in **Fig. 2**.[106] Pasteurized human donor milk or hydrolysate formula can be used if maternal milk is not available; volumes for appropriate supplementation are in **Table 1**.[29,85,106] Further suggestions for supporting breastfeeding during hyperbilirubinemia are provided in **Box 4**.

Hypoglycemia

Standards for screening for and treatment of neonatal hypoglycemia are available.[27,28] In a manner analogous to hyperbilirubinemia, hypoglycemia should be managed with an aim to preserve exclusive breastfeeding. For infants with moderate hypoglycemia in the first 3 hours after delivery (28–39 mg/dL), the first intervention can be direct breastfeeding at the breast. If the latch or suckle are ineffective, or a repeat measure indicates persistent hypoglycemia, the next intervention should be 3–10 mL of expressed mother's milk,[28] if available. In the immediate postpartum period, hand expression is most effective and rapid method of milk expression.[26] For severe hypoglycemia (<28 mg/dL), 10% dextrose should be administered intravenously without delay. While intravenous dextrose is being administered, unrestricted breastfeeding should continue.[28] See **Box 4** for a summary of hypoglycemia interventions.

Box 4
Suggestions for common newborn nursery medial issues that affect breastfeeding

Hyperbilirubinemia

- Only use supplementation as part of therapy if poor intake and/or poor stool output in the context of excessive weight loss is part of the clinical picture.
- Permit continued breastfeeding during phototherapy.
- Consider overhead bilirubin lights over mother and baby while they remain skin-to-skin, or breastfeeding.
- If providing supplemental feeds, use mother's own milk preferentially, followed by pasteurized human donor milk or hydrolysate formula.
- Use a non-bottle method of supplementation, either a cup, dropper, or supplemental nursing system.

Hypoglycemia

- For mild to moderate hypoglycemia, have infant feed directly at the breast, maintaining skin-to-skin contact.
- If direct breastfeeding not successful, use 3–10 mL of hand-expressed colostrum fed by spoon or cup.
- If expressed human milk feeding is not successful, yet glucose remains between 28 and 40 mg/dL, attempt feeding with commercially available infant formula via spoon, cup, or dropper.
- If there is severe hypoglycemia (<28 mg/dL), or all above oral efforts fail, begin intravenous 10% dextrose.
- During IV therapy, allow for unrestricted skin-to-skin contact and continued breastfeeding.

Late preterm infant

- In the absence of respiratory distress, altered thermoregulation, or need for apnea monitoring, allow for rooming-in and encourage skin-to-skin contact.
- If monitoring required, permit unrestricted skin-to-skin contact as medical condition permits.
- Do not restrict breastfeeding if there are no respiratory or other medical issues and the infant is willing to feed.
- Begin milk expression efforts early, as direct breastfeeding can slow after 2–3 day of life.
- Milk expression in days 1–2 should be via hand expression, after this with a hospital-grade double electric pump.
- Provide supplemental feeds with mother's own milk preferentially.
- Consult **Table 2** for appropriate supplement volumes.
- Pay particular attention to increased risks for hypoglycemia, hyperbilirubinemia, and hypothermia.
- Consider the use of an ultra-thin silicone nipple shield for those with poor sustained latch.

Late Preterm Infant

A full review of feeding issues for the late preterm infant is beyond the scope of this article; detailed information is available elsewhere.[107] Hospitals should have specific policies and procedures for both the general care of and the support of breastfeeding for infants born between 34 0/7 and 36 6/7 weeks' gestation. Particular attention to screening for and treatment of hypoglycemia, hyperbilirubinemia, and thermoregulation is critical for this population. Skin-to-skin contact is particularly important for both breastfeeding success and for physiologic stability for late preterm neonates.[31,107]

Breastfeeding should not be at all limited for physiologically stable late preterm infants who can effectively latch and suckle. There should be 8–12 feedings in 24 hours; it may be necessary to awaken the newborn for these feeds.[107,108] If the neonate cannot feed effectively at the breast, the mother may need to express her milk and feed it by an alternative method (see **Fig. 2**); at times a nasogastric tube may be required. For some infants, an ultra-thin silicone nipple shield can assist in effective latch.[109,110] See **Box 4** for further suggestions.

READINESS FOR GOING HOME

Breastfeeding should be assessed and supported during the hospital discharge process, with an array of supports put in place for continued breastfeeding resources and support once the mother and infant are home. A trained staff member should observe at least 1 successful breastfeeding within 8 hours before discharge.[111] All breastfeeding issues should have been already attended to during the birth hospitalization, with a follow-up plan in place for unresolved issues. All medical professionals should emphasize the importance of 6 months of exclusive breastfeeding.[1–4]

Clinicians should give appropriate anticipatory guidance about likely issues within the coming week, such as management of engorgement, the transition of normal intake and output patterns, normal infant sleep patterns, safe sleep practices, and signs of excessive jaundice.[111] If an infant is not discharged with his mother (ill newborn), all possible arrangements should be made for the mother to be able to remain in the hospital with her baby 24 hours a day.[89–91] All newborns should have a follow-up appointment with a primary care provider familiar with the medical management of breastfeeding within 48–72 hours of discharge.[112]

Summary of Learning Objectives

The reader of this review on establishing successful breastfeeding in the newborn period should have learned the following:

- How to counsel, inform, support, and prepare women about breastfeeding during pregnancy;
- How to anticipate potential medical issues that can effect breastfeeding before delivery, and how to provide appropriate medical management of those issues in the newborn nursery;
- The importance of skin-to-skin, early and unrestricted breastfeeding, and 24-hour rooming-in during the newborn hospitalization;
- How the Ten Steps of the BFHI can improve rates of breastfeeding initiation, duration, and exclusivity; and
- How to extend the breastfeeding successes of the newborn hospitalization through discharge and into the home environment.

REFERENCES

1. Eidelman AI, Schanler RJ, Johnston M, et al, American Academy of Pediatrics Section on Breastfeeding. Breastfeeding and the use of human milk. Pediatrics 2012;129(3):e827–84.
2. World Health Organization. The optimal duration of exclusive breastfeeding: report of an expert consultation. Available at: www.who.int/nutrition/publications/optimal_duration_of_exc_bfeeding_report_eng.pdf. Accessed July 13, 2012.

3. U.S. Department of Health and Human Services [homepage on the internet]. Washington (DC). Healthy people 2020; proposed HP2020 objectives; maternal, infant and child health. 2009. Available at: http://healthypeople.gov/2020/topicsobjectives2020/objectiveslist.aspx?topicId=26. Accessed August 20, 2012.

4. US Department of Health, Human Services. The surgeon general's call to action to support breastfeeding. Washington (DC): US Department of Health and Human Services, Office of the Surgeon General; 2011.

5. Whalen B, Cramton R. Overcoming barriers to breastfeeding continuation and exclusivity. Curr Opin Pediatr 2010;22(5):655–63.

6. Philipp BL, Radford A. Baby-friendly: snappy slogan or standard of care? Arch Dis Child Fetal Neonatal Ed 2006;91(2):F145–9.

7. Earle S. Factors affecting the initiation of breastfeeding: implications for breast-feeding promotion. Health Promot Int 2002;17(3):205–14.

8. Henderson J, Redshaw M. Midwifery factors associated with successful breastfeeding. Child Care Health Dev 2011;37(5):744–53.

9. Bentley ME, Caulfield LE, Gross SM, et al. Sources of influence on intention to breastfeed among African- American women at entry to WIC. J Hum Lact 1999;15(1):27–34.

10. Lu MC, Lange L, Slusser W, et al. Provider encouragement of breastfeeding: evidence from a national survey. Obstet Gynecol 2001;97:290–5.

11. Guise JM, Palda V, Westhoff C, et al. The effectiveness of primary care-based interventions to promote breastfeeding: systematic evidence review and meta-analysis for the US preventive services task force. Ann Fam Med 2003;1(2):70–8.

12. Merewood A, Mehta SD, Chamberlain LB, et al. Breastfeeding rates in US baby-friendly hospitals: results of a national survey. Pediatrics 2005;116:628–34.

13. Martens PJ. What do Kramer's Baby-friendly hospital initiative PROBIT studies tell us? A review of a decade of research. J Hum Lact 2012;28(3):335–42.

14. Dyson L, McCormick F, Renfrew MJ. Interventions for promoting the initiation of breastfeeding. Cochrane Database Syst Rev 2005;(2):CD001688.

15. Chung M, Raman G, Trikalinos T, et al. Interventions in primary care to promote breastfeeding: an evidence review for the U.S. preventive services task force. Ann Intern Med 2008;149(8):565–82.

16. Kandiah J, Burian C, Amend V. Teaching new mothers about infant feeding cues may increase breastfeeding duration. Food Nutr Sci 2011;2:259–64.

17. Merewood A, Heinig J. Efforts to promote breastfeeding in the United States: development of a national breastfeeding awareness campaign. J Hum Lact 2004;20(2):140–5.

18. Gupta N, Katende C, Bessinger R. An evaluation of post-campaign knowledge and practices of exclusive breastfeeding in Uganda. J Health Popul Nutr 2004;22(4):429–39.

19. The CDC guide to breastfeeding interventions—media and social marketing. Available at: http://www.cdc.gov/breastfeeding/pdf/BF_guide_6.pdf. Accessed July 23, 2012.

20. Cohen GJ. Committee on psychosocial aspects of child and family health. The prenatal visit. Pediatrics 2009;124(4):1227–32.

21. Pérez-Escamilla R, Chapman DJ. Breastfeeding protection, promotion, and support in the United States: a time to nudge, a time to measure. J Hum Lact 2012;28(2):118–21.

22. Cricco-Lizza R. The milk of human kindness: environmental and human interactions in a WIC clinic that influence infant-feeding decisions of black women. Qual Health Res 2005;15(4):525–38.

23. Holmes AV, Chin NP, Kaczorowski J, et al. A barrier to exclusive breastfeeding for WIC enrollees: limited use of exclusive breastfeeding food package for mothers. Breastfeed Med 2009;4(1):25–30.

24. Finch C, Daniel EL. Breastfeeding education program with incentives increases exclusive breastfeeding among urban WIC participants. J Am Diet Assoc 2002; 102(7):981–4.

25. Wilde P, Wolf A, Fernandes M, et al. Food-package assignments and breastfeeding initiation before and after a change in the special supplemental nutrition program for women, infants, and children. Am J Clin Nutr 2012;96(3): 560–6.

26. Morton J, Hall JY, Wong RJ, et al. Combining hand techniques with electric pumping increases milk production in mothers of preterm infants. J Perinatol 2009;29(11):757–64.

27. The American Academy of Pediatrics, Committee on Fetus and Newborn. Postnatal glucose homeostasis in late-preterm and term infants. Pediatrics 2011; 127(3):575–9.

28. Wight N, Marinelli K, The Academy of Breastfeeding Medicne Protocol Committee. Academy of Breastfeeding Medicine clinical protocol #1: guidelines for glucose monitoring and treatment of hypoglycemia in breastfed infants [revised 2006]. Breastfeed Med 2006;1(3):178–84.

29. The Academy of Breastfeeding Medicne Protocol Committee. Academy of Breastfeeding Medicine Clinical Protocol #3: hospital guidelines for the use of supplementary feedings in the healthy term breastfed neonate. Breastfeed Med 2009;4(3):175–82.

30. Miracle DJ, Szucs KA, Torke AM, et al. Contemporary ethical issues in human milk-banking in the United States. Pediatrics 2011;128(6):1186–91.

31. Moore ER, Anderson GC, Bergman N, et al. Early skin-to-skin contact for mothers and their healthy newborn infants. Cochrane Database Syst Rev 2012;(5):CD003519.

32. Raimbault C, Saliba E, Porter RH. The effect of the odour of mother's milk on breastfeeding behaviour of premature neonates. Acta Paediatr 2007;96(3): 368–71.

33. Righard L, Alade MO. Effect of delivery room routines on success of first breastfeed. Lancet 1990;336(8723):1105–7.

34. The breast crawl. Available at: www.breastcrawl.org. Accessed September 20, 2012.

35. Bystrova K, Widström AM, Matthiesen AS, et al. Early lactation performance in primiparous and multiparous women in relation to different maternity home practices. A randomised trial in St. Petersburg. Int Breastfeed J 2007;8(2):9.

36. Murray EK, Ricketts S, Dellaport J. Hospital practices that increase breastfeeding duration: results from a population-based study. Birth 2007;34(3):202–11.

37. DiGirolamo A, Grummer-Strawn L. Effect of maternity care practices on breastfeeding. Pediatrics 2008;122:S43.

38. American Academy of Pediatrics Committee on Fetus, Newborn. Controversies concerning vitamin K and the newborn. Pediatrics 2003;112(1):191–2.

39. Okan F, Ozdil A, Bulbul A, et al. Analgesic effects of skin-to-skin contact and breastfeeding in procedural pain in healthy term neonates. Ann Trop Paediatr 2010;30(2):119–28.

40. Uga E, Candriella M, Perino A, et al. Heel lance in newborn during breastfeeding: an evaluation of analgesic effect of this procedure. Ital J Pediatr 2008;34(1):3.
41. Dilli D, Küçük IG, Dallar Y, et al. Interventions to reduce pain during vaccination in infancy. J Pediatr 2009;154(3):385–90.
42. U.S. Preventive Services Task Force. Ocular prophylaxis for gonococcal ophthalmia neonatorum: reaffirmation recommendation statement. Am Fam Physician 2012;85(2):195–6.
43. Academy of Breastfeeding Medicine Board of Directors. Position on breastfeeding. Breastfeed Med 2008;3(4):267–70.
44. American Academy of Family Physicians Breastfeeding Advisory Committee. Position paper on family physicians supporting breastfeeding. 2008. Available at: http://www.aafp.org/online/en/home/policy/policies/b/breastfeedingposition paper.html. Accessed September 1, 2012.
45. American College of Obstetricians and Gynecologists, Committee on health care for underserved women, committee on obstetric practice. Breastfeeding: maternal and infant aspects. Obstet Gynecol 2007;361:1–2.
46. Ip S, Chung M, Raman G, et al. A summary of the agency for healthcare research and quality's evidence report on breastfeeding in developed countries. Breastfeed Med 2009;4:S17–30.
47. McCann MF, Baydar N, Williams RL. Breastfeeding attitudes and reported problems in a national sample of WIC participants. J Hum Lact 2007;23(4):314–24.
48. Bunik M, Shobe P, O'Connor ME, et al. Are 2 weeks of daily breastfeeding support insufficient to overcome the influences of formula? Acad Pediatr 2010;10(1):21–8.
49. Powers NG, Slusser W. Breastfeeding update. 2: clinical lactation management. Pediatr Rev 1997;18:147–61.
50. Blythe R, Creedy D, Dennis C, et al. Effect of maternal confidence on breastfeeding duration: an application of breastfeeding self-efficacy theory. Birth 2002;29:278–84.
51. Damota K, Bañuelos J, Goldbronn J, et al. Maternal request for in-hospital supplementation of healthy breastfed infants among low-income women. J Hum Lact 2012 Jun 6. [Epub ahead of print].
52. Emde RN, Swedberg J, Suzuki B. Human wakefulness and biological rhythms after birth. Arch Gen Psychiatr 1975;32(6):780–3.
53. Stern E, Parmalee A, Akiyama Y, et al. Sleep cycle characteristics in infants. Pediatrics 1969;43:67–71.
54. Lawrence RA, Lawrence RM. Breastfeeding: a guide for the medical profession. 7th edition. Philadelphia: Elsevier/Mosby; 2011.
55. Saint L, Smith M, Hartmann P, et al. The yield and nutrient content of colostrum and milk of women form giving birth to one month post-partum. Br J Nutr 1984; 52:87–95.
56. Casey CE, Neifert MR, Seacat JM, et al. Nutrient intake by breastfed infants during the first five days after birth. Am J Dis Child 1986;140:933–6.
57. Yamauchi Y, Yamanouchi I. Breast-feeding frequency during the first 24 hours after birth in full-term neonates. Pediatrics 1990;86(2):171–5.
58. Dollberg S, Lavav S, Mamouni FB. A comparison on intakes of breast-fed and bottle-fed infants during the first two days of life. J Am Coll Nutr 2001;20:209–11.
59. Tunc VT, Camurdan AD, Ilhan MN, et al. Factors associated with defecation patterns in 0-24-month-old children. Eur J Pediatr 2008;167(12):1357–62.
60. McNeilly AS, Robinson IC, Houston MJ, et al. Release of oxytocin and prolactin in response to suckling. Br Med J (Clin Res Ed) 1983;286(6361):257–9.

61. BFHI USA: baby-friendly hospitals and birth centers. 2012. Available at: http://www.babyfriendlyusa.org/eng/03.html. Accessed August 27, 2012.
62. Levitt C, Hanvey L, Kaczorowski J, et al. Breastfeeding policies and practices in Canadian hospitals: comparing 1993 with 2007. Birth 2011;38(3):228–37.
63. Hofvander Y. Breastfeeding and the Baby Friendly Hospitals Initiative (BFHI): organization, response and outcome in Sweden and other countries. Acta Paediatr 2005;94(8):1012–6.
64. American Academy of Pediatrics Section on Breastfeeding. Sample hospital breastfeeding policy for newborns. 2009. Available at: http://www2.aap.org/breastfeeding/curriculum/documents/pdf/Hospital%20Breastfeeding%20Policy_FINAL.pdf. Accessed August 25, 2012.
65. The Academy of Breastfeeding Medicine Protocol Committee. ABM clinical protocol #7: model breastfeeding policy (Revision 2010). Breastfeed Med 2010;5(4):173–7.
66. Fairbank L, O'Meara S, Renfrew MJ, et al. A systematic review to evaluate the effectiveness of interventions to promote the initiation of breastfeeding. Health Technol Assess 2000;4(25):1–171.
67. Rosenberg KD, Stull JD, Adler MR, et al. Impact of hospital policies on breastfeeding outcomes. Breastfeed Med 2008;3(2):110–6.
68. BFHI USA: information for health professionals. 2012. Available at: http://www.babyfriendlyusa.org/eng/06.html. Accessed August 15, 2012.
69. Cattaneo A, Buzzetti R. Effect on rates of breastfeeding of training for the baby friendly hospital initiative. BMJ 2001;323(7325):1358–62.
70. Renfrew MJ, McCormick FM, Wade A, et al. Support for healthy breastfeeding mothers with healthy term babies. Cochrane Database Syst Rev 2012;(5):CD001141.
71. Freed GL, Clark SJ, Sorenson J, et al. National assessment of physicians' breast-feeding knowledge, attitudes, training and experience. JAMA 1995; 273(6):472–6.
72. Feldman-Winter LB, Schanler RJ, O'Connor KG, et al. Pediatricians and the promotion and support of breastfeeding. Arch Pediatr Adolesc Med 2008; 162(12):1142–9.
73. Feldman-Winter L, Barone L, Milcarek B, et al. Residency curriculum improves breastfeeding care. Pediatrics 2010;126(2):289–97.
74. Taveras EM, Capra AM, Braverman AP, et al. Clinician Support and psychosocial risk factors associated with breastfeeding discontinuation. Pediatrics 2003;112:108.
75. Taveras EM, Li R, Grummer-Strawn L, et al. Opinions and practices of clinicians associated with continuation of exclusive breastfeeding. Pediatrics 2004;113(4): e283–90.
76. Sakha K, Behbahan AG. Training for perfect breastfeeding or metoclopramide: which one can promote lactation in nursing mothers? Breastfeed Med 2008;3(2): 120–3.
77. Righard L, Alade MO. Sucking technique and its effect on success of breastfeeding. Birth 1992;19(4):185–9.
78. Santo LC, de Oliveira LD, Giugliani ER. Factors associated with low incidence of exclusive breastfeeding for the first 6 months. Birth 2007;34(3):212–9.
79. Becker GE, McCormick FM, Renfrew MJ. Methods of milk expression for lactating women. Cochrane Database Syst Rev 2008;(4):CD006170.
80. Flaherman VJ, Gay B, Scott C, et al. Randomised trial comparing hand expression with breast pumping for mothers of term newborns feeding poorly. Arch Dis Child Fetal Neonatal Ed 2012;97(1):F18–23.

81. The Academy of Breastfeeding Medicine Protocol Committee. ABM clinical protocol #8: human milk storage information for home use for full-term infants (original protocol march 2004; revision #1 march 2010). Breastfeed Med 2010;5(3):127–30.
82. Grummer-Strawn LM, Scanlon KS, Fein SB. Infant feeding and feeding transitions during the first year of life. Pediatrics 2008;122(Suppl 2):S36–42.
83. Nylander G, Lindemann R, Helsing E, et al. Unsupplemented breastfeeding in the maternity ward. Positive long-term effects. Acta Obstet Gynecol Scand 1991;70(3):205–9.
84. Semenic S, Loiselle C, Gottlieb L. Predictors of the duration of exclusive breastfeeding among first-time mothers. Res Nurs Health 2008;31(5):428–41.
85. Gourley GR, Kreamer B, Cohnen M, et al. Neonatal jaundice and diet. Arch Pediatr Adolesc Med 1999;153:184–8.
86. Sadacharan R, Grossman X, Sanchez E, et al. Trends in US hospital distribution of industry-sponsored infant formula sample packs. Pediatrics 2011;128(4):702–5.
87. Rosenberg KD, Eastham CA, Kasehagen LJ, et al. Marketing infant formula through hospitals: the impact of commercial hospital discharge packs on breastfeeding. Am J Public Health 2008;98(2):290–5.
88. Howard C, Howard F, Lawrence R, et al. Office prenatal formula advertising and its effect on breast-feeding patterns. Obstet Gynecol 2000;95(2):296–303.
89. Yamauchi Y, Yamanouchi I. The relationship between rooming-in/not rooming-in and breast-feeding variables. Acta Paediatr Scand 1990;79(11):1017–22.
90. Keefe MR. Comparison of neonatal nighttime sleep-wake patterns in nursery versus rooming-in environments. Nurse Res 1987;36(3):140–4.
91. Keefe MR. The impact of infant rooming-in on maternal sleep at night. J Obstet Gynecol Neonatal Nurs 1988;17(2):122–6.
92. Hawdon JM, Ward Platt MP, Aynsley-Green A. Patterns of metabolic adaptation for preterm and term infants in the first neonatal week. Arch Dis Child 1992;67(4 Spec No):357–65.
93. De Carvalho M, Robertson S, Friedman A, et al. Effect of frequent breast-feeding on early milk production and infant weight gain. Pediatrics 1983;72(3):307–11.
94. Hill PD, Humenick SS. The occurrence of breast engorgement. J Hum Lact 1994;10(2):79–86.
95. O'Connor NR, Tanabe KO, Siadaty MS, et al. Pacifiers and breastfeeding: a systematic review. Arch Pediatr Adolesc Med 2009;163(4):378–82.
96. Howard CR, Howard FM, Lanphear B, et al. Randomized clinical trial of pacifier use and bottle-feeding or cupfeeding and their effect on breastfeeding. Pediatrics 2003;111:511–8.
97. Centers for Disease Control and Prevention. 2009 National Survey of Maternity Practices in Infant Nutrition and Care. 2010. Available at: http://www.cdc.gov/breastfeeding/data/mpinc/index.htm. Accessed May 26, 2012.
98. Su LL, Chong YS, Chan YH, et al. Antenatal education and postnatal support strategies for improving rates of exclusive breast feeding: randomised controlled trial. BMJ 2007;335(7620):596.
99. Kronborg H, Vaeth M, Olsen J, et al. Effect of early postnatal breastfeeding support: a cluster-randomized community based trial. Acta Paediatr 2007;96(7):1064–70.
100. Dennis CL, Kingston D. A systematic review of telephone support for women during pregnancy and the early postpartum period. J Obstet Gynecol Neonatal Nurs 2008;37(3):301–14.

101. Abrahams SW, Labbok MH. Exploring the impact of the baby-friendly hospital initiative on trends in exclusive breastfeeding. Int Breastfeed J 2009;4:11.

102. Merten S, Dratva J, Ackermann-Liebrich U. Do baby-friendly hospitals influence breastfeeding duration on a national level? Pediatrics 2005;116(5):e702–8.

103. Kramer MS, Chalmers B, Hodnett ED, et al. Promotion of Breastfeeding Intervention Trial (PROBIT): a randomized trial in the Republic of Belarus. JAMA 2001; 285(4):413–20.

104. American Academy of Pediatrics Subcommittee on Hyperbilirubinemia. Management of hyperbilirubinemia in the newborn infant 35 or more weeks of gestation. Pediatrics 2004;114:297–316.

105. Maisels MJ, Bhutani VK, Bogen D, et al. Hyperbilirubinemia in the newborn infant > or 1/4 35 weeks' gestation: an update with clarifications. Pediatrics 2009;124:1193–8.

106. The Academy of Breastfeeding Medicine Protocol Committee. ABM clinical protocol #22: guidelines for management of jaundice in the breastfeeding infant equal to or greater than 35 weeks' gestation. Breastfeed Med 2010;5(2):87–93.

107. The Academy of Breastfeeding Medicine Protocol Committee. ABM clinical protocol #10: breastfeeding the late preterm infant (340/7 to 366/7 weeks gestation) (first revision June 2011). Breastfeed Med 2011;6(3):151–6.

108. Walker M. Breastfeeding the late preterm infant. J Obstet Gynecol Neonatal Nurs 2008;37:692–701.

109. Meier PP, Brown LP, Hurst NM, et al. Nipple shields for preterm infants: effect on milk transfer and duration of breastfeeding. J Hum Lact 2000;16:106–14.

110. Chertok IR. Reexamination of ultra-thin nipple shield use, infant growth and maternal satisfaction. J Clin Nurs 2009;18:2949–55.

111. The Academy of Breastfeeding Medicine Protocol Committee. ABM clinical protocol #2 (2007 revision): guidelines for hospital discharge of the breastfeeding term newborn and mother: "the going home protocol". Breastfeed Med 2007;2(3):158–65.

112. American Academy of Pediatrics. Committee on fetus and newborn. Hospital stay for healthy term newborns. Pediatrics 2010;125:405–9.

Evidence-based Interventions to Support Breastfeeding

Lori Feldman-Winter, MD, MPH

KEYWORDS

- Breastfeeding • Pregnant • Lactation • Postpartum • Breastfeeding support

KEY POINTS

- Considerable progress has been made in the past decade in developing comprehensive support systems to enable more women to reach their breastfeeding goals.
- Given that most women in the United States participate in some breastfeeding, it is essential that each of these support systems be rigorously tested and if effective replicated.
- Additional research is needed to determine the best methods of support during the preconception period to prepare women to exclusively breastfeed as a cultural norm.

INTRODUCTION

Breastfeeding is arguably one of the most important decisions a mother can make after making the decision to have children. The decision to breastfeed, as opposed to formula feed, has the potential to influence numerous health outcomes for mother, child, and society.[1,2] Promoting breastfeeding has been the focus of public health campaigns during the last several decades, and these campaigns and a shifting of the cultural norm have resulted in a dramatic increase in the overall incidence of breastfeeding. Although some women cannot breastfeed or choose to not breastfeed, most in the United States do breastfeed, at least to some extent. In 2010, more than 75% of US mothers started breastfeeding in the early postpartum period, according to data collected as part of the Centers for Disease Control and Prevention National Immunization Survey (NIS) (**Fig. 1**). However, most women in the United States do not breastfeed either exclusively or long enough to meet the American Academy of Pediatrics (AAP) recommendations for breastfeeding. According to data from the NIS, merely 14.8% of women exclusively breastfed to 6 months in 2008. Furthermore, multiple significant disparities continue to exist, and many Americans lose the potential to realize optimal health and wellness. Therefore, focusing on the decision to breastfeed is not sufficient, and a newer public health priority has instead focused on protection and support of breastfeeding.

Department of Pediatrics, Children's Regional Hospital at Cooper University Hospital, 401 Haddon Avenue, Camden, NJ 08103, USA
E-mail address: Winter-Lori@CooperHealth.edu

Pediatr Clin N Am 60 (2013) 169–187
http://dx.doi.org/10.1016/j.pcl.2012.09.007
pediatric.theclinics.com
0031-3955/13/$ – see front matter © 2013 Elsevier Inc. All rights reserved.

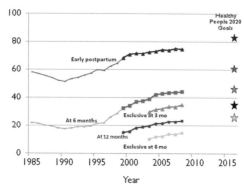

Fig. 1. Centers for Disease Control and Prevention NIS on breastfeeding.

When one considers a mother's experience from the time she becomes pregnant to her child's first birthday and beyond, it is not surprising that most women end up breastfeeding partially, combining infant formula with breastfeeding, and weaning sooner than intended or recommended. Beginning with the first visit to the physician, nurse midwife, or nurse practitioner or the first visit to a local store to order newborn infant products, attending newborn classes, and touring the maternity care facility, families are bombarded with messages, both obvious and subtle, that influence infant feeding decisions. Some of the bias about infant feeding, specifically about exclusive breastfeeding and timing of the introduction of complementary solid food, comes from messages seen even before entering the childbearing years. The decisions about feeding, however, are flexible, may change from one birth to the next, and can be optimized with good support.[3] Mothers and families continue to be affected by environmental support or barriers in the intrapartum and postpartum periods. Availability of community support for breastfeeding varies widely, such that breastfeeding support "deserts (areas that are barren in breastfeeding support services)" exist in communities that are least likely to breastfeed. This review is intended to follow how a family may experience breastfeeding through their life cycle and describe evidence-based practices that have been established to support breastfeeding. Barriers and challenges to breastfeeding support will also be described in light of persistent disparities. Some specific support strategies affect the life cycle and will be addressed separately. Finally, implications for future research to continue expansion and impact of breastfeeding support will be identified.

SUPPORT FOR PREGNANT WOMEN

Given the time most women have with their prenatal health care practitioner, there is potentially ample opportunity for breastfeeding support to be provided while women are pregnant and during their prenatal care visits. The types of messages and education and the methods of delivering this information have been studied extensively, yet results have been mixed. It seems that peer counseling, formal lactation consultations, and breastfeeding education result in increased initiation of breastfeeding. Results of prenatal education on long-term breastfeeding continuation and exclusivity are mixed and more limited.[4] Furthermore, studies of peer counseling and lactation support programs often include a time-frame not only focused on the prenatal period but also transcending the prenatal, in-hospital, and postpartum periods, so the effect of the prenatal component is difficult to decipher.

Mothers with targeted need, or who are at high risk of not breastfeeding, may have more to gain from prenatal support; conversely, minority women may be more at risk for not having received breastfeeding advice.[5] Consistent prenatal education that addresses the benefits of breastfeeding, the management of breastfeeding including positioning and latch, feeding on cue, the importance of skin-to-skin contact after delivery, rooming-in, and the importance of exclusive breastfeeding and risks of supplementing within the first 6 months are elements of Step 3 of the Baby-Friendly Hospital Initiative (BFHI). Hospitals designated as part of the BFHI and that have their own prenatal services are responsible for delivering prenatal education that meets these requirements. The requirement includes education about breastfeeding for all women, not only those who specifically intend to breastfeed. Hospitals that do not have affiliated prenatal clinics are responsible for either offering this education in prenatal or birth classes or helping to foster community-based programs that offer prenatal classes providing comprehensive breastfeeding education and support.[6] These strategies underscore that infant feeding decisions are often changing, not fixed, and may be influenced by support at any time.

Prenatal clinical education about the techniques and management of breastfeeding produce the most significant change in postnatal breastfeeding, especially when combined with postnatal support.[7] These interventions increase breastfeeding initiation, duration, and exclusivity. Educational programs conducted by nurses or lactation specialists in the antenatal setting may increase breastfeeding initiation and short-term duration. Additional support offered by peers provided modest effects when combined with formal education.[8] Content of effective sessions included the benefits of breastfeeding, principles of lactation, myths, common problems, solutions, and skills training. In a number-needed-to-treat analysis, it was estimated that for every 3 to 5 women receiving education, 1 woman would breastfeed for up to 3 months.[7,9]

Prenatal breastfeeding education delivered in a workshop format has been shown to increase self-efficacy, a potential mechanism for increasing breastfeeding initiation and continuation.[10] Prenatal clinics with teaching devices such as model infants and breasts and videos and visual displays will be more successful in delivering hands-on education. Using the primary care setting is reasonable, especially if the primary care practitioners are trained in delivering education about breastfeeding benefits and techniques.[11] Group prenatal instruction, breastfeeding-specific clinic appointments, and peer counseling were among the interventions that were especially effective among minority women and increased breastfeeding initiation, duration, and exclusivity.[12] Further consideration needs to be given to support women at higher risk of breastfeeding problems. One growing problem is the impact of the obesity epidemic. Obesity complicates fertility and delivery and makes breastfeeding problems more likely. Obese women are more likely to have delayed lactogenesis and reduced lactation[13]; therefore, weight-control strategies should be offered both before gestation and throughout the prenatal period.

Considering the positive effect of prenatal education and support programs on breastfeeding, one must also consider the potential negative effect of infant formula company marketing on breastfeeding initiation, duration, and exclusivity. In a randomized trial of formula-marketing educational materials versus noncommercial educational materials, the industry materials resulted in increased breastfeeding cessation during the first 2 weeks after delivery.[14] Although additional marketing strategies have not been systematically studied, it is not difficult to imagine the negative effects of multiple outlets for direct-to-consumer formula marketing. Beginning with the first trip to the infant furniture store or choosing a layette, families are bombarded with advertising of infant formula, bottles, teats, and pacifiers. Purchase of baby products or registering for prenatal classes may result in shipments of infant formula or related marketing materials directly to the home. Prenatal care offices may be stocked with diaper bags containing formula samples and marketing brochures, the ones that used to be given out free in most hospitals. During the past few years the practice of giving commercial sample packs at the time of hospital discharge has changed,[15,16] and companies have shifted their efforts to ambulatory settings and the Internet. Health care practitioners should be aware that breastfeeding support, beginning with the prenatal period, is most effective when combined with the elimination of infant formula marketing. International evidence suggests maternal care practitioners may need further education about the effects of industry marketing and may not be aware of how their practice contributes to the marketing of infant formula.[17] Furthermore, one study suggests that mothers cared for by midwives and family physicians are more likely than mothers cared for by obstetricians to exclusively breastfeed at hospital discharge.[18] This may reflect differences in training (addressed later) or more attention to eliminating the negative influences of industry marketing. For mothers who intend to exclusively formula feed, it is important to deliver individualized education about formula preparation as opposed to group sessions, minimizing the perception by potential breastfeeding patients that using infant formula is a social norm.

SUPPORT FOR WOMEN IN THE PERIPARTUM SETTING

The World Health Organization/United Nations Children's Fund BFHI, a program launched in 1991, has largely shaped improvements in breastfeeding support within the peripartum setting,[19] yet the number of US hospitals that have achieved designation remains low. With national funding and organized initiatives, more hospitals than ever have been entering the pipeline to become designated as Baby-Friendly hospitals, and more deliveries than ever are occurring in US designated facilities (**Fig. 2**). The BFHI, which is based on the Ten Steps to Successful Breastfeeding, provides support by providing optimal evidence-based practices in the hospital and extending support through continuity of care in Steps 3 and 10 prenatally and postpartum (**Box 1**). The BFHI has been shown to increase breastfeeding initiation, continuation, and exclusivity, which are all sustainable over time.[20–23] The Ten Steps seem to have a dose-dependent effect, such that the more steps that are in place, the less likely a mother is to stop breastfeeding during the 2 months following hospital discharge.[24] Given the dose effect, many delivery hospitals are improving the support of breastfeeding women by adopting some, if not all, of the Ten Steps without pursuing Baby-Friendly designation. One of the ways the Ten Steps increase breastfeeding exclusivity is by training the staff and developing evidence-based protocols. Maternity care staff who were adequately trained in effective breastfeeding support led to more nighttime breastfeeding, decreased supplementation especially at night, and more effective breastfeeding assessments.[25]

The BFHI has also been applied globally to sick and premature newborns,[26–28] and the focus has extended beyond the immediate peripartum period to the concept of

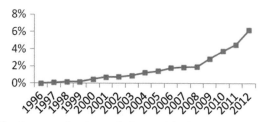

Fig. 2. Rate of deliveries occurring in US designated facilities, 1996–2012.

Box 1
The WHO/UNICEF Ten Steps to Successful Breastfeeding with author's summary of the US Baby-Friendly Guidelines and Evaluation Criteria

Step 1: Have a written infant feeding policy that is routinely communicated to all health care staff (policy includes the International Code of Marketing of Breast Milk Substitutes, being readily available, and having effectiveness monitored regularly).

Step 2: Train all health care staff on the policy (including 20 hours for nursing staff according to 15 lessons, 5 hours of supervised experience, and demonstrating 4 competencies; physicians and advanced practice nurses will be trained with a minimum of 3 hours and achieve similar competencies).

Step 3: Inform all pregnant women on the benefits and management of breastfeeding (beginning preferably in the first trimester, and including education on elements of the Ten Steps including skin-to-skin care, rooming-in, cue-based feedings, and the risks of supplementation in the first 6 months).

Step 4: Help mothers initiate breastfeeding within the first hour after birth: (1) step now interpreted as placing babies in skin-to-skin contact with their mothers immediately following birth for at least an hour and encouraging mothers to recognize when their babies are ready to breastfeed, offering help if needed, (2) this step now applies to all mothers regardless of feeding method.

Step 5: Show mothers how to breastfeed and how to maintain lactation even if they are separated from their infants: (1) education and assistance: (i) the importance of exclusive breastfeeding, (ii) how to maintain lactation for exclusive breastfeeding for about 6 months, (iii) criteria to assess if the baby is getting enough breast milk, (iv) how to express, handle, and store breast milk, including manual expression, and (v) how to sustain lactation if the mother is separated from her infant or will not be exclusively breastfeeding after discharge; (2) if mothers and infants are separated: (i) ensure that milk expression is begun within 6 hours of birth, (ii) expressed milk is given to the baby as soon as the baby is medically ready, (iii) the mother's expressed milk is used before any supplementation with breastmilk substitutes when medically appropriate; and (3) mothers who are formula feeding should receive: (i) individualized written instruction, (ii) not specific to a particular brand, (iii) verbal information about safe preparation, handling, storage and feeding of infant formula, and (iv) this advice should be documented.

Step 6: Give infants no food or drink other than breastmilk unless medically indicated: (1) understanding the rationale for medical contraindications to breastfeed and the acceptable medical indications to supplement breastfeeding, (2) the facility will track exclusive breastfeeding according to The Joint Commission definition for the Perinatal Care Core Measure, (3) track supplemented breastfeeding and compare with the Centers for Disease Control and Prevention NIS rate of supplementation, (4) if a mother requests supplementation of her breastfeeding infant, before this request is granted and documented the health care staff should first explore the reasons for this request, address the concerns raised and educate her about the possible consequences to the health of her baby and/or the success of breastfeeding.

Step 7: Practice rooming-in; allow mothers and infants to remain together 24 hours per day (applies to all infants regardless of feeding method; infants stay with their mothers throughout the day and night except for up to 1 hour for facility procedures or for as long as medically necessary).

Step 8: Encourage breastfeeding on demand [now interpreted for all newborns regardless of feeding method as "encourage feeding on cue" with the following guidelines: (1) understand that no restrictions should be placed on the frequency or length of feeding, (2) understand that newborns usually feed a minimum of 8 times in 24 hours, (3) recognize cues that infants use to signal readiness to begin and end feeds, and (4) understand that physical contact and nourishment are both important].

Step 9: Give no pacifiers or artificial nipples to breastfeeding infants: (1) applies to any fluid supplementation, whether medically indicated or following informed decision of the mothers should be given by tube, syringe, spoon, or cup in preference to an artificial nipple or bottle; and (2) staff should educate all breastfeeding mothers about how the use of bottles and artificial nipples may interfere with the development of optimal breastfeeding.

Step 10: Foster the establishment of breastfeeding support groups and refer mothers to them on discharge from the hospital or birth center (the facility should establish in-house breastfeeding support services if no adequate source of support is available for referral (eg, support group, lactation clinic, home health services, help line, etc).

Adapted from the Baby-Friendly USA, Inc. Guidelines and Evaluation Criteria. For more information please see the Guidelines and Evaluation Criteria found at http://www. babyfriendlyusa.org/get-started/the-guidelines-evaluation-criteria.

Baby-Friendly office practices.[29] Changes and improvements to the Ten Steps during the past 20 years have shifted attention from breastfeeding mothers to all mothers. Now, all mothers have an opportunity to access optimal evidence based maternity care practices, such as skin-to-skin and rooming-in, and have the potential to breastfeed. But even if the mother is not breastfeeding, the benefits of optimal peripartum care support are provided. Furthermore, the BFHI partially offsets the negative impact of marketing of breastmilk substitutes, bottles, teats, and pacifiers by implementing the International Code of Marketing of Breast Milk Substitutes in hospitals and associated prenatal clinics. Several studies have demonstrated the negative effect of specific marketing tactics such as discharge bags and free formula distribution on the initiation, duration, and exclusivity of breastfeeding.[30–32] One additional study demonstrated that eliminating the distribution of sample packs alone was less effective in preserving exclusive breastfeeding than was combining these activities with breastfeeding support policies, staff training, and the restricted availability of infant formula on the pastpartum ward.[33]

Additional support in the peripartum period may include individuals who provide patient-focused care such as doulas and peer counselors. Although the evidence on doula care is limited, one prospective cohort study demonstrated that doula care resulted in earlier timing of lactogenesis II and increased prevalence of 6-week duration of breastfeeding in mothers with and without prenatal stressors.[34] Doulas may also be beneficial in high-risk or underserved mothers, as one study suggested doula care improved exclusive breastfeeding outcomes among Latina women.[35] Doulas may also improve the birth experience, result in fewer interventions, and promote more natural childbirth, all secondarily increasing breastfeeding outcomes.[36] The doula is traditionally a nonmedical person who assists a woman before, during, or after childbirth by providing information, physical assistance, and emotional support. Therefore, this type of breastfeeding support transcends the peripartum period and affects prenatal and postpartum periods.[37]

Peer counselors have also been used in the hospital to provide support and a secure link to community based care. Peer support provided consistently throughout the perinatal period improves breastfeeding initiation and duration.[38,39] The combination of peer support and skilled professional support was most effective in enhancing breastfeeding outcomes and may offset the lack of available professional support services.[40] Peers may be hired as components of hospital-based breastfeeding support systems or may be available for in-hospital support from the local Special Supplemental Nutrition Program for Women, Infants and Children (WIC) program for women who qualify and in states that permit coordination of WIC services with delivery of hospital care. Peer support offered through the WIC program has been successful, and is cost effective, despite national efforts to eliminate this component of the program altogether in proposed budget cuts.[41]

SUPPORT FOR POSTPARTUM WOMEN IN THE COMMUNITY

As previously mentioned, many of the support services available in the community to postpartum breastfeeding women have played a role in prenatal promotion and support, and some have affected the peripartum period. The care provided in the postpartum setting can be categorized as professional and nonprofessional support services.[42] The best outcomes occur when nonprofessional support is combined with effective professional support. Mechanisms of delivery vary and may be in the home, at local agencies, or by telephone, yet all seem to be effective in supporting continuation of exclusive breastfeeding.[43,44]

SUPPORT BY PHYSICIANS AND ADVANCED PRACTICE NURSES

Professional support services include those provided in a clinical setting such as the offices of an obstetrician, family physician, pediatrician, or nurse midwife. One key paradigm shift to the delivery of clinical care is that the provider addresses the mother–infant dyad as a unit. This requires a shift in the usual approach of the pediatrician, obstetrician, and nurse midwife but may be more standard of care for the family practitioner and includes implications for coding and billing. The AAP Section on Breastfeeding has developed a guide for coding and billing as one way to encourage continuity of breastfeeding care.[45] Nevertheless, breastfeeding care delivered by physicians and advanced practice nurses in the clinical setting is often limited by the lack of knowledge, skills, time, and cultural sensitivity.[46–51]

PHYSICIAN EDUCATION

Physicians often lack the necessary education and training and may have insufficient attitudes to provide optimal breastfeeding care.[46] Although attitudes among some physicians seem to be more positive toward breastfeeding than in the past[52] and most maternal care and pediatric care practitioners consider breastfeeding counseling to be an important part of their care, preparation to provide skilled support is lacking.[53] A residency curriculum developed for pediatricians, obstetricians, and family physicians was shown to be effective in increasing knowledge, confidence, and practice patterns among those trained.[54] Training residents in breastfeeding care affected breastfeeding outcomes including increased exclusive breastfeeding for as long as 6 months postpartum. However, the integration into primary care training programs is variable, and there is a need for faculty development and clinician leaders to champion the integration of such curriculum. In a randomized controlled trial of physician education, merely 5 hours of education resulted in improved practices and support, exclusive breastfeeding at 4 weeks, continued breastfeeding for 18 versus 13 weeks, and fewer breastfeeding problems compared with the situation in mothers seen by untrained physicians.[55]

Continuing education courses on breastfeeding for practicing physicians have been offered by a variety of sources. One Web-based curriculum has been shown to increase physician knowledge about breastfeeding.[56] Other opportunities offered at programs sponsored by physician organizations, such as the AAP, Section on Breastfeeding, the combined AAP La Leche League Physician's Seminar, AAP chapter meetings, the Breastfeeding Promotion in Physicians' Office Practices Programs, and the annual meeting of the Academy of Breastfeeding Medicine, including the "What Every Physician Needs to Know About Breastfeeding" precourse, have presumably increased knowledge and improved practice, yet none have been rigorously tested. Now that many physicians, particularly pediatricians, must complete a quality improvement project as part of Maintenance of Certification, several programs have become available on breastfeeding to help physicians comply with this newer requirement. There are online options offered by the University of Virginia Health System and Virginia Department of Health,[57] the American Board of Pediatrics, and the AAP EQIPP

Module: Safe and Health Beginnings.[58] Recognizing the role of health care professionals in supporting breastfeeding throughout the life cycle, core competencies were developed by the United States Breastfeeding Committee (**Box 2**) and endorsed by the AAP.[59] Physicians can also become experts in breastfeeding care and serve as consultants to their colleagues. Experts may be identified as being fellows of the Academy of Breastfeeding Medicine or Chapter Breastfeeding coordinators of the AAP, and they may be board certified as lactation consultants. Some physicians have limited the scope of their practice to breastfeeding care.[60] They often provide online support and consultative services for colleagues with less training and expertise.[61] Given the growing knowledge and sophistication of breastfeeding care, breastfeeding medicine as a specialty has evolved over recent years and in the future may become recognized as a uniquely defined medical specialty.

PROFESSIONAL SUPPORT BY OTHER (NONPHYSICIAN) HEALTH CARE PROFESSIONALS

Another level of professional support is health care nurse support in the postpartum setting. Adequately trained community health workers can deliver breastfeeding support to at-risk inner-city mothers in the home environment and have a unique opportunity to offset multiple challenges and positively influence the lives of their clients.[62] Yet, many community health workers have had their own, personal problems

---

Box 2
United States Breastfeeding Committee core competencies

At a minimum, every health professional should understand the role of lactation, human milk, and breastfeeding in:

- The optimal feeding of infants and young children
- Enhancing health and reducing
  - ○ Long-term morbidities in infants and young children
  - ○ Morbidities in women

All health professionals should be able to facilitate the breastfeeding care process by:

- Preparing families for realistic expectations
- Communicating pertinent information to the lactation care team
- Following up with the family, when appropriate, in a culturally competent manner after breastfeeding care and services have been provided

The United States Breastfeeding Committee proposes to accomplish this by recommending that health professional organizations:

- Understand and act on the importance of protecting, promoting, and supporting breastfeeding as a public health priority
- Educate their practitioners to
  - ○ Appreciate the limitations of their breastfeeding care expertise
  - ○ Know when and how to make a referral to a lactation care professional
- Regularly examine the care practices of their practitioners and establish core competencies related to breastfeeding care and services

Adapted from United States Breastfeeding Committee. Core competencies in breastfeeding care and services for all health professionals. Revised edition. Washington, DC: United States Breastfeeding Committee; 2010.

with breastfeeding and/or have not been adequately trained. In a well-designed randomized controlled trial of home nursing visits compared with traditional office-based postpartum care for healthy mother–infant dyads, the intervention group was more likely to continue breastfeeding for up to 2 months and had a better reported self-efficacy in parenting skills.[43]

Skilled lactation support by internationally board-certified lactation consultants is another form of postpartum support that may be delivered in a variety of settings. Lactation consultants may operate a hospital-based breastfeeding clinic, they may be in a fee-for-service private practice or independent practice, they may be hired as part of the team in an inpatient maternity setting or an ambulatory physician practice, they may be hired by WIC, or they may be available for telephone consultations in any of these settings. Many lactation consultants are also nurses with the ability to make clinical decisions and may already function in an ambulatory office setting performing triage duties. Proactive telephone follow-up support is effective in increasing breastfeeding exclusivity and duration.[44]

Lactation consulting as a profession grew largely out of the need for professional level support during a time when physician and nursing support was generally lacking.[63] More recently, with the advent of more breastfeeding curricula during health professional training, along with training incorporated as part of the BFHI, the lactation consultant professional has assumed different roles that include managerial tasks, health education, curriculum development, and direct breastfeeding care for difficult or complex cases. Serving as a senior manager or consultant to nurses or physicians requires similar referral patterns to other consultants using the 3 "Rs." The consult must be referred by the primary care team, care must be rendered by the consultant, and a letter of care must be sent back in reply. Given new proposals to include lactation consultation services as a component of health reform, lactation consultants may need to develop a new set of skills including documentation and communication with primary care providers. Office practices that coordinate the pediatric office visit with direct lactation consultation may provide the best long-term support with effects on exclusivity and duration of breastfeeding to 9 months postpartum.[64] In the absence of such arrangements, coordination of care will likely produce better outcomes.

Additional health care professionals who have an opportunity to provide support, particularly in complex situations and for vulnerable infants and their mothers, include dietitians,[65] speech pathologists,[66] social workers, and psychologists.[42] Although studies on outcomes from these forms of professional support are limited, it is clear that preprofessional education and training should be considered in a wide variety of health profession curricula.

PEER (LAY) SUPPORT

Continued support for postpartum women requires more than professional care. Support groups such as La Leche League, Baby Cafés, text messages on mobile devices (such as text-for-baby), hospital led support groups, and other community-based support programs all offer added support for the mother, the father, and other family members. Modifiable factors that affect continuation of breastfeeding include breastfeeding intent, self-efficacy, and social support.[67] The last 2 issues are positively affected by lay support. However, many of the support systems identified by mothers are not available to them for a long enough time postpartum and mothers eventually rely on their partners and family members to fill the gap.[68] Several strategies for enhancement of social support have been tried. These include programs to improve the father's self-efficacy in parenting and supporting the mother,[69] those emphasizing person-centered communication skills and ongoing relationships with community support persons,[70] and breast pump information being delivered in classes, support groups, or by relatives or friends (as opposed to by physicians/physicians assistants).[71] Vulnerable mothers and families, particularly those served by WIC, identify numerous reasons for early cessation of breastfeeding: return to work or school, sore nipples, lack of access to breast pumps, and free formula provided by WIC.[72] Finally, timing of peer support is critical for WIC participants, and the sooner the peer counselors can provide services, the more likely the mother is to breastfeed at all in addition to exclusively.[73]

EMPLOYMENT

Many more workplaces now than 25 years ago offer accommodations to breastfeeding employees. These patterns were evolving even before health reform and the Patient Protection and Affordable Care Act (ACA) of 2010, which includes the requirement for workplaces to provide appropriate space and reasonable break time to breastfeed or express milk. It has been estimated that, annually, 165,000 new mothers continue to breastfeed beyond 6 months directly as a result of the provisions set forth in the ACA.[74] To facilitate employer compliance with the law, the Maternal and Child Health Bureau in collaboration with the Department of Health and Human Services Office on Women's Health developed the "Business Case for Breastfeeding" toolkit with brochures, policies, and recommendations on implementing workplace support for lactation.[75] Despite such progress, there are still many employees who cannot access these accommodations, such as teachers, fast food workers, and toll booth operators, to name a few. The US Department of Labor regularly monitors telephone calls to track types of employment and anecdotes of employees who cannot access appropriate accommodations.

Studies have shown part-time employment may be as supportive of an environment as not working at all, and both are more supportive toward sustaining breastfeeding than full-time employment.[76] Furthermore, professionals have a greater likelihood of sustaining breastfeeding than managers or other positions, because they may be more in control of their workplace environment with potential availability of direct breastfeeding and contact with their child. With the digital age, many women have options such as telecommuting, working from home, and flexible hours. Paid maternity leave and consideration of mother's "work" as part of the gross national productivity are considerations for enhancements to breastfeeding support.

CHILD CARE

The First Lady's Let's Move! Campaign to prevent obesity in the United States includes a program called Let's Move Child Care. In addition to strategies targeted at physical exercise and proper nutrition, there are provisions to increase breastfeeding and breast milk feeding among child care attendees. Education of child care workers on methods of being supportive to breastfeeding mothers and the proper storage, handling, and feeding of breastmilk is now being conducted routinely. Many states have received grants to educate child care workers, revise child care regulations, and update child care facilities to meet these guidelines. On-site and nearby child care arrangements facilitate direct breastfeeding and, combined with effective workplace support, may be more effective in supporting the continuation of breastfeeding after return to work.[77] Evidence to support child care interventions is accumulating and should provide guidance for national policy and local strategies.

SCHOOLS AND PRECONCEPTION EDUCATION

Schools serve as an important environment to potentially support breastfeeding. As mentioned earlier, school teachers have some of the worst employment provisions regarding their own breastfeeding support. Schools must also change to accommodate adolescents who return to school breastfeeding. Finally, schools play an important role in educating youth about breastfeeding. School nurses and teachers generally agree that inclusion of breastfeeding into school curricula for middle and high school students is appropriate[78]; however, the efficacy of this education on future breastfeeding experiences has not been studied.

FOUNDATIONAL SUPPORT TRANSCENDING THE TIMELINE
Support for Adolescent Mothers

Given that adolescents have the lowest reported rates of breastfeeding in the United States, support for breastfeeding among adolescents requires special attention. Social supports for the adolescent must be tailored to the developmental and individual needs of the mother and potentially the father or identified peer support person.[79] Breastfeeding adolescents may benefit most from emotional, self-esteem, and network support.[80] Furthermore, adolescents have a demonstrated need for information about breastfeeding, have limited knowledge about breastfeeding, and may have opportunities to access breastfeeding information in prenatal classes. Similar to adult women, adolescents need instrumental or practical advice on how to breastfeed. Finally, adolescents may respond to support for autonomy and privacy. In one trial of telephone contact with adolescents, the peer support offered by telephone resulted in increased exclusivity of breastfeeding but not increased duration of breastfeeding.[81] Assessment of adolescents' social support needs may be ascertained using a new instrument providing the opportunity to facilitate optimal care in the early postpartum period.[82]

Culturally and Linguistically Sensitive Support

Given the growing diversity among Americans, there have been multiple studies examining the cultural influences and culturally sensitive provision of breastfeeding care. Certain cultures adhere to specific rituals, practices, and diets in the peripartum period; however, it is important to remember there may be variations on how a particular family interprets or practices these cultural practices. One example is in the Cambodian population. In one delivery hospital, mothers did not breastfeed because of the lack of culturally appropriate food available in the postpartum period. Cultural beliefs required these mothers to eat certain foods to breastfeed and provide their colostrum. Once the hospital adapted menu options that included foods often consumed by this population, these mothers went on to exclusively breastfeed.[83] The mechanism used to understand cultural beliefs and preferences involve asking open-ended questions, validating feelings, and providing education and guidance that is tailored to the individual needs of the patient and family. Linguistic support is a federal requirement, yet implementation with communities that speak multiple languages can be challenging. Trained and certified interpreters either in-person or via the telephone should be used in all cases, as opposed to using family members or other parts of the health care team not directly involved in the care. Educational materials produced by hospitals, offices, and other programs should be translated into commonly spoken languages at a literacy level of about 5th grade. Health care professionals need to recognize that language barriers are often compounded by literacy issues.

GOVERNMENT AND LEGISLATION

There have been multiple developments during the past several years to increase public support for breastfeeding encompassing multiple federal agencies and departments. Laying the groundwork was the 2011 Surgeon General's Call to Action to Support Breastfeeding (SGCTA).[84] As the highest ranking health official in the United States, Dr Regina Benjamin outlined 20 action steps to support breastfeeding. These action steps should be performed in 6 domains: mothers and families, communities, health care, employment, research, and public health infrastructure. The SGCTA has sparked numerous additional federal activities with additional funding, manpower, and coordination of federal agencies to support breastfeeding at multiple levels. Soon after the launch of the SGCTA, the First Lady Michelle Obama's Let's Move! Campaign outlined provisions to support breastfeeding as a strategy to combat childhood obesity. She announced the importance of breastfeeding support to thousands of pediatricians at a plenary session at the AAP annual meeting in 2011, raising awareness of the pediatrician's role in supporting breastfeeding. During the same period, the *Healthy People 2020* goals were released, and for the first time since breastfeeding targets were first set in 1979, the targets were raised for initiation and 6-month and 12-month duration. Additional targets were set for exclusive breastfeeding at 3 and 6 months, and goals were added for decreasing the supplementation of breastfed newborns in the early postpartum period, and increasing the number of newborns delivered at hospitals that implement the Ten Steps to Successful Breastfeeding. The Centers for Disease Control and Prevention followed with grant support to fund the National Initiative for Children's Healthcare Quality in the Best Fed Beginning project with an aim to add 90 new hospitals to the already 143 designated Baby-Friendly hospitals in the United States (as of May 2012). Additional encouragement came from The Joint Commissions Perinatal Care Core Measure (PC-05), which measures the rate of exclusive breast milk feeding within the delivery hospital. Furthermore, recent changes to the WIC package were developed to encourage exclusive breastfeeding and decrease the incentive to supplement with infant formula. However, with all of these new and exciting federal strategies to increase support for breastfeeding comes an even more urgent need to measure the evidence.[85]

In the near future there will be 2 additional federal campaigns to increase awareness and support for breastfeeding. The US Department of Agriculture has commissioned the Institute of Medicine to determine the best social marketing campaign to follow up on the prior WIC "Loving Support Makes Breastfeeding Work campaign." The Office of Women's Health has been developing another campaign targeting African American women in an attempt to decrease racial disparities in breastfeeding initiation and continuation. Similarly, rigorous evaluations must be part of these plans to determine the most effective method of messaging and using social media.

Finally, there are several legislative strategies undertaken by states to protect a woman's right to breastfeed in public and to provide support in the workplace. Federally, the ACA law provides further support in the workplace, but there are still a few provisions lacking. These are proposed as the Breastfeeding Promotion Act (BPA) of 2011. The BPA of 2011 has been proposed in the House as H. R. 2758 and Senate as S. 1463 to amend the Civil Rights Act of 1964 to protect new breastfeeding mothers from being fired or discriminated in the workplace and to provide reasonable break time for nursing mothers. Despite many states having laws to protect breastfeeding mothers' rights, the effects of these laws on overall support and breastfeeding exclusivity and duration have yet to be determined.[86]

FUTURE RESEARCH

As many more US hospitals seek Baby-Friendly designation, breastfeeding will become more apparent in the community. Additional research is needed to determine the best methods of support during the preconception period to prepare women to exclusively breastfeed as a cultural norm and to enter pregnancy with the intent to breastfeed according to public health recommendations. In addition to outcomes-focused research, studies are needed to determine the cost-benefit analyses of breastfeeding support programs and interventions in various health care settings. Rigorous evaluation of government activities and programs aimed at supporting

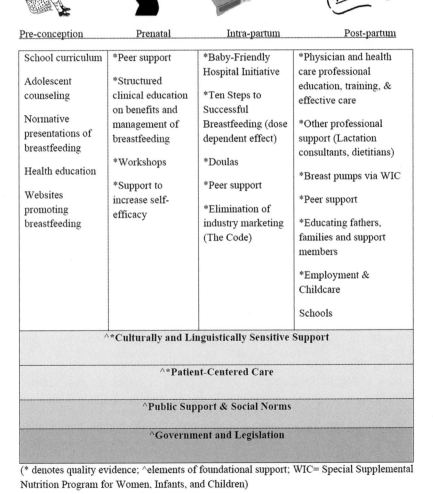

Pre-conception	Prenatal	Intra-partum	Post-partum
School curriculum	*Peer support	*Baby-Friendly Hospital Initiative	*Physician and health care professional education, training, & effective care
Adolescent counseling	*Structured clinical education on benefits and management of breastfeeding	*Ten Steps to Successful Breastfeeding (dose dependent effect)	*Other professional support (Lactation consultants, dietitians)
Normative presentations of breastfeeding			
Health education	*Workshops	*Doulas	*Breast pumps via WIC
Websites promoting breastfeeding	*Support to increase self-efficacy	*Peer support	*Peer support
		*Elimination of industry marketing (The Code)	*Educating fathers, families and support members
			*Employment & Childcare
			Schools

^*Culturally and Linguistically Sensitive Support
^*Patient-Centered Care
^Public Support & Social Norms
^Government and Legislation

(* denotes quality evidence; ^elements of foundational support; WIC= Special Supplemental Nutrition Program for Women, Infants, and Children)

Fig. 3. Schematic approach using a life cycle timeline to identify potential evidence-based opportunities for interventions.

breastfeeding must also be conducted to determine the most effective strategies. For programs that involve multiple dimensions of support, research study designs should allow for evaluation of individual components. Finally, it is important to determine ways to create public support for women to exclusively breastfeed for 6 months and continue to breastfeed for at least 1 year, so that the nation can reach *Healthy People 2020* goals for breastfeeding.

SUMMARY

Considerable progress has been made in the past decade in developing comprehensive support systems to enable more women to reach their breastfeeding goals. Given that most women in the United States participate in some breastfeeding, it is essential that each of these support systems be rigorously tested and, if effective, replicated. To summarize the domains of support, **Fig. 3** provides a schematic approach using a life cycle timeline to identify potential evidence-based opportunities for interventions.

REFERENCES

1. American Academy of Pediatrics, Section on Breastfeeding. Breastfeeding and the use of human milk. Pediatrics 2012;129(3):e827.
2. Ip S, Chung M, Raman G, et al. Breastfeeding and maternal and infant health outcomes in developed countries. Evid Rep Technol Assess (Full Rep) 2007;(153):1–186.
3. Kruse L, Denk CE, Feldman-Winter L, et al. Longitudinal patterns of breastfeeding initiation. Matern Child Health J 2006;10(1):13–8. http://dx.doi.org/10.1007/s 10995-005-0027-1.
4. Lumbiganon P, Martis R, Laopaiboon M, et al. Antenatal breastfeeding education for increasing breastfeeding duration. Cochrane Database Syst Rev 2011;(11):CD006425. http://dx.doi.org/10.1002/14651858.CD006425.pub2.
5. Beal AC, Kuhlthau K, Perrin JM. Breastfeeding advice given to African American and white women by physicians and WIC counselors. Public Health Rep 2003; 118(4):368–76.
6. Baby-Friendly USA INC. Guidelines and evaluation criteria for facilities seeking Baby-Friendly designation. 2011. Available at: http://www.babyfriendlyusa.org/eng/docs/2010_Guidelines_Criteria_4.19.11.pdf. Accessed September 15, 2012.
7. Guise JM, Palda V, Westhoff C, et al. The effectiveness of primary care-based interventions to promote breastfeeding: systematic evidence review and meta-analysis for the US Preventive Services Task Force. Ann Fam Med 2003;1(2): 70–8.
8. Ingram L, MacArthur C, Khan K, et al. Effect of antenatal peer support on breastfeeding initiation: a systematic review. CMAJ 2010;182(16):1739–46. http://dx.doi.org/10.1503/cmaj.091729.
9. Chung M, Raman G, Trikalinos T, et al. Interventions in primary care to promote breastfeeding: an evidence review for the U.S. Preventive Services Task Force. Ann Intern Med 2008;149(8):565–82.
10. Noel-Weiss J, Bassett V, Cragg B. Developing a prenatal breastfeeding workshop to support maternal breastfeeding self-efficacy. J Obstet Gynecol Neonatal Nurs 2006;35(3):349–57. http://dx.doi.org/10.1111/j.1552-6909.2006.00053.x.

11. U.S. Preventive Services Task Force. Primary care interventions to promote breastfeeding: U.S. Preventive Services Task Force recommendation statement. Ann Intern Med 2008;149(8):560–4.

12. Chapman DJ, Perez-Escamilla R. Breastfeeding among minority women: moving from risk factors to interventions. Adv Nutr 2012;3(1):95–104. http://dx.doi.org/10.3945/an.111.001016.

13. Lepe M, Bacardi Gascon M, Castaneda-Gonzalez LM, et al. Effect of maternal obesity on lactation: systematic review. Nutr Hosp 2011;26(6):1266–9. http://dx.doi.org/10.1590/S0212-16112011000600012.

14. Howard C, Howard F, Lawrence R, et al. Office prenatal formula advertising and its effect on breast-feeding patterns. Obstet Gynecol 2000;95(2):296–303.

15. Merewood A, Grossman X, Cook J, et al. US hospitals violate WHO policy on the distribution of formula sample packs: results of a national survey. J Hum Lact 2010;26(4):363–7. http://dx.doi.org/10.1177/0890334410376947.

16. Sadacharan R, Grossman X, Sanchez E, et al. Trends in US hospital distribution of industry-sponsored infant formula sample packs. Pediatrics 2011;128(4):702–5. http://dx.doi.org/10.1542/peds.2011-0983.

17. Salasibew M, Kiani A, Faragher B, et al. Awareness and reported violations of the WHO international code and Pakistan's national breastfeeding legislation; a descriptive cross-sectional survey. Int Breastfeed J 2008;3:24. http://dx.doi.org/10.1186/1746-4358-3-24.

18. McDonald SD, Pullenayegum E, Chapman B, et al. Prevalence and predictors of exclusive breastfeeding at hospital discharge. Obstet Gynecol 2012;119(6):1171–9. http://dx.doi.org/10.1097/AOG.0b013e318256194b.

19. World Health Organization. Baby-Friendly Hospital Initiative: revised, updated, and expanded for integrated care. 2009. Available at: http://www.who.int/nutrition/publications/infantfeeding/9789241594950/en/index.html. Accessed September 14, 2012.

20. Merewood A, Mehta SD, Chamberlain LB, et al. Breastfeeding rates in US Baby-Friendly hospitals: results of a national survey. Pediatrics 2005;116(3):628–34. http://dx.doi.org/10.1542/peds.2004-1636.

21. Merewood A, Patel B, Newton KN, et al. Breastfeeding duration rates and factors affecting continued breastfeeding among infants born at an inner-city US Baby-Friendly hospital. J Hum Lact 2007;23(2):157–64. http://dx.doi.org/10.1177/0890334407300573.

22. Philipp BL, Merewood A, Miller LW, et al. Baby-Friendly Hospital Initiative improves breastfeeding initiation rates in a US hospital setting. Pediatrics 2001;108(3):677–81.

23. Philipp BL, Malone KL, Cimo S, et al. Sustained breastfeeding rates at a US baby-friendly hospital. Pediatrics 2003;112(3 Pt 1):e234–6.

24. DiGirolamo AM, Grummer-Strawn LM, Fein SB. Effect of maternity-care practices on breastfeeding. Pediatrics 2008;122(Suppl 2):S43–9. http://dx.doi.org/10.1542/peds.2008-1315e.

25. Mellin PS, Poplawski DT, Gole A, et al. Impact of a formal breastfeeding education program. MCN Am J Matern Child Nurs 2011;36(2):82–8. http://dx.doi.org/10.1097/NMC.0b013e318205589e [quiz: 89–90].

26. Chalmers B. The Baby Friendly Hospital Initiative: where next? BJOG 2004;111(3):198–9.

27. Nyqvist KH, Haggkvist AP, Hansen MN, et al. Expansion of the Ten Steps to successful breastfeeding into neonatal intensive care: expert group

recommendations for three guiding principles. J Hum Lact 2012;28(3):289–96. http://dx.doi.org/10.1177/0890334412441862.

28. Merewood A, Philipp BL, Chawla N, et al. The Baby-Friendly Hospital Initiative increases breastfeeding rates in a US neonatal intensive care unit. J Hum Lact 2003;19(2):166–71.

29. Bettinelli ME, Chapin EM, Cattaneo A. Establishing the Baby-Friendly community initiative in Italy: development, strategy, and implementation. J Hum Lact 2012; 28(3):297–303. http://dx.doi.org/10.1177/0890334412447994.

30. Donnelly A, Snowden HM, Renfrew MJ, et al. Commercial hospital discharge packs for breastfeeding women. Cochrane Database Syst Rev 2000;(2):CD002075. http://dx.doi.org/10.1002/14651858.CD002075.

31. Dungy CI, Losch ME, Russell D, et al. Hospital infant formula discharge packages. Do they affect the duration of breast-feeding? Arch Pediatr Adolesc Med 1997;151(7):724–9.

32. Rosenberg KD, Eastham CA, Kasehagen LJ, et al. Marketing infant formula through hospitals: the impact of commercial hospital discharge packs on breastfeeding. Am J Public Health 2008;98(2):290–5. http://dx.doi.org/10.2105/AJPH.2006.103218.

33. Feldman-Winter L, Grossman X, Palaniappan A, et al. Removal of industry-sponsored formula sample packs from the hospital: does it make a difference? J Hum Lact 2012;28(3):380–8. http://dx.doi.org/10.1177/0890334412444350.

34. Nommsen-Rivers LA, Mastergeorge AM, Hansen RL, et al. Doula care, early breastfeeding outcomes, and breastfeeding status at 6 weeks postpartum among low-income primiparae. J Obstet Gynecol Neonatal Nurs 2009;38(2): 157–73. http://dx.doi.org/10.1111/j.1552-6909.2009.01005.x.

35. Newton KN, Chaudhuri J, Grossman X, et al. Factors associated with exclusive breastfeeding among Latina women giving birth at an inner-city baby-friendly hospital. J Hum Lact 2009;25(1):28–33. http://dx.doi.org/10.1177/0890334408329437.

36. Scott KD, Klaus PH, Klaus MH. The obstetrical and postpartum benefits of continuous support during childbirth. J Womens Health Gend Based Med 1999;8(10): 1257–64.

37. Gilliland AL. Beyond holding hands: the modern role of the professional doula. J Obstet Gynecol Neonatal Nurs 2002;31(6):762–9.

38. Haider R, Ashworth A, Kabir I, et al. Effect of community-based peer counsellors on exclusive breastfeeding practices in Dhaka, Bangladesh: a randomised controlled trial [see comments]. Lancet 2000;356(9242):1643–7.

39. Kistin N, Abramson R, Dublin P. Effect of peer counselors on breastfeeding initiation, exclusivity, and duration among low-income urban women. J Hum Lact 1994;10(1):11–5.

40. Kaunonen M, Hannula L, Tarkka MT. A systematic review of peer support interventions for breastfeeding. J Clin Nurs 2012;21(13–14):1943–54. http://dx.doi.org/10.1111/j.1365-2702.2012.04071.x.

41. Frick KD, Pugh LC, Milligan RA. Costs related to promoting breastfeeding among urban low-income women. J Obstet Gynecol Neonatal Nurs 2011. http://dx.doi.org/10.1111/j.1552-6909.2011.01316.x.

42. Joanna Briggs Institute. Best practice information sheet: women's perceptions and experiences of breastfeeding support. Nurs Health Sci 2012;14(1):133–5. http://dx.doi.org/10.1111/j.1442-2018.2012.00679.x.

43. Paul IM, Beiler JS, Schaefer EW, et al. A randomized trial of single home nursing visits vs office-based care after nursery/maternity discharge: the Nurses for Infants Through Teaching and Assessment after the Nursery (NITTANY) study.

Arch Pediatr Adolesc Med 2012;166(3):263–70. http://dx.doi.org/10.1001/archpediatrics.2011.198.

44. Dennis CL, Kingston D. A systematic review of telephone support for women during pregnancy and the early postpartum period. J Obstet Gynecol Neonatal Nurs 2008;37(3):301–14. http://dx.doi.org/10.1111/j.1552-6909.2008.00235.x.

45. American Academy of Pediatrics. Supporting breastfeeding and lactation: the primary care pediatrician's guide to getting paid. 2010. Available at: http://www2.aap.org/breastfeeding/files/pdf/coding.pdf. Accessed September 14, 2012.

46. Feldman-Winter LB, Schanler RJ, O'Connor KG, et al. Pediatricians and the promotion and support of breastfeeding. Arch Pediatr Adolesc Med 2008; 162(12):1142–9. http://dx.doi.org/10.1001/archpedi.162.12.1142.

47. Freed GL, Clark SJ, Sorenson J, et al. National assessment of physicians' breastfeeding knowledge, attitudes, training, and experience. JAMA 1995;273(6):472–6.

48. Taveras EM, Li R, Grummer-Strawn L, et al. Mothers' and clinicians' perspectives on breastfeeding counseling during routine preventive visits. Pediatrics 2004; 113(5):e405–11.

49. Taveras EM, Li R, Grummer-Strawn L, et al. Opinions and practices of clinicians associated with continuation of exclusive breastfeeding. Pediatrics 2004;113(4): e283–90.

50. Noble LM, Noble A, Hand IL. Cultural competence of healthcare professionals caring for breastfeeding mothers in urban areas. Breastfeed Med 2009;4(4): 221–4. http://dx.doi.org/10.1089/bfm.2009.0020.

51. Hellings P, Howe C. Breastfeeding knowledge and practice of pediatric nurse practitioners. J Pediatr Health Care 2004;18(1):8–14.

52. Anchondo I, Berkeley L, Mulla ZD, et al. Pediatricians', obstetricians', gynecologists', and family medicine physicians' experiences with and attitudes about breast-feeding. South Med J 2012;105(5):243–8. http://dx.doi.org/10.1097/SMJ.0b013e3182522927.

53. Power ML, Locke E, Chapin J, et al. The effort to increase breast-feeding. Do obstetricians, in the forefront, need help? J Reprod Med 2003;48(2):72–8.

54. Feldman-Winter L, Barone L, Milcarek B, et al. Residency curriculum improves breastfeeding care. Pediatrics 2010;126(2):289–97. http://dx.doi.org/10.1542/peds.2009-3250.

55. Labarere J, Gelbert-Baudino N, Ayral AS, et al. Efficacy of breastfeeding support provided by trained clinicians during an early, routine, preventive visit: a prospective, randomized, open trial of 226 mother-infant pairs. Pediatrics 2005;115(2): e139–46. http://dx.doi.org/10.1542/peds.2004-1362.

56. O'Connor ME, Brown EW, Lewin LO. An Internet-based education program improves breastfeeding knowledge of maternal-child healthcare providers. Breastfeed Med 2011;6(6):421–7. http://dx.doi.org/10.1089/bfm.2010.0061.

57. University of Virginia Health System and Virginia Department of Health. Breastfeeding Friendly Performance Improvement Project. 2011. Available at: http://www.breastfeedingpi.org/Login.aspx?lgt=1. Accessed September 14, 2012.

58. American Academy of Pediatrics. Education in quality improvement for pediatric practice: safe and healthy beginnings. 2011. Available at: http://www.eqipp.org/. Accessed September 14, 2012.

59. United States Breastfeeding Committee, editor. Core competencies in breastfeeding care for all health professionals. Washington, DC: United States Breastfeeding Committee; 2009. Available at: http://www.usbreastfeeding.org/Portals/0/Publications/Core-Competencies-2010-rev.pdf. Accessed October 23, 2012.

60. Shaikh U, Smillie CM. Physician-led outpatient breastfeeding medicine clinics in the United States. Breastfeed Med 2008;3(1):28–33. http://dx.doi.org/10.1089/bfm.2007.0011.

61. Thomas JR, Shaikh U. Use of electronic communication by physician breastfeeding experts for support of the breastfeeding mother. Breastfeed Med 2012. http://dx.doi.org/10.1089/bfm.2011.0133.

62. Furman LM, Dickinson C. Community health workers: collaborating to support breastfeeding among high-risk inner-city mothers. Breastfeed Med 2012. http://dx.doi.org/10.1089/bfm.2012.0027.

63. Wambach K, Campbell SH, Gill SL, et al. Clinical lactation practice: 20 years of evidence. J Hum Lact 2005;21(3):245–58. http://dx.doi.org/10.1177/0890334405279001.

64. Witt AM, Smith S, Mason MJ, et al. Integrating routine lactation consultant support into a pediatric practice. Breastfeed Med 2012;7(1):38–42. http://dx.doi.org/10.1089/bfm.2011.0003.

65. James DC, Lessen R, American Dietetic Association. Position of the American Dietetic Association: promoting and supporting breastfeeding. J Am Diet Assoc 2009;109(11):1926–42.

66. Sheppard JJ, Fletcher KR. Evidence-based interventions for breast and bottle feeding in the neonatal intensive care unit. Semin Speech Lang 2007;28(3):204–12. http://dx.doi.org/10.1055/s-2007-984726.

67. Meedya S, Fahy K, Kable A. Factors that positively influence breastfeeding duration to 6 months: a literature review. Women Birth 2010;23(4):135–45. http://dx.doi.org/10.1016/j.wombi.2010.02.002.

68. Razurel C, Bruchon-Schweitzer M, Dupanloup A, et al. Stressful events, social support and coping strategies of primiparous women during the postpartum period: a qualitative study. Midwifery 2011;27(2):237–42. http://dx.doi.org/10.1016/j.midw.2009.06.005.

69. de Montigny F, Lacharite C, Devault A. Transition to fatherhood: modeling the experience of fathers of breastfed infants. ANS Adv Nurs Sci 2012;35(3):E11–22. http://dx.doi.org/10.1097/ANS.0b013e3182626167.

70. Schmied V, Beake S, Sheehan A, et al. Women's perceptions and experiences of breastfeeding support: a metasynthesis. Birth 2011;38(1):49–60. http://dx.doi.org/10.1111/j.1523-536X.2010.00446.x.

71. Chen PG, Johnson LW, Rosenthal MS. Sources of education about breastfeeding and breast pump use: what effect do they have on breastfeeding duration? An analysis of the infant feeding practices survey II. Matern Child Health J 2011. http://dx.doi.org/10.1007/s10995-011-0908-4.

72. Haughton J, Gregorio D, Perez-Escamilla R. Factors associated with breastfeeding duration among Connecticut Special Supplemental Nutrition Program for Women, Infants, and Children (WIC) participants. J Hum Lact 2010;26(3):266–73. http://dx.doi.org/10.1177/0890334410365067.

73. Gross SM, Resnik AK, Nanda JP, et al. Early postpartum: a critical period in setting the path for breastfeeding success. Breastfeed Med 2011;6(6):407–12. http://dx.doi.org/10.1089/bfm.2010.0089.

74. Drago R, Hayes J, Yi Y, editors. Better health care for mothers and children: breastfeeding accommodations under the Affordable Care Act. Washington, DC: Institute for Women's Policy Research; 2010. p.1-20. Available at: http://www.iwpr.org. Accessed October 23, 2012.

75. US Department of Health and Human Services (DHSS), Health Resources and Services Administration (HRSA), Maternal and Child Health Bureau. The business

case for breastfeeding. 2008. Available at: http://mchb.hrsa.gov/pregnancy andbeyond/breastfeeding/. Accessed September 14, 2012.

76. Ogbuanu C, Glover S, Probst J, et al. Balancing work and family: effect of employment characteristics on breastfeeding. J Hum Lact 2011;27(3):225–38. http://dx.doi.org/10.1177/0890334410394860 [quiz: 293–5].

77. Bettinelli ME. Breastfeeding policies and breastfeeding support programs in the mother's workplace. J Matern Fetal Neonatal Med 2012;25(Suppl 4):73–4. http://dx.doi.org/10.3109/14767058.2012.715033.

78. Spear HJ. School nurses and teachers: attitudes regarding inclusion of breast-feeding education in school curricula. J Sch Nurs 2010;26(2):137–46. http://dx.doi.org/10.1177/1059840509350739.

79. Feldman-Winter L, Shaikh U. Optimizing breastfeeding promotion and support in adolescent mothers. J Hum Lact 2007;23(4):362–7. http://dx.doi.org/10.1177/0890334407308303.

80. Grassley JS. Adolescent mothers' breastfeeding social support needs. J Obstet Gynecol Neonatal Nurs 2010;39(6):713–22. http://dx.doi.org/10.1111/j.1552-6909.2010.01181.x.

81. Meglio GD, McDermott MP, Klein JD. A randomized controlled trial of telephone peer support's influence on breastfeeding duration in adolescent mothers. Breastfeed Med 2010;5(1):41–7. http://dx.doi.org/10.1089/bfm.2009.0016.

82. Grassley JS, Spencer BS, Bryson D. The development and psychometric testing of the supportive needs of adolescents breastfeeding scale. J Adv Nurs 2012. http://dx.doi.org/10.1111/j.1365-2648.2012.06119.x.

83. Galvin S, Grossman X, Feldman-Winter L, et al. A practical intervention to increase breastfeeding initiation among cambodian women in the US. Matern Child Health J 2008;12(4):545–7. http://dx.doi.org/10.1007/s10995-007-0263-7.

84. US Department of Health and Human Services, editor. The surgeon general's call to action to support breastfeeding. Washington, DC: US Department of Health and Human Services, Office of the Surgeon General; 2011. p. 1-87. Available at: http://www.surgeongeneral.gov/library/calls/breastfeeding/calltoactiontosupport breastfeeding.pdf. Accessed October 23, 2012.

85. Perez-Escamilla R, Chapman DJ. Breastfeeding protection, promotion, and support in the united states: a time to nudge, a time to measure. J Hum Lact 2012;28(2):118–21. http://dx.doi.org/10.1177/0890334412436721.

86. Nguyen TT, Hawkins SS. Current state of US breastfeeding laws. Matern Child Nutr 2012. http://dx.doi.org/10.1111/j.1740-8709.2011.00392.x.

Human Milk for the Premature Infant

Mark A. Underwood, MD, MAS

KEYWORDS

• Human milk • Premature infant • Necrotizing enterocolitis • Donor milk • Lactation

KEY POINTS

- Fortified mother's own milk is the optimal diet for the premature infant to maximize growth, development, and protection against necrotizing enterocolitis and infection.
- Fortified pasteurized human donor milk is recommended by the American Academy of Pediatrics Section on Breastfeeding as the preferred alternative for premature infants whose mothers are unable to provide a sufficient volume of their own milk.
- Pasteurized donor human milk does not provide the same nutrient or biologically active molecules as unpasteurized own mother's milk.
- Careful attention to establishing and maintaining milk production in women delivering preterm has significant benefits.

Human milk provides the optimal nutrition for term infants. Human milk is also recommended for preterm infants, but does not alone provide optimal nutrition. The growth and neurodevelopmental needs of the evolutionarily new population of very premature infants are best met by appropriate fortification of human milk. To explore the role of human milk in the care of premature infants, it is appropriate to begin with a comparison of amniotic fluid (the optimal beverage of the fetus), milk from mothers delivering preterm, and milk from mothers delivering at term. We then consider the benefits and challenges of providing human milk to premature infants, approaches to human milk fortification, the advantages and challenges of donor human milk products, and finally some practical approaches to increasing human milk consumption in premature infants.

In the United States, approximately 12% of infants are born preterm (<37 weeks gestation).[1] This is a very heterogeneous population with widely diverse nutritional

Funding sources: Eunice K. Shriver National Institute of Child Health and Human Development Grant HD059127. The author has received nutritional products from Prolacta Bioscience for clinical trials.
Disclosure: The authors have nothing to disclose.
Department of Pediatrics, University of California Davis, 2516 Stockton Boulevard, Sacramento, CA 95817, USA
E-mail address: munderwood@ucdavis.edu

Pediatr Clin N Am 60 (2013) 189–207
http://dx.doi.org/10.1016/j.pcl.2012.09.008
0031-3955/13/$ – see front matter © 2013 Elsevier Inc. All rights reserved.

requirements and highly different stages of immunocompetence. A 2.5-kg neonate born at 34 weeks gestation differs from a 500-g neonate born at 24 weeks gestation in essentially every physiologic aspect of the gastrointestinal system and the innate and adaptive immune systems. Consequently, the current body of knowledge about nutrition and host defense of premature infants has many gaps. Studies performed on larger, older premature infants may not be applicable to the extremely low birth weight infants (<1000 g) that now survive routinely.

AMNIOTIC FLUID, "PREMATURE" HUMAN MILK, AND "TERM" HUMAN MILK

Amniotic fluid contains amino acids, proteins, vitamins, minerals, hormones, and growth factors. Although the concentration of these nutrients is much lower than that found in human milk, the large volumes of amniotic fluid swallowed in utero (up to 1 liter a day late in gestation, considerably more than the newborn consumes after birth) have a significant impact on growth and maturation of both the fetus and the fetal intestine.[2] Animal studies and limited human observations suggest that swallowed amniotic fluid accounts for about 15% of fetal growth.[3–5]

Milk from women who deliver prematurely differs from that of women who deliver at term. Preterm milk is initially higher in protein, fat, free amino acids, and sodium, but over the first few weeks following delivery these levels decrease (**Fig. 1**A). The mineral content (including trace minerals) of preterm milk is similar to that of term milk, with the following exceptions: Calcium is significantly lower in preterm milk than term milk and does not seem to increase over time, whereas copper and zinc content are both higher in preterm milk than term milk and decrease over the time of lactation.[6,7]

Lactose is the major carbohydrate in human milk. This disaccharide is an important energy source, is relatively low in colostrum, and increases over time with more dramatic increases in preterm milk (see **Fig. 1**A). Complex oligosaccharides are the second most abundant carbohydrate in human milk. These human milk oligosaccharides (HMOs) are not digestible by host glycosidases and yet are produced in large amounts with highly variable structures by the mother.[8] HMOs seem to have 3 important functions: Prebiotic (stimulation of commensal bacteria containing the bacterial glycosidases to deconstruct and consume the HMOs),[9,10] decoy (structural similarity to the glycans on enterocytes allows HMOs to competitively bind to pathogens),[11] and provision of fucose and sialic acid, which seem to be important in host defense and neurodevelopment, respectively.[12] Preterm milk is highly variable in HMO content with differences between populations[13] and significant variability over time in content of fucosylated HMOs in individual mothers delivering preterm.[14] Glycosaminoglycans also seem to act as decoys, providing binding sites for pathogenic bacteria to prevent adherence to the enterocyte. Premature milk is richer in glycosaminoglycans than term milk.[15]

Bioactive molecules in human milk are important components of the innate immune system. Differences in cytokines, growth factors, and lactoferrin between preterm and term milk are most dramatic in colostrum and early milk and mostly resolve by 4 weeks after delivery (see **Fig. 1**B). Leptin is produced by mammary glands, secreted into human milk, and may be important in post-natal growth. Human milk leptin does not seem to differ between preterm and term milk.[16] Bile salt-stimulated lipase activity is similar in term and preterm milk, whereas lipoprotein lipase activity is higher in term milk.[17]

BENEFITS OF HUMAN MILK FOR PREMATURE INFANTS

The most recent policy statement from the Section on Breastfeeding of the American Academy of Pediatrics represents a significant shift from previous statements in its

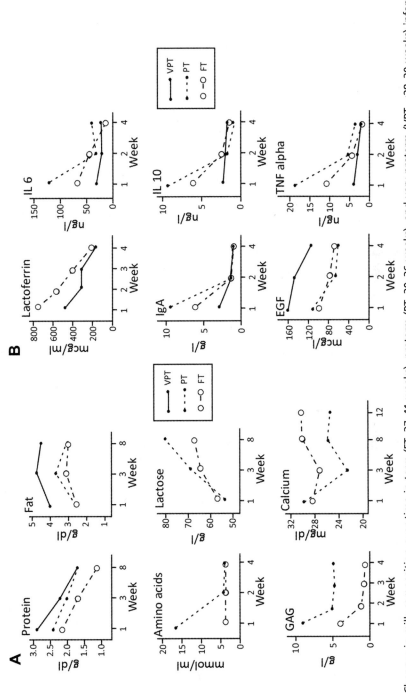

Fig. 1. Changes in milk composition over time in term (FT, 37–41 weeks), preterm (PT, 30–36 weeks), and very preterm (VPT, <28–30 weeks) infants. Nutrients (A); Bioactive molecules (B). EGF, epidermal growth factor; GAG, glycosaminoglycans; IL-6, interleukin 6; IgA, immunoglobulin A; IL-10, interleukin 10; TNF-alpha, tumor necrosis factor alpha. (*Data from* Refs.[15,82,115–122])

recommendation that all preterm infants should receive human milk, with pasteurized donor milk rather than premature infant formula the preferred alternative if a mother is unable to provide an adequate volume.[18] The current recommendation is based on an impressive array of benefits that human milk provides to this highly vulnerable population, including decreased rates of late-onset sepsis,[19] necrotizing enterocolitis (NEC),[20,21] and retinopathy of prematurity,[22,23] fewer re-hospitalizations in the first year of life,[24] and improved neurodevelopmental outcomes.[24–26] In addition, premature infants who receive human milk have lower rates of metabolic syndrome, lower blood pressure[27] and low-density lipoprotein levels,[28] and less insulin and leptin resistance[29] when they reach adolescence, compared with premature infants receiving formula.

Among these benefits, perhaps the most compelling benefit of human milk feeding is the observed decrease in NEC, given its high prevalence (5%–10% of all infants with birth weight <1500 g), high case fatality, and long-term morbidity owing to complications like strictures, cholestasis, short-bowel syndrome, and poor growth and neurodevelopment.[30] For many of these outcomes, there seems to be a dose response effect of human milk feeding. For instance, a dose of mother's own milk of more than 50 mL/kg per day decreases the risk of late-onset sepsis and NEC compared with less than 50 mL/kg per day,[21,31] and for each 10 mL/kg per day increase in human milk in the diet there is a 5% reduction in hospital readmission rate.[26] The mechanisms by which human milk protects the premature infant against NEC are likely multifactorial. Human milk secretory immunoglobulin A, lactoferrin, lysozyme, bile salt-stimulating lipase, growth factors, and HMOs all provide protective benefits that could potentially contribute to reduction in NEC. In a multicenter, randomized clinical trial, bovine lactoferrin treatment decreased late-onset sepsis but not NEC in premature infants.[32] Recombinant human lactoferrin trials are currently in progress in premature infants (clinicaltrials.gov NCT00854633). In animal models, epidermal growth factor[33] and pooled HMOs[34] prevent NEC, but these have not yet been tested in premature infants.

Microbial colonization is thought to play an important role in risk of NEC.[35,36] Breastfeeding is one of many factors that influence the composition of the intestinal microbiota in term infants[37]; limited studies suggest that diet may have less of an effect on the composition of the intestinal microbiota in the premature infant than other factors (such as antibiotic administration).[38] New bioinformatic tools to correlate the extensive array of fecal metabolites and the fecal microbiota offer great promise in understanding the factors that influence the microbiota of the premature infant. Studies to date suggest that the metabolites differing between human milk-fed and formula-fed infants that are most closely associated with shaping the microbiota include sugars and fatty acids.[39] Whether and how these metabolites differ functionally in the extremely premature infant is unknown.

Other potential benefits of human milk to premature infants have been studied with mixed results. There do not seem to be consistent benefits of human milk in premature infants in relation to feeding tolerance,[19] time to full enteral feeding,[24] or allergic/atopic outcomes.[40] Providing human milk has been postulated to decrease parental anxiety, and increase skin-to-skin contact and parent–infant bonding, but data to support these hypotheses are limited. The provision of human colostrum in the form of oral care for intubated premature infants has been proposed as a method of stimulating the oropharyngeal-associated lymphatic tissue and altering the oral microbiota, but data to support this intervention are lacking.[41]

Studies of the benefits of human milk in premature infants to date have predominantly compared mother's own milk with premature infant formula. Whether pasteurized donor human milk (which generally is provided by women who delivered at term) provides similar or superior protection is unclear. In premature infants receiving only mother's own milk or pasteurized donor human milk (no formula), increasing amounts of mother's own milk correlate with better weight gain and less NEC.[42] A meta-analysis in 2007 concluded that formula feeding was associated with both increased short-term growth and increased incidence of NEC compared with donor human milk feeding (relative risk, 2.5; 95% confidence interval [CI], 1.2–5.1), number needed to harm 33 (95% CI, 17–100) with no differences in long-term growth or neurodevelopment.[43] However, of the 8 studies included in the meta-analysis, 7 were published before 1990, during which time nutritional comparisons were limited. For example, several of the reviewed studies did not include formulas designed for premature infants and none included nutrient-enriched donor milk. One study, initiated in 1982, followed a cohort of premature infants who received either premature infant formula or unfortified donor human milk with the latter group showing decreased blood pressure[27] and improved lipoprotein profiles as adolescents.[28] In the single included study published since 1990, infants whose mothers were unable to provide sufficient milk for their extremely premature infants (<30 weeks' gestation) were randomly assigned to receive supplementation with either premature infant formula or nutrient-enriched donor human milk; donor human milk led to slower weight gain, but did not decrease episodes of sepsis, or retinopathy of prematurity, length of hospital stay, or mortality compared with supplementation with premature infant formula. The incidence of NEC was decreased in the donor human milk group by almost half compared with the formula group, but this did not attain significance owing to the small sample size.[44] It is noteworthy in this study that, despite increased supplementation in the donor milk group, 20% of the infants were changed to formula because of poor growth. A more recent comparison of mother's own milk with pasteurized human donor milk demonstrated improved growth and less NEC with the former.[42]

CHALLENGES OF PROVIDING HUMAN MILK TO PREMATURE INFANTS

Providing human milk to very premature infants presents a variety of challenges. To maximize milk supply, new mothers should begin frequent pumping shortly after delivery. Mothers whose babies are in the neonatal intensive care unit (NICU) should be encouraged to begin pumping within 6 to 12 hours of delivery and to pump 8 to 12 times per day, ensuring that they empty the breast each time. These interventions significantly increase the likelihood that a premature infant will receive his mother's own milk.[45]

Perhaps the greatest concern in providing human milk to premature infants is growth. Term infants undergo rapid growth in the third trimester of pregnancy, receiving nutrition through the placenta and swallowed amniotic fluid with no need to expend calories for temperature regulation or gas exchange. Premature infants miss out on much or all of the third trimester and thus have higher nutritional requirements on a per kilogram basis than term infants. Human milk evolved/was designed to nourish the term infant who can tolerate large fluid volumes, whereas premature infants are less tolerant of high fluid volumes.

For these reasons, human milk is generally fortified for premature infants with birth weights of less than 1500 g. Human milk fortifier powders were developed from bovine milk to supplement key nutrients with particular emphasis on protein, calcium, phosphorus, and vitamin D. Fortification of human milk leads to improved growth in weight,[46] length, and head circumference[47]; however, improvements in bone mineralization and neurodevelopmental outcomes are unclear.[47] Recent studies suggest that higher protein intake is beneficial for premature infants.[48] There is large variation in the energy and protein content of human milk (between mothers, over time in a given mother, and between foremilk and hindmilk).[49] Protein content decreases over time of lactation and is likely to be much lower in donor human milk than milk from mothers delivering prematurely. Current NICU practices are often based on the clearly misleading assumption that human milk has approximately 0.67 kcal/mL with stable protein content. "Assumed" protein intake from standard fortification is significantly lower than actual protein intake.[50] These observations have led to clinical trials of "individualized" fortification, that is, adjusting the amount of added protein based on actual measurements of milk samples[51] or based on metabolic parameters indicative of protein accretion in the neonate (eg, blood urea nitrogen).[52] Both methods led to increased protein intake and improved growth. A recent trial of a human milk fortifier with higher protein content demonstrated increased growth and fewer infants with weight below the 10th percentile.[53]

Use of commercial human milk fortifiers, however, is not without complications, as demonstrated by the observation of a marked increase in metabolic acidosis associated with the introduction of a new fortifier.[54] Human milk fortifiers have also been associated with increased markers of oxidative stress compared with unfortified human milk and with infant formula.[55] In addition, bacterial contamination[56] of powdered infant formulas and associated sepsis[57] has been well documented, resulting in more than 100 cases of neonatal Cronobacter (Enterobacter sakazakii) infections leading to high mortality rates. This association has led to calls for "powder-free" NICUs and the development of new liquid human milk fortifiers. Unfortunately, one of the challenges of liquid fortifiers is displacement of the volume of mother's own milk, so that the infant receives less total volume of human milk. **Table 1** provides a comparison of the nutrient content and volume of human milk displaced by the liquid formulations of several commercial human milk fortifiers. Note that the use of the bovine liquid fortifiers means that 17% to 50% of the volume ingested is formula. The table also demonstrates the significant variation in macro- and micronutrients among these products.

PASTEURIZED DONOR HUMAN MILK FOR PREMATURE INFANTS

There are significant challenges in providing donor human milk for all premature infants whose mothers are unable to provide an adequate supply of their own milk: Nutrition, safety, supply, and immune protection. First, most donor human milk is provided by women who have delivered at term and have weaned their own infant but continue to pump and donate their milk in later lactation. As noted in **Fig. 1**, this milk from mothers of term infants, several months after delivery, is low in protein, fat, and many bioactive molecules compared with preterm milk provided in the first few weeks after delivery. A second challenge of providing donor milk is to minimize the potential to transmit infectious agents. For this reason, milk banks have rigid standards for screening and testing potential donors, for pasteurization, and for testing milk before distribution.[58,59] Pasteurization is highly effective at decreasing the risk of transmission of HIV, cytomegalovirus (CMV), hepatitis B, and hepatitis C. The costs involved in establishing and maintaining a milk bank are considerable; however, the feasibility of providing pasteurized donor milk in developing countries has been demonstrated.[60] Unpasteurized donor milk has been advocated for premature infants in areas where religious beliefs preclude the use of milk from unknown donors.[61,62] Further, "mother-to-mother milk-sharing" through Internet-based communities is a rapidly growing practice in more than 50 countries,[63] but health officials recommend against this practice owing to safety risks, including lack of pasteurization, uncertain storage and shipping processes, and uncertain medication and substance use in the donor.[64]

Unfortunately, although pasteurization safeguards against transmission of infectious agents, it also has detrimental effects on the bioactive components of human milk. The currently recommended Holder pasteurization method (62.5°C for 30 minutes) results in significant decreases in secretory immunoglobulin A, lactoferrin, lysozyme, insulin-like growth factors, hepatocyte growth factor, water-soluble vitamins, bile salt-stimulated lipase, lipoprotein lipase, and anti-oxidant activity, but does not decrease oligosaccharides, long-chain polyunsaturated fatty acids, gangliosides, lactose, fat-soluble vitamins, or epidermal growth factor.[65–69] Holder pasteurization increases some medium chain saturated fatty acids, decreases some cytokines (tumor necrosis factor-α, interferon-γ, interleukin (IL)-1β, and IL-10), and increases others (IL-8).[70] High-temperature, short-time pasteurization (72°C–75°C for 15–16 seconds) has been demonstrated to eliminate bacteria and many viruses[71,72] with less protein loss (including maintenance of bile salt stimulating lipase, lactoferrin, and some immunoglobulins),[73] less severe loss of antioxidant activity, but greater loss of antimicrobial activity.[66,74] In resource-poor countries, flash-heat treatment (temperature >56°C for 6 minutes 15 seconds) does not alter milk antibacterial activity against *Escherichia coli* and *Staphylococcus aureus*, only minimally decreases lactoferrin antibacterial activity, but significantly diminishes lysozyme antibacterial activity.[75] Further research to determine the optimal pasteurization method to minimize risk and maximize bioactivity has great potential benefit for premature infants.

A fundamental concern is that the supply of donor human milk is currently limited. There are 12 milk banks in the United States and Canada that form the Human Milk Banking Association of North America (www.hmbana.org). In 2011, Human Milk Banking Association of North America milk banks distributed more than 2 million ounces of donor milk (a 5-fold increase from 2000), and the International Breast Milk Project (www.breastmilkproject.org) has distributed more than 280,000 ounces of donor milk to infants in South Africa since its founding in 2006, but such distributions represent only a fraction of the potential demand. The scarcity of this precious resource raises questions about how to increase the supply and equitably allocate human milk.[76]

AN "ALL-HUMAN" DIET FOR PREMATURE INFANTS

The development of a human milk fortifier formulated by concentrating pasteurized donor human milk and then adding vitamins and minerals has created the possibility of providing an "all-human diet" to premature infants. Various caloric densities of this fortifier allow for individual adjustment based on growth or blood urea nitrogen. A small study demonstrated a decrease in both moderate and severe NEC in small premature infants (birth weight <1250 g) receiving the "all-human diet."[77] Unfortunately, this study was not adequately powered to study NEC as an outcome and the comparison group received formula if mother's milk supply was not adequate, whereas the "all-human" infants received donor human milk in such a situation (ie, the increase in NEC in the comparison group could be related to either the powdered bovine human milk fortifier or the premature infant formula). This study underscores the fundamental question of whether components of human milk are protective against NEC or components of bovine milk somehow induce NEC. These 2 possibilities are, of course, not mutually exclusive. The cost of providing a fortifier made from donor human milk is significant. A recent cost-benefit analysis suggested that the savings in NEC prevention outweigh the costs of the "all-human" strategy; however, this analysis was based

Table 1
Nutrient content of commonly used human milk fortifiers in North America

	Enfamil Human Milk Fortifier Acidified Liquid (4 Vials = 20 mL) Add to 100 mL EBM	Similac Special Care 30 Cal/oz (50 mL) Add to 50 mL EBM	Prolact +4 H²MF (20 mL)[a] Add to 80 mL EBM	Similac Human Milk Fortifier (4 Packets = 3.6 g) Add to 100 mL EBM	Enfamil Human Milk Fortifier (4 Packets = 2.8 g) Add to 100 mL EBM
Formulation	Liquid	Liquid	Liquid	Powder	Powder
Protein source	Bovine	Bovine	Human	Bovine	Bovine
Calories	30	50	28	14	14
Protein (g)	2.2	1.5	1.2	1.0	1.1
Fat (g)	2.3	3.3	1.8	0.36	1
Carbohydrate (g)	<1.2	3.9	1.8	1.8	<0.4
Vitamin A (IU)	1160	625	61	620	950
Vitamin D (IU)	188	75	26	120	150
Vitamin E (IU)	5.6	2.0	0.4	3.2	4.6
Vitamin K (μg)	5.7	6.0	<0.2	8.3	4.4
Vitamin B1 (μg)	184	125	4	233	150
Vitamin B2 (μg)	260	310	15	417	220

Vitamin B6 (μg)	140	125	4.1	211	115
Vitamin B12 (μg)	0.64	0.27	0.05	0.64	0.18
Niacin (μg)	3700	2500	52.4	3570	3000
Folic acid (μg)	31	18.5	5.4	23	25
Pantothenic acid (μg)	920	950	74.8	1500	730
Biotin (μg)	3.4	18.5	Not available	26	2.7
Vitamin C (mg)	15.2	18.5	<0.2	25	12
Calcium (mg)	116	90	103	117	90
Phosphorus (mg)	63	50	53.8	67	50
Iron (mg)	1.76	0.9	0.1	0.35	1.44
Zinc (mg)	0.96	0.75	0.7	1.0	0.72
Copper (μg)	60	125	64	170	44
Manganese (μg)	10	6	<12	7.2	10
Sodium (mg)	27	22	37	15	16
Potassium (mg)	45	65	50	63	29
Chloride (mg)	28	41	29	38	13

Abbreviation: EBM, expressed breast milk.
[a] Values are averages and may vary.

on assumptions generated from the clinical trial described and may therefore overestimate the protective effect of this approach.[78] The ethical issues of marketing human milk for profit have recently been reviewed.[76]

IMPROVING BREASTFEEDING RATES FOR PREMATURE INFANTS

Premature labor and delivery are highly stressful to parents. Education regarding the importance and value of breastfeeding should begin during pregnancy and be reemphasized when premature delivery seems likely. As noted, pumping with an electric pump should be initiated within 6 to 12 hours of delivery and continued 8 to 12 times per 24 hours until the milk supply is well established.[45] Reassurance and encouragement are valuable, because new mothers are often worried and discouraged by the initial small volumes obtained. Early assistance by a nurse or lactation consultant is helpful in establishing an effective pumping regimen. Regular questioning by the NICU nurse or physician regarding milk supply is valuable to encourage early intervention when milk production decreases. Milk production decreases with maternal depression and increases with increased frequency of pumping and time spent skin-to-skin with the premature infant.[79]

Parents should be instructed in the proper labeling, storage, and transport of milk so that milk pumped at home arrives frozen in the NICU. Color-coded labeling of colostrum to ensure its early/immediate use is valuable. A recent study demonstrated that fresh human milk is stable in a 4°C refrigerator for 96 hours and does not need to be discarded after 24 or 72 hours as previously practiced.[80] Freezing and thawing of human milk may rupture fat globules, leading to adherence of lipid to plastic surfaces. For this reason, there may be benefit in avoiding continuous feedings of human milk when possible and positioning syringe pumps so that the syringe is near vertical.[81]

Differences in nutrient content between foremilk and hindmilk are well established. Hindmilk from women delivering preterm is higher in protein, fatty acids, energy, and fat-soluble vitamins than foremilk.[82,83] The practice of discarding the foremilk and feeding premature infants predominantly hindmilk has been shown to increase weight gain.[84,85] Hindmilk has higher viscosity and may be more difficult to express with an electric pump. The combination of hand expression and electric pumping has been shown to increase milk production[86] and fat content of expressed milk.[87] The benefits of increased hindmilk include not only increased calories, but increased polyunsaturated fats and increased absorption of fat-soluble vitamins.

It is common for women delivering prematurely to experience a decrease in milk production. Interventions to increase production include increased skin-to-skin time, stress reduction, careful attention to diet, sleep, and pumping schedule, and medications.[88] Domperidone is effective in increasing milk production.[89,90] Metoclopramide has also been studied as a galactogogue; however, studies to date are of limited quality and enthusiasm for this product is dampened by concerns about tardive dyskinesia. Herbal galactagogues are popular, with more than 15% of lactating women reporting use. Fenugreek (*Trigonella foenumgraexum*) is widely used with several anecdotal reports of increased milk supply within 24 to 72 hours in most women.[91] Two small, randomized, blinded, placebo-controlled trials are available in the medical literature. The first showed no difference in milk supply in women receiving capsules of fenugreek compared with the reference group.[92] The second showed an increase in milk production of almost double in women receiving tea containing fenugreek, fennel, raspberry leaf, and goat's rue compared with a placebo tea.[93] Maternal side effects include nausea, diarrhea, and exacerbation of asthma. Because fenugreek is a member of the pea family, mothers allergic to chickpeas, soybeans, or peanuts should avoid this remedy. It is worth noting that fenugreek can impart a maple syrup odor to the sweat and urine of both mother and infant. Studies of milk composition and amount of fenugreek in expressed milk have not been published. Milk thistle (*Silbum marianum*) has been demonstrated in a placebo-controlled trial to almost double milk production with no change in nutrient content of the milk or detectable levels of the active ingredient (silymarin).[94] Side effects seem to be rare and include nausea, diarrhea, and anaphylaxis. Shatavari (dried powdered *Asparagus racemosus* root) has been studied in 2 randomized, placebo-controlled, blinded studies, with 1 study demonstrating increased maternal prolactin levels and increased infant weight gain[95] and the other showing no benefit.[96] Side effects include runny nose, conjunctivitis, and contact dermatitis. Torbangun leaves (*Coleus amboinicus* Lour) added to a soup increased milk production in a randomized, blinded, placebo-controlled trial[92]; however, side effects were not mentioned and a commercial preparation is not available. Evidence of safety and efficacy of other herbal galactogogues including blessed thistle, fennel, and chasteberry is lacking. Detailed reviews of the existing data for herbal galactogogues are available.[88,97]

Successful transition from tube feedings to breastfeeding can be challenging. Skin-to-skin care begun as soon as the baby is stable improves hemodynamic stability without increasing energy expenditure.[98,99] Non-nutritive sucking (mother pumps first and then places the baby to the breast) can be attempted as soon as the baby is extubated and stable with success noted as early as 28 weeks corrected gestational age.[100] Most premature infants can begin nutritive sucking at about 32 weeks gestation. Assistance from an experienced nurse or lactation consultant is invaluable. Positioning that supports the mother's breast and the baby's head and neck are essential, with the cross-cradle and football holds being most effective. Early use of nipple shields increases milk intake and duration of breastfeeding.[101]

WITHHOLDING MOTHER'S OWN MILK FROM PREMATURE INFANTS

In most instances, provision of mother's own milk is optimal. The few circumstances in which mother's own milk should not be provided are discussed in Chapter 15. Although it is certainly plausible that premature infants with their immature immune systems are more vulnerable to infection, in most cases data regarding differences between premature and term infants in susceptibility to milk-associated infections are lacking. This section focuses on contraindications specific to premature infants.

Post-natal transmission of CMV through breast milk is a frequent occurrence given that approximately 50% of adults are carriers of CMV. Symptomatic post-natal CMV infection is rare in term infants, likely because of maternal antibody transfer in the third trimester. A recent meta-analysis found wide variation among studies with overall mean rate of CMV transmission via breast milk of 23%, a mean risk of symptomatic CMV infection of 3.7%, and a mean risk of sepsis-like symptoms of 0.7% with most symptomatic infections in premature infants.[102] Low birth weight and early transmission after birth are risk factors for symptomatic disease.[103] Whether CMV infection increases the severity of the diseases of prematurity (eg, chronic lung disease, NEC, periventricular leukomalacia) is unknown. Long-term studies of premature infants infected with CMV through mother's own milk are few, but suggest that hearing loss and severe neurodevelopmental delays are uncommon.[104,105] Pasteurization inactivates CMV; freezing may decrease but does not eliminate transmission of CMV.[106] There is no consensus among neonatologists and pediatricians regarding the best balance between the benefits of human milk and the risks of CMV infection.

Recommendations vary from pasteurizing all human milk until corrected gestational age of 32 weeks, to screening all mothers who deliver preterm and withholding colostrum and pasteurizing milk of women who are CMV IgG positive, to freezing all CMV-positive milk for premature infants younger than 32 weeks.

Drug abuse is common among pregnant and nursing women and increases the risk of premature delivery.[107,108] Long-term effects of in utero and post-natal exposure to these substances are unclear, but studies to date are concerning.[109,110] Whether the risks of continued exposure to these substances outweigh the benefits of human milk for the premature infant with its rapidly developing central nervous system is unclear. Current guidelines are to encourage mothers who abuse substances other than opiates to obtain counseling and to refrain from providing milk for their infants until they are free of the abused drugs.[111]

Treatment of depression in pregnancy and in breastfeeding women is an area of particular relevance given the reported associations between maternal antidepressant use and preterm labor,[112] neonatal seizures,[112] and neonatal primary pulmonary hypertension. Causality and the mechanisms underlying these associations are unknown. It is unclear whether the latter association in a small number of studies is related to the medications or to risk factors associated with both maternal depression and pulmonary hypertension (eg, obesity, smoking, prematurity, and cesarean delivery).[113] A recent review of antidepressant medication use in lactating women suggested caution in the use of fluoxetine and avoidance of doxepine and nefazodone.[114] Data specific to preterm infants or neonates with pulmonary hypertension are not available.

It is likely that in situations where mother's own milk should not be given, donor human milk would be advantageous. There are rare exceptions wherein an infant should receive no (eg, galactosemia) or limited volumes (eg, some inborn errors of metabolism and human milk protein intolerance) of human milk. These are particularly relevant to premature infants in whom the brain is developing rapidly.

SUMMARY

Fortified human milk has tremendous benefits in improving the growth and short- and long-term outcomes for the premature infant. Mother's own milk has clear advantages to donor human milk both owing to its composition and the lack of necessity for pasteurization. Increased efforts to establish and maintain milk supply in women delivering preterm are likely to have greater benefits than providing pasteurized donor human milk. Improved pasteurization protocols and carefully performed trials of galactogogues may be of particular value to this highly vulnerable population.

ACKNOWLEDGMENTS

The author wishes to thank Sarah Lueders, UC Davis Children's Hospital NICU dietitian, for assistance in compiling **Table 1**.

REFERENCES

1. Martin J, Hamilton B, Ventura S, et al. Births: final data for 2010. Natl Vital Stat Rep 2012;61(1):1–100.
2. Underwood MA, Gilbert WM, Sherman MP. Amniotic fluid: not just fetal urine anymore. J Perinatol 2005;25(5):341–8.

3. Pitkin RM, Reynolds WA. Fetal ingestion and metabolism of amniotic fluid protein. Am J Obstet Gynecol 1975;123(4):356–63.
4. Cellini C, Xu J, Buchmiller TL. Effect of esophageal ligation on small intestinal development in normal and growth-retarded fetal rabbits. J Pediatr Gastroenterol Nutr 2006;43(3):291–8.
5. Burjonrappa SC, Crete E, Bouchard S. The role of amniotic fluid in influencing neonatal birth weight. J Perinatol 2010;30(1):27–9.
6. de Figueiredo CS, Palhares DB, Melnikov P, et al. Zinc and copper concentrations in human preterm milk. Biol Trace Elem Res 2010;136(1):1–7.
7. O'Brien CE, Krebs NF, Westcott JL, et al. Relationships among plasma zinc, plasma prolactin, milk transfer, and milk zinc in lactating women. J Hum Lact 2007;23(2):179–83.
8. Ruhaak LR, Lebrilla CB. Advances in analysis of human milk oligosaccharides. Adv Nutr 2012;3(3):406S–14S.
9. Sela DA, Mills DA. Nursing our microbiota: molecular linkages between bifidobacteria and milk oligosaccharides. Trends Microbiol 2010;18(7):298–307.
10. Coppa GV, Gabrielli O, Zampini L, et al. Oligosaccharides in 4 different milk groups, Bifidobacteria, and Ruminococcus obeum. J Pediatr Gastroenterol Nutr 2011;53(1):80–7.
11. Newburg DS, Ruiz-Palacios GM, Morrow AL. Human milk glycans protect infants against enteric pathogens. Annu Rev Nutr 2005;25:37–58.
12. Bode L. Human milk oligosaccharides: every baby needs a sugar mama. Glycobiology 2012;22:1147–62.
13. Gabrielli O, Zampini L, Galeazzi T, et al. Preterm milk oligosaccharides during the first month of lactation. Pediatrics 2011;128(6):e1520–31.
14. De Leoz ML, Gaerlan SC, Strum JS, et al. Lacto-N-tetraose, fucosylation, and secretor status are highly variable in human milk oligosaccharides from women delivering preterm. J Proteome Res 2012;11:4662–72.
15. Coppa GV, Gabrielli O, Zampini L, et al. Glycosaminoglycan content in term and preterm milk during the first month of lactation. Neonatology 2012;101(1): 74–6.
16. Eilers E, Ziska T, Harder T, et al. Leptin determination in colostrum and early human milk from mothers of preterm and term infants. Early Hum Dev 2011; 87(6):415–9.
17. Freed LM, Berkow SE, Hamosh P, et al. Lipases in human milk: effect of gestational age and length of lactation on enzyme activity. J Am Coll Nutr 1989;8(2): 143–50.
18. American Academy of Pediatrics Section on Breastfeeding. Breastfeeding and the use of human milk. Pediatrics 2012;129:e827–41.
19. Schanler RJ, Shulman RJ, Lau C. Feeding strategies for premature infants: beneficial outcomes of feeding fortified human milk versus preterm formula. Pediatrics 1999;103(6 Pt 1):1150–7.
20. Sisk PM, Lovelady CA, Dillard RG, et al. Early human milk feeding is associated with a lower risk of necrotizing enterocolitis in very low birth weight infants. J Perinatol 2007;27(7):428–33.
21. Meinzen-Derr J, Poindexter B, Wrage L, et al. Role of human milk in extremely low birth weight infants' risk of necrotizing enterocolitis or death. J Perinatol 2009;29(1):57–62.
22. Okamoto T, Shirai M, Kokubo M, et al. Human milk reduces the risk of retinal detachment in extremely low-birthweight infants. Pediatr Int 2007;49(6): 894–7.

23. Maayan-Metzger A, Avivi S, Schushan-Eisen I, et al. Human milk versus formula feeding among preterm infants: short-term outcomes. Am J Perinatol 2012; 29(2):121–6.
24. Vohr BR, Poindexter BB, Dusick AM, et al. Beneficial effects of breast milk in the neonatal intensive care unit on the developmental outcome of extremely low birth weight infants at 18 months of age. Pediatrics 2006;118(1):e115–23.
25. Isaacs EB, Fischl BR, Quinn BT, et al. Impact of breast milk on intelligence quotient, brain size, and white matter development. Pediatr Res 2010;67(4): 357–62.
26. Vohr BR, Poindexter BB, Dusick AM, et al. Persistent beneficial effects of breast milk ingested in the neonatal intensive care unit on outcomes of extremely low birth weight infants at 30 months of age. Pediatrics 2007;120(4):e953–9.
27. Singhal A, Cole TJ, Lucas A. Early nutrition in preterm infants and later blood pressure: two cohorts after randomised trials. Lancet 2001;357(9254):413–9.
28. Singhal A, Cole TJ, Fewtrell M, et al. Breastmilk feeding and lipoprotein profile in adolescents born preterm: follow-up of a prospective randomised study. Lancet 2004;363(9421):1571–8.
29. Singhal A, Farooqi IS, O'Rahilly S, et al. Early nutrition and leptin concentrations in later life. Am J Clin Nutr 2002;75(6):993–9.
30. Hintz SR, Kendrick DE, Stoll BJ, et al. Neurodevelopmental and growth outcomes of extremely low birth weight infants after necrotizing enterocolitis. Pediatrics 2005;115(3):696–703.
31. Furman L, Taylor G, Minich N, et al. The effect of maternal milk on neonatal morbidity of very low-birth-weight infants. Arch Pediatr Adolesc Med 2003; 157(1):66–71.
32. Manzoni P, Rinaldi M, Cattani S, et al. Bovine lactoferrin supplementation for prevention of late-onset sepsis in very low-birth-weight neonates: a randomized trial. JAMA 2009;302(13):1421–8.
33. Dvorak B. Milk epidermal growth factor and gut protection. J Pediatr 2010; 156(Suppl 2):S31–5.
34. Jantscher-Krenn E, Zherebtsov M, Nissan C, et al. The human milk oligosaccharide disialyllacto-N-tetraose prevents necrotising enterocolitis in neonatal rats. Gut 2012;61:1417–25.
35. Wang Y, Hoenig JD, Malin KJ, et al. 16S rRNA gene-based analysis of fecal microbiota from preterm infants with and without necrotizing enterocolitis. ISME J 2009;3(8):944–54.
36. Mai V, Young CM, Ukhanova M, et al. Fecal microbiota in premature infants prior to necrotizing enterocolitis. PLoS One 2011;6(6):e20647.
37. Adlerberth I, Wold AE. Establishment of the gut microbiota in Western infants. Acta Paediatr 2009;98(2):229–38.
38. Cilieborg MS, Boye M, Sangild PT. Bacterial colonization and gut development in preterm neonates. Early Hum Dev 2012;88(Suppl 1):S41–9.
39. Poroyko V, Morowitz M, Bell T, et al. Diet creates metabolic niches in the "immature gut" that shape microbial communities. Nutr Hosp 2011;26(6): 1283–95.
40. Zachariassen G, Faerk J, Esberg BH, et al. Allergic diseases among very preterm infants according to nutrition after hospital discharge. Pediatr Allergy Immunol 2011;22(5):515–20.
41. Rodriguez NA, Meier PP, Groer MW, et al. Oropharyngeal administration of colostrum to extremely low birth weight infants: theoretical perspectives. J Perinatol 2009;29(1):1–7.

42. Montjaux-Regis N, Cristini C, Arnaud C, et al. Improved growth of preterm infants receiving mother's own raw milk compared with pasteurized donor milk. Acta Paediatr 2011;100(12):1548–54.
43. Quigley MA, Henderson G, Anthony MY, et al. Formula milk versus donor breast milk for feeding preterm or low birth weight infants. Cochrane Database Syst Rev 2007;(4):CD002971.
44. Schanler RJ, Lau C, Hurst NM, et al. Randomized trial of donor human milk versus preterm formula as substitutes for mothers' own milk in the feeding of extremely premature infants. Pediatrics 2005;116(2):400–6.
45. Spatz DL. Ten steps for promoting and protecting breastfeeding for vulnerable infants. J Perinat Neonatal Nurs 2004;18(4):385–96.
46. Kashyap S, Schulze KF, Forsyth M, et al. Growth, nutrient retention, and metabolic response of low-birth-weight infants fed supplemented and unsupplemented preterm human milk. Am J Clin Nutr 1990;52(2):254–62.
47. Kuschel CA, Harding JE. Multicomponent fortified human milk for promoting growth in preterm infants. Cochrane Database Syst Rev 2004;(1):CD000343.
48. Premji SS, Fenton TR, Sauve RS. Higher versus lower protein intake in formula-fed low birth weight infants. Cochrane Database Syst Rev 2006;(1):CD003959.
49. Weber A, Loui A, Jochum F, et al. Breast milk from mothers of very low birth-weight infants: variability in fat and protein content. Acta Paediatr 2001;90(7):772–5.
50. Arslanoglu S, Moro GE, Ziegler EE. Preterm infants fed fortified human milk receive less protein than they need. J Perinatol 2009;29(7):489–92.
51. Polberger S, Raiha NC, Juvonen P, et al. Individualized protein fortification of human milk for preterm infants: comparison of ultrafiltrated human milk protein and a bovine whey fortifier. J Pediatr Gastroenterol Nutr 1999;29(3):332–8.
52. Arslanoglu S, Moro GE, Ziegler EE. Adjustable fortification of human milk fed to preterm infants: does it make a difference? J Perinatol 2006;26(10):614–21.
53. Miller J, Makrides M, Gibson RA, et al. Effect of increasing protein content of human milk fortifier on growth in preterm infants born at <31 wk gestation: a randomized controlled trial. Am J Clin Nutr 2012;95(3):648–55.
54. Rochow N, Jochum F, Redlich A, et al. Fortification of breast milk in VLBW infants: metabolic acidosis is linked to the composition of fortifiers and alters weight gain and bone mineralization. Clin Nutr 2011;30(1):99–105.
55. Friel JK, Diehl-Jones B, Cockell KA, et al. Evidence of oxidative stress in relation to feeding type during early life in premature infants. Pediatr Res 2011;69(2):160–4.
56. Reich F, Konig R, von Wiese W, et al. Prevalence of Cronobacter spp. in a powdered infant formula processing environment. Int J Food Microbiol 2010;140(2–3):214–7.
57. Friedemann M. Epidemiology of invasive neonatal Cronobacter (Enterobacter sakazakii) infections. Eur J Clin Microbiol Infect Dis 2009;28(11):1297–304.
58. Guidelines for the establishment and operation of a donor human milk bank. Available at: http://www.hmbana.org/. Accessed October 12, 2012.
59. Centre for Clinical Practice at NICE. Donor Breast Milk Banks: The Operation of Donor Milk Bank Services. London: National Institute for Health and Clinical Excellence 2010. Available at: http://www.ncbi.nlm.nih.gov/books/NBK66142/.
60. Coutsoudis I, Adhikari M, Nair N, et al. Feasibility and safety of setting up a donor breastmilk bank in a neonatal prem unit in a resource limited setting: an observational, longitudinal cohort study. BMC Public Health 2011;11:356.

61. al-Naqeeb NA, Azab A, Eliwa MS, et al. The introduction of breast milk donation in a Muslim country. J Hum Lact 2000;16(4):346–50.
62. Hsu HT, Fong TV, Hassan NM, et al. Human milk donation is an alternative to human milk bank. Breastfeed Med 2012;7(2):118–22.
63. Akre JE, Gribble KD, Minchin M. Milk sharing: from private practice to public pursuit. Int Breastfeed J 2011;6:8.
64. Use of donor human milk. 2012. Available at: http://www.fda.gov/ScienceResearch/SpecialTopics/PediatricTherapeuticsResearch/ucm235203.htm. Accessed October 12, 2012.
65. Ewaschuk JB, Unger S, Harvey S, et al. Effect of pasteurization on immune components of milk: implications for feeding preterm infants. Appl Physiol Nutr Metab 2011;36(2):175–82.
66. Silvestre D, Miranda M, Muriach M, et al. Antioxidant capacity of human milk: effect of thermal conditions for the pasteurization. Acta Paediatr 2008;97(8):1070–4.
67. Bertino E, Coppa GV, Giuliani F, et al. Effects of Holder pasteurization on human milk oligosaccharides. Int J Immunopathol Pharmacol 2008;21(2):381–5.
68. Goelz R, Hihn E, Hamprecht K, et al. Effects of different CMV-heat-inactivation-methods on growth factors in human breast milk. Pediatr Res 2009;65(4):458–61.
69. Van Zoeren-Grobben D, Schrijver J, Van den Berg H, et al. Human milk vitamin content after pasteurisation, storage, or tube feeding. Arch Dis Child 1987;62(2):161–5.
70. Ewaschuk JB, Unger S, O'Connor DL, et al. Effect of pasteurization on selected immune components of donated human breast milk. J Perinatol 2011;31(9):593–8.
71. Goldblum RM, Dill CW, Albrecht TB, et al. Rapid high-temperature treatment of human milk. J Pediatr 1984;104(3):380–5.
72. Terpstra FG, Rechtman DJ, Lee ML, et al. Antimicrobial and antiviral effect of high-temperature short-time (HTST) pasteurization applied to human milk. Breastfeed Med 2007;2(1):27–33.
73. Baro C, Giribaldi M, Arslanoglu S, et al. Effect of two pasteurization methods on the protein content of human milk. Front Biosci (Elite Ed) 2011;3:818–29.
74. Silvestre D, Ruiz P, Martinez-Costa C, et al. Effect of pasteurization on the bactericidal capacity of human milk. J Hum Lact 2008;24(4):371–6.
75. Chantry CJ, Wiedeman J, Buehring G, et al. Effect of flash-heat treatment on antimicrobial activity of breastmilk. Breastfeed Med 2011;6(3):111–6.
76. Miracle DJ, Szucs KA, Torke AM, et al. Contemporary ethical issues in human milk-banking in the United States. Pediatrics 2011;128(6):1186–91.
77. Sullivan S, Schanler RJ, Kim JH, et al. An exclusively human milk-based diet is associated with a lower rate of necrotizing enterocolitis than a diet of human milk and bovine milk-based products. J Pediatr 2010;156(4):562–7.e1.
78. Ganapathy V, Hay JW, Kim JH. Costs of necrotizing enterocolitis and cost-effectiveness of exclusively human milk-based products in feeding extremely premature infants. Breastfeed Med 2012;7(1):29–37.
79. Lau C, Hurst NM, Smith EO, et al. Ethnic/racial diversity, maternal stress, lactation and very low birthweight infants. J Perinatol 2007;27(7):399–408.
80. Slutzah M, Codipilly CN, Potak D, et al. Refrigerator storage of expressed human milk in the neonatal intensive care unit. J Pediatr 2010;156(1):26–8.
81. Brennan-Behm M, Carlson GE, Meier P, et al. Caloric loss from expressed mother's milk during continuous gavage infusion. Neonatal Netw 1994;13(2):27–32.

82. Charpak N, Ruiz JG. Breast milk composition in a cohort of pre-term infants' mothers followed in an ambulatory programme in Colombia. Acta Paediatr 2007;96(12):1755–9.

83. Bishara R, Dunn MS, Merko SE, et al. Nutrient composition of hindmilk produced by mothers of very low birth weight infants born at less than 28 weeks' gestation. J Hum Lact 2008;24(2):159–67.

84. Valentine CJ, Hurst NM, Schanler RJ. Hindmilk improves weight gain in low-birth-weight infants fed human milk. J Pediatr Gastroenterol Nutr 1994; 18(4):474–7.

85. Ogechi AA, William O, Fidelia BT. Hindmilk and weight gain in preterm very low-birthweight infants. Pediatr Int 2007;49(2):156–60.

86. Morton J, Hall JY, Wong RJ, et al. Combining hand techniques with electric pumping increases milk production in mothers of preterm infants. J Perinatol 2009;29(11):757–64.

87. Morton J, Wong RJ, Hall JY, et al. Combining hand techniques with electric pumping increases the caloric content of milk in mothers of preterm infants. J Perinatol 2012;32(10):791–6.

88. Jackson PC. Complementary and alternative methods of increasing breast milk supply for lactating mothers of infants in the NICU. Neonatal Netw 2010;29(4): 225–30.

89. Donovan TJ, Buchanan K. Medications for increasing milk supply in mothers expressing breastmilk for their preterm hospitalised infants. Cochrane Database Syst Rev 2012;(3):CD005544.

90. Gabay MP. Galactogogues: medications that induce lactation. J Hum Lact 2002; 18(3):274–9.

91. Huggins K. Fenugreek: one remedy for low milk production. 2012. Available at: http://www.breastfeedingonline.com/fenuhugg.shtml. Accessed October 12, 2012.

92. Damanik R, Wahlqvist ML, Wattanapenpaiboon N. Lactagogue effects of Torbangun, a Bataknese traditional cuisine. Asia Pac J Clin Nutr 2006;15(2):267–74.

93. Turkyilmaz C, Onal E, Hirfanoglu IM, et al. The effect of galactagogue herbal tea on breast milk production and short-term catch-up of birth weight in the first week of life. J Altern Complement Med 2011;17(2):139–42.

94. Di Pierro F, Callegari A, Carotenuto D, et al. Clinical efficacy, safety and tolerability of BIO-C (micronized Silymarin) as a galactagogue. Acta Biomed 2008; 79(3):205–10.

95. Gupta M, Shaw B. A double-blind randomized clinical trial for evaluation of galactogogue activity of asparagus racemosus wild. Iranian J Pharm Res 2011; 10(1):167–72.

96. Sharma S, Ramji S, Kumari S, et al. Randomized controlled trial of Asparagus racemosus (Shatavari) as a lactogogue in lactational inadequacy. Indian Pediatr 1996;33(8):675–7.

97. Zapantis A, Steinberg JG, Schilit L. Use of herbals as galactagogues. J Pharm Pract 2012;25(2):222–31.

98. Fohe K, Kropf S, Avenarius S. Skin-to-skin contact improves gas exchange in premature infants. J Perinatol 2000;20(5):311–5.

99. Bauer J, Sontheimer D, Fischer C, et al. Metabolic rate and energy balance in very low birth weight infants during kangaroo holding by their mothers and fathers. J Pediatr 1996;129(4):608–11.

100. Nyqvist KH, Sjoden PO, Ewald U. The development of preterm infants' breastfeeding behavior. Early Hum Dev 1999;55(3):247–64.

101. Meier PP, Brown LP, Hurst NM, et al. Nipple shields for preterm infants: effect on milk transfer and duration of breastfeeding. J Hum Lact 2000;16(2):106–14 [quiz: 129–31].

102. Kurath S, Halwachs-Baumann G, Muller W, et al. Transmission of cytomegalovirus via breast milk to the prematurely born infant: a systematic review. Clin Microbiol Infect 2010;16(8):1172–8.

103. Hamprecht K, Maschmann J, Jahn G, et al. Cytomegalovirus transmission to preterm infants during lactation. J Clin Virol 2008;41(3):198–205.

104. Bevot A, Hamprecht K, Krageloh-Mann I, et al. Long-term outcome in preterm children with human cytomegalovirus infection transmitted via breast milk. Acta Paediatr 2012;101(4):e167–72.

105. Bryant P, Morley C, Garland S, et al. Cytomegalovirus transmission from breast milk in premature babies: does it matter? Arch Dis Child Fetal Neonatal Ed 2002; 87(2):F75–7.

106. Maschmann J, Hamprecht K, Weissbrich B, et al. Freeze-thawing of breast milk does not prevent cytomegalovirus transmission to a preterm infant. Arch Dis Child Fetal Neonatal Ed 2006;91(4):F288–90.

107. Hayatbakhsh MR, Flenady VJ, Gibbons KS, et al. Birth outcomes associated with cannabis use before and during pregnancy. Pediatr Res 2012;71(2): 215–9.

108. Gouin K, Murphy K, Shah PS. Effects of cocaine use during pregnancy on low birthweight and preterm birth: systematic review and metaanalyses. Am J Obstet Gynecol 2011;204(4):340.e1–12.

109. Bandstra ES, Morrow CE, Accornero VH, et al. Estimated effects of in utero cocaine exposure on language development through early adolescence. Neurotoxicol Teratol 2011;33(1):25–35.

110. Ackerman JP, Riggins T, Black MM. A review of the effects of prenatal cocaine exposure among school-aged children. Pediatrics 2010;125(3):554–65.

111. American Academy of Pediatrics Committee on Drugs. Transfer of drugs and other chemicals into human milk. Pediatrics 2001;108(3):776–89.

112. Hayes RM, Wu P, Shelton RC, et al. Maternal antidepressant use and adverse outcomes: a cohort study of 228,876 pregnancies. Am J Obstet Gynecol 2012;207(1):49.e1–9.

113. Occhiogrosso M, Omran SS, Altemus M. Persistent pulmonary hypertension of the newborn and selective serotonin reuptake inhibitors: lessons from clinical and translational studies. Am J Psychiatry 2012;169(2):134–40.

114. Davanzo R, Copertino M, De Cunto A, et al. Antidepressant drugs and breast-feeding: a review of the literature. Breastfeed Med 2011;6(2):89–98.

115. Bauer J, Gerss J. Longitudinal analysis of macronutrients and minerals in human milk produced by mothers of preterm infants. Clin Nutr 2011;30(2): 215–20.

116. Molto-Puigmarti C, Castellote AI, Carbonell-Estrany X, et al. Differences in fat content and fatty acid proportions among colostrum, transitional, and mature milk from women delivering very preterm, preterm, and term infants. Clin Nutr 2011;30(1):116–23.

117. Chuang CK, Lin SP, Lee HC, et al. Free amino acids in full-term and pre-term human milk and infant formula. J Pediatr Gastroenterol Nutr 2005;40(4): 496–500.

118. Friel JK, Andrews WL, Jackson SE, et al. Elemental composition of human milk from mothers of premature and full-term infants during the first 3 months of lactation. Biol Trace Elem Res 1999;67(3):225–47.

119. Coppa GV, Gabrielli O, Pierani P, et al. Changes in carbohydrate composition in human milk over 4 months of lactation. Pediatrics 1993;91(3):637–41.
120. Mehta R, Petrova A. Biologically active breast milk proteins in association with very preterm delivery and stage of lactation. J Perinatol 2011;31(1): 58–62.
121. Castellote C, Casillas R, Ramirez-Santana C, et al. Premature delivery influences the immunological composition of colostrum and transitional and mature human milk. J Nutr 2011;141(6):1181–7.
122. Dvorak B, Fituch CC, Williams CS, et al. Increased epidermal growth factor levels in human milk of mothers with extremely premature infants. Pediatr Res 2003;54(1):15–9.

Supporting Breastfeeding in the Neonatal Intensive Care Unit

Rush Mother's Milk Club as a Case Study of Evidence-Based Care

Paula P. Meier, PhD, RN[a,b,*], Aloka L. Patel, MD[a],
Harold R. Bigger, MD[a], Beverly Rossman, PhD, RN[b],
Janet L. Engstrom, PhD, RN, CNM, WHNP-BC[b,c]

KEYWORDS

- Human milk • Breastfeeding • Breast pump • Lactation

KEY POINTS

- The evidence for the use of human milk (HM) in the neonatal intensive care unit (NICU) is compelling, but the translation of this evidence into best practices, toolkits, policies and procedures, talking points, and parent information packets is limited.
- HM feedings are not yet prioritized in a manner comparable with that of other NICU therapies, and NICU staff members and families have inconsistent information and a lack of lactation technologies to optimize the dose and exposure period of HM feedings.
- Stimulating a culture of using the evidence about HM in the NICU can change this circumstance, and requires use of evidence-based quality indicators to benchmark the use of HM, consistent messaging by the entire NICU team about the importance of HM for infants in the NICU, establishing procedures that protect maternal milk supply, and incorporating lactation technologies that take the guesswork out of HM feedings and facilitate milk transfer during breastfeeding.

INTRODUCTION

Human milk (HM) feedings from the infant's own mother reduce the risk of numerous short-term and long-term morbidities, their associated sequelae, and costs of care for premature and other at-risk infants.[1] For premature infants, higher doses of HM are associated with a lower risk of enteral feeding intolerance, late-onset sepsis,

Supported by National Institutes of Health Grant NR010009, The Kenneth and Anne Griffin Foundation and the Rossman Family Foundation.
[a] Department of Pediatrics, Section of Neonatology, Rush University Medical Center, Chicago, IL 60612, USA; [b] Department of Women, Children and Family Nursing, Rush University Medical Center, Chicago, IL 60612, USA; [c] Frontier Nursing University, Hyden, KY 41749, USA
* Corresponding author.
E-mail address: paula_meier@rush.edu

Pediatr Clin N Am 60 (2013) 209–226
http://dx.doi.org/10.1016/j.pcl.2012.10.007
0031-3955/13/$ – see front matter © 2013 Published by Elsevier Inc.

pediatric.theclinics.com

necrotizing enterocolitis, chronic lung disease, retinopathy of prematurity, neurocognitive delay, and rehospitalization at 18 and 30 months of age.[2–10] Further, the postnatal timing of high doses of HM may be important, because several studies suggest that high doses of HM during the first 14 to 28 days of life are associated with lower risk of various adverse outcomes in the neonatal intensive care unit (NICU).[2–4,7] A separate line of research also suggests that the presence of bovine products (not merely the absence of HM feedings) negatively affects intestinal permeability and gut colonization,[11–15] making the relationship between HM feedings and morbidities even more complex. However, the rapidly accumulating evidence suggests that the bioactive components of HM provide morbidity-specific protection via different mechanisms during different exposure periods in the NICU hospitalization.

Although these outcomes of HM feedings are well documented for infants in the NICU, families and health care providers struggle to translate this evidence into actionable policies, procedures, guidelines, and resource allocation to improve the use of HM in the NICU. This article summarizes the processes for creating a culture of evidence for increasing the dose and exposure period of HM feedings in the NICU, including the implementation of evidence-based quality indicators for measuring and benchmarking HM use. Best NICU practices for encouraging mothers to initiate and maintain lactation, protecting the maternal milk supply, caring for pumped HM, transferring from gavage to at-breast feeding, and using lactation technologies to solve common NICU problems with HM feedings are summarized.

A CULTURE OF USING THE EVIDENCE ABOUT HM IN THE NICU

The Rush Mothers' Milk Club is an evidence-based lactation program in the 57-bed NICU at Rush University in Chicago, in which 98% of mothers provide milk for their infants in the NICU, and the average daily dose of HM received during the NICU hospitalization by very low birth weight (VLBW; <1500 g birth weight) infants exceeds 60 mL/kg/d. This program translates the evidence about HM into understandable concepts and teaching materials for health care providers and families, and allocates resources, such as industrial freezers to store HM and the use of breastfeeding peer counselors (BPCs), to optimize the dose and exposure period of HM feedings for all infants in the NICU. Most fundamentally, the Rush program has established a culture of using the evidence, which has in turn led to high rates of HM feeding.

Of the various therapies used routinely in the NICU, HM use has among the most empiric support for safety, efficacy, availability and cost-effectiveness.[1] When conceptualized within a culture of using the evidence, HM feedings are a therapeutic priority for compromised infants, implemented in a manner like other evidence-based practices that improve outcomes in the NICU. Specifically, this process entails engaged practitioners who knowledgeably discuss the evidence for use of HM in the NICU, policies and guidelines that translate the evidence into routine clinical practices, and quality improvement efforts that provide feedback about the achievement of evidence-based benchmarks. In the context of a culture of using the evidence, infrastructure or resource needs are addressed for HM feedings (eg, storage freezers and waterless milk warmers) and considered in the same manner as other evidence-based interventions known to improve neonatal health outcomes.

In contrast, we do not advocate conceptualizing the NICU as having a culture of breastfeeding, which may lead to use of non-evidenced strategies based on emotional or sociopolitical rationale and avoidance of lactation technologies (eg, creamatocrits, test weights, nipple shields, and special bottle units for feeding

HM), making breastfeeding unnatural. The culture of using the evidence regarding breastfeeding is not based on changing staff attitudes and beliefs, does not accept staff indicating that they cannot help a mother feed her infant at the breast because they have not breastfed themselves, but is based on consistent dissemination of evidence that provides the highest standards of care for staff and families.

EVIDENCE-BASED QUALITY INDICATORS FOR THE USE OF HM IN THE NICU

A first step in translating the evidence about HM feedings in the NICU is to establish evidence-based quality indicators against which practice improvements can be benchmarked.[1] Currently used quality indicators do not reflect the research that demonstrates the relationship between the dose and exposure period of HM feedings and the reduction in the risk of morbidities for infants in the NICU. Current indicators measure only the proportion of infants in the NICU who ever received HM and the proportion who were still receiving any HM at the time of NICU discharge, which does not adequately reflect the evidence about risk reduction.[1] For example, the following 2 clinical scenarios both result in classification of an extremely low-birth-weight infant as receiving any HM in the NICU and no HM at discharge: (1) received exclusive HM feedings for 60 days followed by exclusive formula in the final week before NICU discharge, versus (2) received a single HM feeding while in NICU hospitalization. Simple-to use quality indicators that measure the amount and timing of HM feedings received by the infant in the NICU are needed in order to make the quality indicators consistent with the research.

The relationship between HM feeding status at the time of NICU discharge was recently explored as a part of an ongoing National Institutes of Health (NIH) cohort study in the Rush NICU that enrolled 400 VLBW infants between 2008 and 2012.[16] Of the 295 VLBW infants for whom data had been analyzed at the time of this writing, 289 (98%) infants received some HM. The average daily dose of HM received during the NICU hospitalization was 60 mL/kg/d (range, 0–156), and total HM intake received during the first 28 days after birth was 51 mL/kg/d (range, 0–135) or 71% (0%–100%) of total enteral feeding volume. Of the infants who were discharged receiving no HM (62% of the cohort), we found that exclusive HM feedings were received for 24% of the NICU hospital days, and partial HM feedings were received for 38% of the NICU hospital days. HM feedings constituted 76% and 58% of total enteral feedings during the first 14 and 28 postnatal days, respectively, for infants in the group who received no HM at discharge.[17] Given that studies have shown a beneficial impact of high doses of HM feedings during the first 14 or 28 days after birth in premature infants,[2–4,7] we propose that evidence-based quality improvement measures incorporate these exposure periods (**Box 1**).

BEST PRACTICES FOR SHARING EVIDENCE ABOUT HM WITH FAMILIES OF BABIES IN THE NICU

A major barrier to the initiation and maintenance of lactation in mothers whose infants are in the NICU is the inconsistent information that they receive regarding the importance of HM for their infants, strategies to pump and store their expressed milk, specific guidelines for transferring the infants to feeding at the breast, and combining pumping and feeding during the late NICU hospitalization and after discharge. When HM is used within a culture of evidence, addressing these issues becomes an NICU responsibility, not the job of a single lactation practitioner. Policies, procedures, and talking points that translate key HM research into understandable words and concepts

---

Box 1
Evidence-based quality improvement measures for the use of HM in the NICU

- Proportion of infants who ever received HM
- Average daily dose of HM, days 1 to 14
- Average daily dose of HM, days 1 to 28
- Average daily dose of HM, NICU hospitalization
- Proportion of feedings from human milk, days 1 to 14
- Proportion of feedings from HM, days 1 to 28
- Proportion of feedings from HM, NICU hospitalization
- Total number of NICU days of any HM feedings
- Total number of NICU days of exclusive HM feedings
- HM feeding status (partial, exclusive, none) at discharge

---

are developed and implemented so that messaging and information are consistent for staff and families.

CONSISTENCY OF INFORMATION

In the Rush Mothers' Milk Club, families receive standardized information about the importance of HM from perinatologists, neonatologists, nurses, nurse practitioners, NICU dietitians, and NICU-based BPCs before an infant's birth and throughout the NICU hospitalization. One consistent message is, "Your milk is a medicine that helps protect your baby from health problems and complications during and after the NICU hospitalization."[1] Other talking points are summarized in **Box 2**. With this strong message, 98% of mothers of infants in the NICU provide their milk although 50% of these women originally intended to feed formula. These mothers changed the decision to provide HM after the initial consultation with the neonatologist. Several studies have

---

Box 2
Sample talking points for sharing evidence about HM

- Your milk contains both food and medicine parts. These parts work together to help protect your baby from health problems during and after the NICU hospitalization.

- The protection from your milk extends past the period of when your baby receives it. This protection is because the milk changes the way that your baby's body fights infections and other health problems. So, the benefits last long after the milk ends.

- The milk that you make during the first couple of weeks is especially protective for your baby. It works to grow your baby's intestines, help develop important digestive juices, and protect your baby's intestines from the growth of harmful germs that can get inside the blood stream and cause infections and other problems.

- You do not need to decide right now about whether you want to pump long-term or even whether you want to feed your baby from the breast. Now, we just need for you to pump and provide your milk. You can decide later how long you want to continue. We can help you make those decisions once you and your baby get settled and you learn more about your milk.

shown that this matter-of-fact messaging does not make mothers feel coerced, pressured, or guilty, and that the women indicate that they depend on NICU care providers to share this evidence with them.[18,19] Further, in all of these studies, low-income African American mothers were disproportionately represented among the women who had initially chosen formula for their infants, but changed the decision to provide HM when the neonatologist indicated the advantages of HM for their own infant. The need for specific education of families at risk for premature birth, but unlikely to provide HM, resulted in the production of an educational DVD (*In Your Hands*, Rush Mothers' Milk Club, Chicago, IL) featuring families who detailed changing the decision to provide milk for their own infants and the beneficial outcomes that they noted.[20,21] This DVD is played in the hospital educational television channel for all families of new infants in the NICU.

PARENTS OF INFANTS WHO WERE IN THE NICU PROVIDE DIRECT LACTATION CARE FOR NEW FAMILIES

Once mothers of infants in the NICU have made the decision to initiate lactation for their infants, lactation care must be consistent, individualized, and highly specialized to address the lactation challenges of breast pump-dependent mothers with fragile infants. In 2005, the Rush Mothers' Milk Club implemented a program wherein parents of infants formerly cared for in the Rush NICU were hired as BPCs.[1,22,23] These parents completed a 5-day training program in generic BPC practice and upon their employment at Rush, also completed a 12-week orientation that included NICU-specific evidence and practices. Contrary to other models of BPC practice, these former parents of infants in the NICU work as an integral part of the health care team, assuming many lactation interventions traditionally performed by lactation consultants, with the bedside nurse serving as their major resource. The BPCs also work as research assistants on the externally funded research projects of the program, manage the NICU milk storage procedures and make home visits after infants in the NICU are discharged from the hospital.

BPCs are available in the Rush NICU 7 days a week, morning to evening, and form peer relationships with new families because of the shared experience of providing HM for an infant in the NICU. The BPCs conduct an initial visit with all mothers of infants in the NICU in the antepartum, intrapartum, or postpartum units, at which time they share the story of their own infants in the NICU and explain the importance of providing HM. The BPCs do all of the initial teaching about pumping, collecting, storing, and labeling HM, and sit with the mother when she uses the breast pump for the first time, adjusting the pump suction pressure and fitting breast shields. The BPCs help mothers solve problems such as low milk volume, sore nipples, lack of family support, and making pumping a priority despite the stress of having an infant in the NICU. Two published studies have detailed the mothers' and the health care providers' experiences with the BPCs in the Rush NICU.[23,24] The mothers reported that they preferred to receive lactation care from the BPCs, whom they perceived as knowledgeable, empathetic, and inspirational.[23] The health care providers reported that the BPCs were a valuable part of the NICU health care team, who made their work easier and more satisfying.[24]

FAMILIES LEARN THE SCIENCE OF HM, LACTATION, AND BREASTFEEDING

Central to the Rush Mothers' Milk Club program is the use of evidence to answer families' questions and address their concerns about HM, lactation, and breastfeeding. To ensure staff consistency and competency with respect to these topics, the program has developed policies, procedure, talking points, and professionally produced products (eg, brochures and parent education sheets) for families that summarize common concerns.[20,25] These products constitute an NICU toolkit for translating the evidence about HM into actionable practices, ensuring that information is shared accurately and consistently.

The Rush Mothers' Milk Club luncheon meeting also provides a forum for group lactation care in which families learn scientific principles about HM and lactation, and can share their own concerns and experiences.[1,26] The discussion is facilitated by staff and attended by the BPCs, current families, and parents whose infants were in the NICU who return to share their stories and seek additional information about providing HM via pumping or feeding at the breast. Although the group provides new families with much-needed support, the focus remains on sharing relevant scientific information, such as why a mother in the group might be at risk for delayed onset of lactation. Initiating lactation and maintaining an adequate milk supply despite the many obstacles to doing so are topics that always emerge, and the experienced mothers in the group share strategies with the newer mothers.

PROTECTING MATERNAL MILK SUPPLY IN PUMP-DEPENDENT MOTHERS WITH INFANTS IN THE NICU

Most mothers who provide HM for their infants in the NICU are breast pump-dependent, meaning that they rely on the breast pump instead of a healthy breastfeeding infant for the initiation and maintenance of lactation.[27,28] Breast pump-dependency, in combination with a myriad of factors that predispose to delayed onset of lactation and low milk volume, make mothers of infants in the NICU at greater risk for insufficient milk when compared with mothers with healthy breastfeeding infants.[27–29] Because milk is medicine for infants in the NICU, the single most important priority in the NICU is to protect the maternal milk supply by applying knowledge of the physiology of lactation to the individual mother's goals for providing her milk. This process is facilitated by the use of milk volume targets, milk diaries, easy-to-use assessment tools, and evidence-based milk expression protocols. Breast pumps, pumping kits, breast shields, and other supplies should be chosen based on their proven effectiveness, efficiency, and comfort in mothers of infants in the NICU.

PHYSIOLOGY OF LACTATION APPLIED TO THE PUMP-DEPENDENT MOTHER OF AN INFANT IN THE NICU

In all mammals, the trigger for secretory activation (lactogenesis II) is the withdrawal of progesterone that occurs with the birth of the placenta, thus removing its inhibitory effect on serum prolactin.[30] Colostrum, the initial milk product, is the transition from intrauterine to extrauterine nutrition for the infant, and is rich in bioactive factors that grow, mature, and protect the immature intestinal tract of the infant.[13,31–33] A healthy term breastfeeding infant removes approximately 15 mL of colostrum in 10 breastfeedings during the first 24 hours after birth and does so using a uniquely human infant sucking pattern characterized by a rapid rate, relatively strong sucking pressures, and intermittent pauses.[28,34] This early suckling on the part of the human infant is believed to provide a type of stimulus or programming during a critical window after birth that protects the maternal milk supply throughout lactation.[28,34] Under the ideal conditions of unrestricted breastfeeds, the mother's milk output increases from 15 mL during the first day of life to 500 to 600 mL of milk by days 4 to 7.[35–38] The challenge in the NICU is to apply this physiology to the breast pump-dependent mother, for whom the early postbirth period is complicated by stress and anxiety about her fragile infant and her own medical and birth complications.

MILK VOLUME TARGETS

Although several lines of evidence suggest that the very early postbirth period is a critical time for the stimulation or programming of subsequent milk yield, mothers of infants in the NICU seldom receive this clear information in words that they can act on. For many mothers and care providers, an adequate maternal milk supply means that there is enough HM for the infant's daily feedings. Mothers have heard that as their infants require more milk, they will make more milk, and health care providers are concerned about pressuring mothers about milk supply during this vulnerable time. However, research indicates that milk output during the first 2 postnatal weeks predicts the adequacy of milk volume during the late NICU hospitalization.[28,38,39] Thus, it is of primary importance that mothers understand from the beginning that there are 2 milk volume targets, which are enough for: (1) their infant in the NICU at the time, which may be very small amounts because of prematurity, surgical complications, or fluid restrictions; and (2) protecting the milk supply by early programming that enables their infants to receive exclusive HM feedings after the NICU hospitalization.[28,40] Protecting the milk supply translates into minimal milk volumes of 350 mL per day (adequate for a 2-kg infant at discharge), and volumes closer to 1000 mL per day ensure enough milk even if mothers experience later problems with their milk supply.

MILK DIARIES

Fig. 1 depicts the milk diary, *My Mom Pumps for Me!*, which is used in the Rush Mothers' Milk Club for all pumping mothers. The user-friendly diary is conceptualized as the mother's breastfeeding memento. In addition to recording the milk output and time spent pumping per session, she places decals (eg, first colostrum, first feeding of HM, first tasting of milk at breast) onto the daily page, commemorating the special events in her infant's stay in the NICU.[20] The bedside nurse or BPC reviews the milk diary each day after birth until the mother's milk output stabilizes at 350 mL per day or greater, and subsequently as needed to troubleshoot milk volume problems. These diaries provide objective, quantifiable information and serve as excellent teaching tools for use with mothers.

COMING TO VOLUME ASSESSMENT TOOL

The breast pump-dependent mother with an infant in the NICU experiences unique challenges to the initial establishment of an adequate milk supply, which differ from those of a mother with a healthy breastfeeding infant. She must learn to use a breast pump, adjust the pump pressures so they are effective but not uncomfortable, ensure that the breast shields (the part of the pump kit that fits over the areola and nipple) are properly sized, and recognize when the breasts are as thoroughly emptied as possible. These activities are the most critical during the first 2 weeks after birth as the mother moves from secretory differentiation into secretory activation and into establishing a complete milk supply or coming to volume.[1] The nurses and BPCs in the Rush Mothers' Milk Club complete a coming to volume assessment tool (**Fig. 2**) daily during the first 14 days after birth for all pump-dependent mothers with infants in the NICU. This form reflects commonly encountered problems during the early days of pump dependency, to ensure that problems such as sore nipples and incomplete breast emptying are averted before they compromise milk supply.

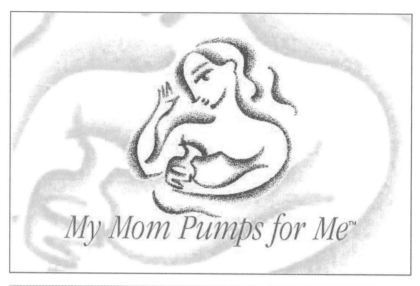

Today's Date: _____

My baby weighs: _____

My baby eats: ☐ every 2 hours
☐ every 3 hours
☐ on demand

Today

Yes or No   I visited the nursery to be with my baby.

Yes or No   We did kangaroo care.

Yes or No   My baby tasted drops of milk at breast.

Yes or No   My baby took a feeding at breast.

Milk Sample	1	2	3	4	5	6	7	8
Time pumping started								
Time pumping ended								
Amount of milk from Left Breast								
Amount of milk from Right Breast								
Number of containers used								
Place pumped: (home, work, NICU)								

Today I pumped a total of _____ times, and got _____ mls of milk for my baby.

Things I want to remember about today: _____

Fig. 1. *My Mom Pumps for Me!* milk diary. Conceptualized as a memento for a mother whose child is in the NICU as well as a record of milk output, the diary features 1 checkbooklike insert page for each NICU day. The mother can record milk output and time spent pumping for each daily pumping session separately for the right and left breasts. The memento also permits recording of events that the mother wants to remember about that NICU day. (*From* Rush Mothers' Milk Club, Rush University Medical Center, Chicago, IL; with permission.)

EVIDENCE-BASED MILK EXPRESSION PROTOCOLS

A breast pump-dependent mother should be assisted with her first milk expression as soon as possible after the birth of her infant. In the Rush Mothers' Milk Club program, a BPC helps a new mother use the breast pump in the delivery room, because it is recommended that healthy term infants feed at breast within the first hour after birth. The freshly expressed colostrum is taken to the NICU and 0.2 mL is administered oropharyngeally to the infant[41,42] as soon as feasible, preferably by the father. Thereafter, effective and frequent breast pumping is essential, and protocols should specifically include the type of breast pump, fitting of breast shields, and instructions for using the pump.

Rush Mothers' Milk Club
Coming to Volume Assessment

1056491826

Mother's Name: _____   Infant's Name: _____

Infant's Date of Birth: ☐ / ☐ / ☐

	Day: 1	Day: 2	Day: 3	Day: 4	Day: 5	Day: 6	Day: 7
	/ /	/ /	/ /	/ /	/ /	/ /	/ /
1. Location of assessment: (NLFC, NICU, Phone, etc.)							
2. Volume recorded in the last 24 hours:	mls	mls	mls	mls	mls	mls	mls
3. Number of pumpings in the last 24 hours:							
4. Longest interval between pumpings in the last 24 hours:	hrs.	hrs.	hrs.	hrs.	hrs.	hrs.	hrs.
5. What are the changes if any on the mother's daily volume?	☐ Increasing ☐ Decreasing ☐ The same ☐ N/A	☐ Increasing ☐ Decreasing ☐ The same ☐ N/A	☐ Increasing ☐ Decreasing ☐ The same ☐ N/A	☐ Increasing ☐ Decreasing ☐ The same ☐ N/A	☐ Increasing ☐ Decreasing ☐ The same ☐ N/A	☐ Increasing ☐ Decreasing ☐ The same ☐ N/A	☐ Increasing ☐ Decreasing ☐ The same ☐ N/A
6. Do mother's breasts feel full between pumpings?	☐ Yes ☐ No	☐ Yes ☐ No	☐ Yes ☐ No	☐ Yes ☐ No	☐ Yes ☐ No	☐ Yes ☐ No	☐ Yes ☐ No
7. Does milk drip or leak between pumpings?	☐ Yes ☐ No	☐ Yes ☐ No	☐ Yes ☐ No	☐ Yes ☐ No	☐ Yes ☐ No	☐ Yes ☐ No	☐ Yes ☐ No
8. Do all areas of both breasts empty thoroughly with pumping?	☐ Yes ☐ No	☐ Yes ☐ No	☐ Yes ☐ No	☐ Yes ☐ No	☐ Yes ☐ No	☐ Yes ☐ No	☐ Yes ☐ No
9. Are both nipples free of discomfort?	☐ Yes ☐ No	☐ Yes ☐ No	☐ Yes ☐ No	☐ Yes ☐ No	☐ Yes ☐ No	☐ Yes ☐ No	☐ Yes ☐ No
10. Are both nipples free of redness and pain at the base of the nipple?	☐ Yes ☐ No	☐ Yes ☐ No	☐ Yes ☐ No	☐ Yes ☐ No	☐ Yes ☐ No	☐ Yes ☐ No	☐ Yes ☐ No
11. Are both nipples free of lacerations and bleeding?	☐ Yes ☐ No	☐ Yes ☐ No	☐ Yes ☐ No	☐ Yes ☐ No	☐ Yes ☐ No	☐ Yes ☐ No	☐ Yes ☐ No
12. Are all medications and doses the same as previous day? (ask specifically about OTC cold remedies and hormonal birth control)	☐ Yes ☐ No	☐ Yes ☐ No	☐ Yes ☐ No	☐ Yes ☐ No	☐ Yes ☐ No	☐ Yes ☐ No	☐ Yes ☐ No
13. Assessment completed by: (initials)							
14. Attempted to reach mother but was unsuccessful.	☐ Attempted	☐ Attempted	☐ Attempted	☐ Attempted	☐ Attempted	☐ Attempted	☐ Attempted

If answers to questions number 8 - 12 are no, please specify finding and plan of care on the back of this page.

Fig. 2. Coming to volume assessment tool. This simple-to-use tool tracks progress with establishing an optimal milk supply for breast pump-dependent mothers with infants in the NICU. It is completed by the BPC or NICU nurse daily until the mother achieves at least 350 mL of milk per day for 5 consecutive days. (*From* Rush Mothers' Milk Club, Rush University Medical Center, Chicago, IL; with permission.)

Despite the fact that the breast pump is a lifeline and surrogate infant for a mother whose infant is in the NICU, few studies have examined the effectiveness, efficiency, comfort, and convenience of electric breast pumps and their associated breast pump suction patterns.[27,28] A recent randomized clinical trial of 105 mothers of premature infants reported significantly greater milk output in less time spent pumping using a breast pump suction pattern (Preemie Plus, Symphony, Medela, McHenry, IL) designed to mimic the sucking rate and rhythm of the human infant during the early days after birth, when milk flow from the breast is limited.[28] These findings and those of other human and animal studies suggest that there is a critical period for development and programming of the mammary epithelium, and that the type of breast pump may help compensate for the lack of an infant feeding at the breast.[43–46]

Breast shields should be fitted on the individual mother while she is pumping to ensure that the sizing is correct. Shields that are too tight compress the milk ducts during pumping and do not permit the release of milk via the normal milk ejection and pump suction pressures, whereas shields that are too large draw too much of the mother's areola into the tunnel, leading to edema in the tissues and subsequent compression of milk ducts.[1] In either case, the results of an incorrectly fitted breast shield are nipple trauma and areas of the breast that do not empty appropriately. In the early postpartum period, milk that remains in the breast triggers feedback mechanisms that downregulate milk synthesis.[47] Because nipple plasticity and degree of areolar edema change over the early postpartum period, a mother may require different sizes of breast shields to remove milk effectively and comfortably. Women may also need different sizes of shields for the left and right breasts.

In the Rush Mothers' Milk Club program, a BPC always sits with a mother the first time that she uses the breast pump and explains how to correctly position the breast shields so that the nipple moves freely and comfortably, how to adjust the suction pressures on the pump, while explaining what the mother should feel (eg, uterine cramping, bleeding, pulling on the nipple vs pain) and validating these sensations as normal. Data indicate that mothers value this assistance with their first pumping, because many mothers whose infant is in the NICU have never seen or used a breast pump.[23] Instructions for breast pump rental and its use in the home are reviewed with the mother several times during her hospitalization. The frequency of daily pumpings is individualized to the mother's breastfeeding goals and her life demands, but generic starting points include beginning breast pump use as soon as physically possible after birth, ideally in the delivery room and using a hospital-grade electric breast pump that is effective, efficient, and comfortable.[28]

PROTECTING PUMPED HM

HM that undergoes expression, collection, storage, warming, and feeding is subjected to environmental pathogens and temperature changes that can compromise its nutritional, immunologic, and microbiological integrity.[48–51] Further, as increasing numbers of mothers provide HM for their infants, the on-site storage of pumped HM poses a challenge for many NICUs. The Rush Mothers' Milk Club program handles approximately 500 containers of HM each day among 14 smaller refrigerator and freezers in the patient care areas and maintains 4 industrial overflow freezers, which are locked and temperature-controlled at all times. These practices ensure that all HM fed in the NICU is under the NICU's safe handling of HM protocol at all times. Other interventions to ensure that pumped milk is protected from bacterial contamination include a program to clean the exterior of the shared NICU breast pumps before each use. In the Rush Mothers' Milk Club, this task is the responsibility of the mother who will use the pump. The bedside nurse or the BPC demonstrates this cleaning procedure for the mother, and laminated instructions in English and Spanish are attached to the breast pump in order to reinforce these steps. Sanitizing wipes for cleaning the pump are kept in a wire basket mounted to the breast pump trolley.

Another documented risk in the handling of pumped HM is thawing and warming HM in water baths consisting of tap water,[52] because it is difficult for even the most seasoned NICU nurse to prepare an HM feeding without inadvertently having the feeding syringe or container come into contact with water. There are commercially available products that warm HM to a specified temperature without direct contact with water, and these should be a funding priority in the NICU because of safety and quality.

DEVELOPMENTALLY BASED TRANSITION TO FEEDING AT BREAST IN THE NICU

Most infants in the NICU receive parenteral nutrition before the introduction of early colostrum feedings. Thus, the initial breastfeeding relationship for mothers and infants in the NICU begins with skin-to-skin (STS) holding (kangaroo care), in which the infant, clothed only in a diaper, is held between the mother's breasts for warmth and stability (**Fig. 3**). Comprehensive literature shows the safety and efficacy of STS holding with respect to infant stability, regardless of weight and maturity.[53,54] In addition, STS holding is also believed to provide the recipient infant with customized HM, in that the mother produces antibodies to NICU-specific pathogens that home to the mammary gland via the enteromammary pathway.[55] Studies also reveal a beneficial impact on the NICU mother's milk output and stress response.[56] STS holding should be offered as a standard of care when the mother is in the NICU, and should not be subject to non–evidence-based practices, such as individual nurses' comfort levels with this intervention. Many routine care practices such as clinical assessments, diaper changes, gavage feedings, and diagnostics can be performed while the infant is in STS holding, and no data indicate that STS holding should be restricted to a certain length of time provided that the infant remains physiologically stable.

Few infants are able to feed orally when first admitted to the NICU, so initial enteral feedings of HM are administered by gavage. Several studies have reported that intermittent bolus feedings are superior to slower continuous feedings of HM with respect

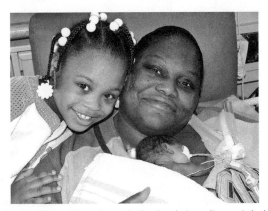

Fig. 3. STS holding in the NICU. The infant, clothed only in a diaper, is held STS between the mother's breasts for warmth and physiologic stability. (*From* Rush Mothers' Milk Club, Rush University Medical Center, Chicago, IL; with permission.)

to delivery of nutrients and minimizing bacterial growth.[1,57] Once an infant has been extubated, tasting milk from the breast can be initiated, whereby the mother removes milk from the breast before an infant is placed STS to suckle nonnutritively (**Fig. 4**). Tasting milk at the breast is technically similar to nonnutritive sucking with a pacifier, and the intent is not that the infant latches onto the breast and consumes milk.[1,58] In the Rush Mothers' Milk Club, a mother removes her milk approximately 15 minutes before the infant's scheduled 2-hourly feeding, and the infant is placed STS around the breast to taste milk for a few minutes before administration of the gavage feeding. The infant suckles nonnutritively and falls asleep, sucking intermittently at the breast as the feeding infuses.

As the infant matures, nonnutritive tasting segues into consuming small amounts of milk at the breast, and the mother pumps only the portion of the milk that flows rapidly at the beginning of milk removal. Developmentally, this practice is consistent with numerous studies that reveal that premature infants can consume oral feedings with maximum safety when the flow of the milk is reduced.[59,60] Gradually, based on the individual infant's maturity and the rate of the mother's milk flow, the mother discontinues prefeed pumping and the infant is allowed to feed nutritively from the breast. Several studies have reported that early breastfeeding is less physiologically stressful than early bottle feedings for premature infants, primarily because of the inability of the infant to control the rate of flow from commercially available bottle units used in the NICU.[61–63]

One of the most common misconceptions on the part of mothers whose infant is in the NICU is that they do not need to use the breast pump after their infant feeds at the breast, because unless they are taught otherwise, they assume that the infant has emptied the breast. Furthermore, mothers want to ensure that they have milk in the breasts in case their infants, who are likely being fed on cue by this point in the NICU hospitalization, awaken again shortly after a completed feeding. Although infant intake during breastfeeding in the NICU is variable, most premature infants consume relatively small amounts of milk at breast during the late NICU hospitalization[61,64–66] and make the final transition to exclusive breastfeeding after NICU discharge.[64] Failure to use the breast pump on a regular basis while feeds at breast are advanced results in milk stasis, with resultant low milk volume and potential mastitis.

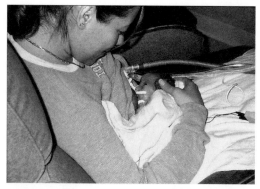

Fig. 4. Tasting milk at the breast as a developmentally based transition to breastfeeding. The mother uses a breast pump to remove the milk approximately 15 minutes before the infant's scheduled feeding. The infant is placed STS around the breast surface to taste milk. The intent is not for the infant to latch on to the breast and consume milk. (*From* Rush Mothers' Milk Club, Rush University Medical Center, Chicago, IL; with permission.)

Breastfeedings for the term infant cared for in the NICU should not be managed based on policies and procedures that are appropriate for premature infants. For many term and some late preterm infants in the NICU, breastfeedings could be started earlier in the NICU hospitalization if test weights (discussed later) were instituted to measure and manage milk intake during breastfeedings.[66,67] As a general rule, if the infant in the NICU is capable of receiving feedings orally (eg, by bottle), the infant should be able to breastfeed. Best NICU practices should make it the exception for an orally fed term infant in the NICU to routinely receive pumped HM by bottle if the mother is available and desires to feed the infant by breast.

LACTATION TECHNOLOGIES OPTIMIZE HM FEEDINGS

Technologies to improve the use of HM in the NICU continue to evolve based on new evidence with respect to clinical need, ease of use, precision and accuracy, and overall acceptance by NICU care providers and families. Such technologies may initially be considered too costly or labor intensive, or NICU staff may initially express concern that mothers may be stressed by such technologies. However, the technologies of creamatocrits or other milk analysis procedures, test weights to measure milk intake, and nipple shields to facilitate milk transfer are grounded in numerous studies that address any such NICU concerns.[66–69] These technologies optimize HM feedings in the NICU, and they should be considered standard NICU equipment.[1]

CREAMATOCRIT TECHNIQUE

The creamatocrit technique is quick, easily used, inexpensive, and an accurate estimate of HM lipid and caloric content.[69–71] The technique has been adapted for ease of use in the clinical setting, making it even simpler to use and interpret by NICU care providers.[69] A 2-phase, blinded trial revealed that mothers of infants in the NICU performed the technique as accurately as advance practice nurses and that they enjoyed assuming this responsibility for their infant's care.[72]

Although technologies that also measure lactose and protein content in HM are available, these techniques are significantly most costly than the creamatocrit, and may be impractical in many NICUs.[73] In addition, the lipid content in HM is the most variable macronutrient, with high within-mother and between-mother variability, and is the component most affected by routine handling and feeding of HM.[73,74] HM is not homogenized, so lipid separates from the aqueous portion of the milk, and is not completely delivered to the recipient infant.[57] The inadequate delivery of lipid can result in infants in the NICU receiving a low-lipid, high-lactose milk, which manifests as slow weight gain and feed intolerance. Thus, the creamatocrit is recommended to troubleshoot these common HM feeding problems for infants in the NICU.[75]

MEASURING MILK INTAKE WITH TEST WEIGHTS

During the late NICU hospitalization, when infants transfer from tasting milk at the breast to actively feeding, measuring milk intake provides NICU clinicians and families with objective information about the adequacy of milk intake during breastfeeding. Few premature and late preterm infants consume adequate volumes of milk directly from the breast until they achieve approximately term, corrected age, despite the fact that their mothers have an adequate milk supply.[61,64,65,76] Thus, it is not safe to discharge these infants from the NICU with instructions to feed on cue; neither is it appropriate to routinely supplement each breastfeeding with a bottle-feeding. Contrary to many assumptions, test weights are accurate, necessary (when knowledge about the amount of milk ingested is important), and easily used and accepted by families of infants in the NICU.[61,65] Test weights can also facilitate continued breastfeeding after NICU discharge when used in the home by families, and an accurate, easy-to-use scale (BabyWeigh, Medela, McHenry, IL) is available in the rental market for this purpose.[65] The use of the scale during the first month after NICU discharge does not make mothers feel more anxious and facilitates transition to complete breastfeeding.[64]

NIPPLE SHIELDS TO FACILITATE MILK TRANSFER

Premature, late preterm, and other compromised infants in the NICU have maturity-limited or medically limited suction pressures that make it difficult or impossible for the infant to sustain an effective latch on the breast. Although suction is not critical to bottle units that incorporate hydrostatic pressure, suction on the part of the infant is essential for creating the nipple shape and transferring milk from the breast.[77,78] Clinically, immature suction pressures result in the infant slipping off the breast, appearing satiated after consuming no or small amounts of milk, and falling asleep early in the feeding. Although these suction-based limitations can be helped with effective breast-feeding positions that support the infant's head, neck, and torso, maturation is the major determinant of feeding effectiveness and efficiency. An ultrathin silicone nipple shield has been shown to compensate for this temporary problem in infants in the NICU by creating the nipple shape and facilitating the transfer of milk to the infant.[68] Most mothers need to use the shield until their premature infants achieve approximately term, corrected age and are gaining weight well on exclusive feeds at breast.

SUMMARY

The evidence for the use of HM in the NICU is compelling, but the translation of this evidence into best practices, toolkits, policies and procedures, talking points, and parent information packets is limited. As a result, HM feedings are not yet prioritized in a manner comparable with that of other NICU therapies, and NICU staff members and families have inconsistent information and a lack of lactation technologies to optimize the dose and exposure period of HM feedings. Stimulating a culture of using the evidence about HM in the NICU can change this circumstance, and requires use of evidence-based quality indicators to benchmark the use of HM, consistent messaging by the entire NICU team about the importance of HM for infants in the NICU, establishing procedures that protect maternal milk supply, and incorporating lactation technologies that take the guesswork out of HM feedings and facilitate milk transfer during breastfeeding.

REFERENCES

1. Meier PP, Engstrom JL, Patel AL, et al. Improving the use of human milk during and after the NICU stay. Clin Perinatol 2010;37(1):217–45.
2. Sisk PM, Lovelady CA, Dillard RG, et al. Early human milk feeding is associated with a lower risk of necrotizing enterocolitis in very low birth weight infants. J Perinatol 2007;27:428–33.
3. Sisk PM, Lovelady CA, Gruber KJ, et al. Human milk consumption and full enteral feeding among infants who weigh ≤ 1250 grams. Pediatrics 2008;121(6): e1528–33.
4. Meinzen-Derr J, Poindexter B, Wrage L, et al. Role of human milk in extremely low birth weight infants' risk of necrotizing enterocolitis or death. J Perinatol 2009; 29(1):57–62.

5. Schanler RJ, Lau C, Hurst NM, et al. Randomized trial of donor human milk versus preterm formula as substitutes for mothers' own milk in the feeding of extremely premature infants. Pediatrics 2005;116(2):400–6.
6. Schanler RJ, Shulman RJ, Lau C. Feeding strategies for premature infants: beneficial outcomes of feeding fortified human milk versus preterm formula. Pediatrics 1999;103(6 Pt 1):1150–7.
7. Furman L, Taylor G, Minich N, et al. The effect of maternal milk on neonatal morbidity of very low-birth-weight infants. Arch Pediatr Adolesc Med 2003; 157(1):66–71.
8. Vohr BR, Poindexter BB, Dusick AM, et al. Beneficial effects of breast milk in the neonatal intensive care unit on the developmental outcome of extremely low birth weight infants at 18 months of age. Pediatrics 2006;118(1):e115–23.
9. Vohr BR, Poindexter BB, Dusick AM, et al. Persistent beneficial effects of breast milk ingested in the neonatal intensive care unit on outcomes of extremely low birth weight infants at 30 months of age. Pediatrics 2007;120(4):e953–9.
10. Hylander MA, Strobino DM, Pezzullo JC, et al. Association of human milk feedings with a reduction in retinopathy of prematurity among very low birthweight infants. J Perinatol 2001;21(6):356–62.
11. Sullivan S, Schanler RJ, Kim JH, et al. An exclusively human milk-based diet is associated with a lower rate of necrotizing enterocolitis than a diet of human milk and bovine milk-based products. J Pediatr 2010;156(4):562–567.e1.
12. Taylor SN, Basile LA, Ebeling M, et al. Intestinal permeability in preterm infants by feeding type: mother's milk versus formula. Breastfeed Med 2009;4(1):11–5.
13. Sangild PT. Gut responses to enteral nutrition in preterm infants and animals. Exp Biol Med 2006;231(11):1695–711.
14. Sangild PT, Siggers RH, Schmidt M, et al. Diet- and colonization-dependent intestinal dysfunction predisposes to necrotizing enterocolitis in preterm pigs. Gastroenterology 2006;130(6):1776–92.
15. Thymann T, Burrin DG, Tappenden KA, et al. Formula-feeding reduces lactose digestive capacity in neonatal pigs. Br J Nutr 2006;95(6):1075–81.
16. Meier PP. Health benefits and cost of human milk for very low birthweight infants. Chicago: Rush Mothers' Milk Club; 2007. Available at: http://www.rushmothers milkclub.com.
17. Bigger H, Fogg L, Patel AL, et al. Discharge-based quality indicators do not adequately reflect the amount of human milk consumed by very low birthweight infants during the neonatal intensive care unit hospitalization [abstract]. Presented at the 16th International Meeting of the Society for Research in Human Milk and Lactation. Trieste (Italy): 2012.
18. Miracle DJ, Meier PP, Bennett PA. Mothers' decisions to change from formula to mothers' milk for very-low-birth-weight infants. J Obstet Gynecol Neonatal Nurs 2004;33(6):692–703.
19. Miracle DJ, Meier PP, Bennett PA. Making my baby healthy: changing the decision from formula to human milk feedings for very-low-birth-weight infants. Adv Exp Med Biol 2004;554:317–9.
20. Rush Mothers' Milk Club. Updated 2009. Available at: http://www.rush mothersmilkclub.com. Accessed November 28, 2009.
21. Rush Mothers' Milk Club. In your hands: the importance of mothers' milk for premature babies. [DVD]. Chicago (IL): 2010.
22. Meier PP. Breastfeeding peer counselors in the NICU: increasing access to care for very low birthweight infants. Illinois Children's Healthcare Foundation; 2005.

23. Rossman B, Engstrom JL, Meier PP, et al. "They've walked in my shoes": mothers of very low birth weight infants and their experiences with breastfeeding peer counselors in the neonatal intensive care unit. J Hum Lact 2011;27(1): 14–24.

24. Rossman. B, Engstrom JL, Meier PP. Healthcare providers' perceptions of breastfeeding peer counselors in the neonatal intensive care unit. Res Nurs Health 2012;35(5):460–74.

25. Rodriguez NA, Miracle DJ, Meier PP. Sharing the science on human milk feedings with mothers of very-low-birth-weight infants. J Obstet Gynecol Neonatal Nurs 2005;34(1):109–19.

26. Meier PP, Engstrom J, Mingolelli SR, et al. The rush mother's milk club: breastfeeding interventions for mothers with very-low-birth-weight infants. J Obstet Gynecol Neonatal Nurs 2004;33(2):164–74.

27. Meier PP, Engstrom JL, Hurst NM, et al. A comparison of the efficiency, efficacy, comfort, and convenience of two hospital-grade electric breast pumps for mothers of very low birthweight infants. Breastfeed Med 2008;3(3):141–50.

28. Meier PP, Engstrom JL, Janes JE, et al. Breast pump suction patterns that mimic the human infant during breastfeeding: greater milk output in less time spent pumping for breast pump-dependent mothers with premature infants. J Perinatol 2012;32: 103–10.

29. Hurst NM. Recognizing and treating delayed or failed lactogenesis II. J Midwifery Womens Health 2007;52(6):588–94.

30. Neville MC, Morton J, Umemura S. Lactogenesis. The transition from pregnancy to lactation. Pediatr Clin North Am 2001;48(1):35–52.

31. Jensen AR, Elnif J, Burrin DG, et al. Development of intestinal immunoglobulin absorption and enzyme activities in neonatal pigs is diet dependent. J Nutr 2001;131(12):3259–65.

32. Bjornvad CR, Schmidt M, Petersen YM, et al. Preterm birth makes the immature intestine sensitive to feeding-induced intestinal atrophy. Am J Physiol Regul Integr Comp Physiol 2005;289(4):R1212–22.

33. Mei J, Zhang Y, Wang T, et al. Oral ingestion of colostrum alters intestinal transforming growth factor-beta receptor intensity in newborn pigs. Livest Sci 2006; 105:214–22.

34. Santoro W Jr, Martinez FE, Ricco RG, et al. Colostrum ingested during the first day of life by exclusively breastfed healthy newborn infants. J Pediatr 2010; 156(1):29–32.

35. Neville M, Keller R, Seacat J, et al. Studies in human lactation: milk volumes in lactating women during the onset of lactation and full lactation. Am J Clin Nutr 1988;48:1375–86.

36. Ingram JC, Woolridge MW, Greenwood RJ, et al. Maternal predictors of early breast milk output. Acta Paediatr 1999;88(5):493–9.

37. Chen DC, Nommsen-Rivers L, Dewey KG, et al. Stress during labor and delivery and early lactation performance. Am J Clin Nutr 1998;68(2):335–44.

38. Hill PD, Aldag JC, Chatterton RT, et al. Comparison of milk output between mothers of preterm and term infants: the first 6 weeks after birth. J Hum Lact 2005;21(1):22–30.

39. Morton J, Hall JY, Wong RJ, et al. Combining hand techniques with electric pumping increases milk production in mothers of preterm infants. J Perinatol 2009;29(11):757–64.

40. Meier PP, Engstrom JL. Evidence-based practices to promote exclusive feeding of human milk in very low-birthweight infants. NeoReviews 2007;8(11):e467–77.

41. Rodriguez NA, Meier PP, Groer MW, et al. Oropharyngeal administration of colostrum to extremely low birth weight infants: theoretical perspectives. J Perinatol 2009;29(1):1–7.
42. Rodriguez NA, Meier PP, Groer MW, et al. A pilot study of the oropharyngeal administration of own mother's colostrum to extremely low birth weight infants. Adv Neonatal Care 2010;10(4):206–12.
43. Drewett RF, Woolridge M. Sucking patterns of human babies on the breast. Early Hum Dev 1979;3(4):315–21.
44. Mathew OP, Bhatia J. Sucking and breathing patterns during breast- and bottle-feeding in term neonates. Effects of nutrient delivery and composition. Am J Dis Child 1989;143(5):588–92.
45. Bowen-Jones A, Thompson C, Drewett RF. Milk flow and sucking rates during breast-feeding. Dev Med Child Neurol 1982;24(5):626–33.
46. Mizuno K, Ueda A. Changes in sucking performance from nonnutritive sucking to nutritive sucking during breast- and bottle-feeding. Pediatr Res 2006;59(5):728–31.
47. Neville MC, Morton J. Physiology and endocrine changes underlying human lactogenesis II. J Nutr 2001;131(11):3005S–8S.
48. Miranda M, Muriach M, Almansa I, et al. Oxidative status of human milk and its variations during cold storage. Biofactors 2004;20(3):129–37.
49. Jocson MA, Mason EO, Schanler RJ. The effects of nutrient fortification and varying storage conditions on host defense properties of human milk. Pediatrics 1997;100(2):240–3.
50. Hamosh M, Ellis LA, Pollock DR, et al. Breastfeeding and the working mother: effect of time and temperature of short-term storage on proteolysis, lipolysis, and bacterial growth in milk. Pediatrics 1996;97(4):492–8.
51. Slutzah M, Codipilly CN, Potak D, et al. Refrigerator storage of expressed human milk in the neonatal intensive care unit. J Hum Lact 2010;26(3):233–4.
52. Buyukyavuz BI, Adiloglu AK, Onal S, et al. Finding the sources of septicemia at a neonatal intensive care unit: newborns and infants can be contaminated while being fed. Jpn J Infect Dis 2006;59(4):213–5.
53. Furman L, Kennell J. Breastmilk and skin-to-skin kangaroo care for premature infants. Avoiding bonding failure. Acta Paediatr 2000;89(11):1280–3.
54. Lawn JE, Mwansa-Kambafwile J, Horta BL, et al. 'Kangaroo mother care' to prevent neonatal deaths due to preterm birth complications. Int J Epidemiol 2011;40(2):521–5.
55. Riskin A, Imog M, Peri R, et al. Changes in immunomodulatory constituents of human milk in response to active infection in the nursing infant. Pediatr Res 2012;71(2):220–5.
56. Hurst NM, Valentine CJ, Renfro L, et al. Skin-to-skin holding in the neonatal intensive care unit influences maternal milk volume. J Perinatol 1997;17:213–7.
57. Brennan-Behm M, Carlson GE, Meier P, et al. Caloric loss from expressed mother's milk during continuous gavage infusion. Neonatal Netw 1994;13(2):27–32.
58. Meier PP. Supporting lactation in mothers with very low birth weight infants. Pediatr Ann 2003;32(5):317–25.
59. Mathew OP. Breathing patterns of preterm infants during bottle feeding: role of milk flow. J Pediatr 1991;119(6):960–5.
60. Lau C, Smith EO, Schanler RJ. Coordination of suck-swallow and swallow respiration in preterm infants. Acta Paediatr 2003;92(6):721–7.
61. Meier PP, Engstrom JL, Fleming BA, et al. Estimating milk intake of hospitalized preterm infants who breastfeed. J Hum Lact 1996;12(1):21–6.

62. Meier PP, Anderson GC. Responses of small preterm infants to bottle and breast-feeding. MCN Am J Matern Child Nurs 1987;12:97–105.

63. Meier PP. Bottle and breastfeeding: effects on transcutaneous oxygen pressure and temperature in small preterm infants. Nurs Res 1988;37:36–41.

64. Hurst NM, Meier PP, Engstrom JL, et al. Mothers performing in-home measurement of milk intake during breastfeeding of their preterm infants: maternal reactions and feeding outcomes. J Hum Lact 2004;20(2):178–87.

65. Meier PP, Engstrom JL, Crichton CL, et al. A new scale for in-home test-weighing for mothers of preterm and high risk infants [see comment]. J Hum Lact 1994;10(3):163–8.

66. Meier PP, Lysakowski TY, Engstrom JL, et al. The accuracy of test weighing for preterm infants. J Pediatr Gastroenterol Nutr 1990;10(1):62–5.

67. Kavanaugh K, Engstrom JL, Meier PP, et al. How reliable are scales for weighing preterm infants? Neonatal Netw 1990;9(3):29–32.

68. Meier PP, Brown LP, Hurst NM, et al. Nipple shields for preterm infants: effect on milk transfer and duration of breastfeeding. J Hum Lact 2000;16(2):106–14 [Quiz 129–31].

69. Meier PP, Engstrom JL, Zuleger JL, et al. Accuracy of a user-friendly centrifuge for measuring creamatocrits on mothers' milk in the clinical setting. Breastfeed Med 2006;1(2):79–87.

70. Meier PP, Engstrom JL, Murtaugh MA, et al. Mothers' milk feedings in the neonatal intensive care unit: accuracy of the creamatocrit technique. J Perinatol 2002;22(8):646–9.

71. Lucas A, Gibbs JA, Lyster RL, et al. Creamatocrit: simple clinical technique for estimating fat concentration and energy value of human milk. Br Med J 1978;1(6119):1018–20.

72. Griffin TL, Meier PP, Bradford LP, et al. Mothers' performing creamatocrit measures in the NICU: accuracy, reactions, and cost. J Obstet Gynecol Neonatal Nurs 2000;29(3):249–57.

73. Weber A, Loui A, Jochum F, et al. Breast milk from mothers of very low birthweight infants: variability in fat and protein content. Acta Paediatr 2001;90(7):772–5.

74. Wang CD, Chu PS, Mellen BG, et al. Creamatocrit and the nutrient composition of human milk. J Perinatol 1999;19(5):343–6.

75. Meier PP, Engstrom JL. Preventing, diagnosing and managing slow weight gain in the human milk-fed very low birthweight infant. In: Davanzo R, editor. Sulla Nutrizione con Latte Materno. Switzerland: Medela, Inc; 2008. p. 33–47.

76. Davanzo R, Ronfani L, Brovedani P, et al, Breastfeeding in Neonatal Intensive Care Unit Study Group. Breast feeding very-low-birthweight infants at discharge: a multicentre study using WHO definitions. Paediatr Perinat Epidemiol 2009;23(6):591–6.

77. Meier PP, Furman LM, Degenhardt M. Increased lactation risk for late preterm infants and mothers: evidence and management strategies to protect breastfeeding. J Midwifery Womens Health 2007;52(6):579–87.

78. Geddes DT, Kent JC, Mitoulas LR. Tongue movement and intra-oral vacuum in breast-feeding infants. Early Hum Dev 2008;84:471–7.

"Breastfeeding" by Feeding Expressed Mother's Milk

Valerie J. Flaherman, MD, MPH[a],*, Henry C. Lee, MD, MS[b]

KEYWORDS

- Breastfeeding • Lactation • Breast pumping • Hand expression

KEY POINTS

- About 85% of breastfeeding mothers have expressed milk.
- Milk may be expressed by hand, hand-powered pumping, or electric pumping.
- For working mothers, bilateral electric pumps are often more convenient than other methods, but individual mothers may prefer alternative methods.
- For mothers of infants who cannot breastfeed directly, including preterm infants, bilateral electric breast pumps are important for developing and maintaining milk supply and may be used in conjunction with hand techniques.
- For mothers of healthy term infants who have not yet experienced lactogenesis II, hand expression may be preferable to pumping.

MILK EXPRESSION

Milk expression, defined as the removal of breast milk from a mother's breast without an infant's mouth at her nipple, is a normal component of breastfeeding for many mothers. Survey data indicate that 85% of breastfeeding mothers express milk at some point within 4 months of delivery.[1] Mothers practice expression for a variety of reasons, including enabling another person to feed their infant, storing milk for unexpected maternal–infant separation, relieving engorgement and/or nipple pain, maintaining milk supply, and obtaining breast milk to mix with cereal or other foods.[1,2] Milk expression is more common for working mothers and for those with higher income and education.

METHODS OF MILK EXPRESSION

Mothers have several options for milk expression. Review of these options also requires some clarification of the terminology used for milk expression (**Box 1**).

[a] Department of Pediatrics, University of California San Francisco, 3333 California Street, Box 0503, San Francisco, CA 94143-0503, USA; [b] Division of Neonatal and Developmental Medicine, Stanford University School of Medicine, Stanford, CA, USA
* Corresponding author.
E-mail address: FlahermanV@peds.ucsf.edu

Pediatr Clin N Am 60 (2013) 227–246
http://dx.doi.org/10.1016/j.pcl.2012.10.003
0031-3955/13/$ – see front matter © 2013 Elsevier Inc. All rights reserved.

Box 1
Terminology of milk expression

Hand expression

- This method is also called manual expression.

- Hand expression is when a mother uses her hands to exert pressure on her breast for milk expression.

Breast pumping

- This method uses a pump to generate a vacuum similar to that generated by the oral cavity of a feeding newborn.

- There are 2 types:

   ○ Electrical pump: powered by battery or direct electrical current

   ○ Hand pump: manual pumping by the mother

Hands-on pumping

- This method combines breast compression/hand expression with simultaneous bilateral electric breast pumping.

- This method may be especially useful for mothers of premature newborns.

Hand expression may also be called manual expression and differs from hand-powered pumping, which may also be called hand pumping or manual pumping. The most commonly used form of milk expression in developed countries is electric-powered pumping. In addition, mothers may use "hands-on pumping," which combines hand expression with electric-powered pumping. In resource-constrained areas, hand expression may be the only available approach, and may often be adequate to address maternal needs.[3–5]

Hand Expression

Hand expression is an easily taught technique in which a mother uses her hand or hands to exert gentle pressure on her breast in such a way that milk is expressed. Manual hand expression with proper hygiene is no different in terms of infection risk than expression using sterile pumping equipment.[6] Several approaches to hand expression may be used, and a mother who hand expresses regularly refines her technique until she finds the approach that is most effective for her. When teaching hand expression, a provider can suggest that the mother form a "C-shape" with her ipsilateral hand, placing her thumb 2 to 3 cm above and her fingers 2 to 3 cm below her areola. To initiate expression, the mother may press gently back toward her chest wall, exerting continuous pressure without eliciting any pain. The thumb and fingers are pressed toward the chest wall and then brought together and pressed gently forward, so that they push on the ducts beneath the areola. Milk is often expressed at this point. Using a cycle of pressing and releasing and rotating her fingers around the areola, a mother can aim to capture all the ducts until a maximum volume of milk has been expressed.

Breast Pumping

Breast pumping simulates infant suck by generating a vacuum similar to that generated by the oral cavity of a feeding newborn. Breast pumps may be bilateral or unilateral and may be powered electrically, manually, or by foot. Electric pumps are the most widely used method of expression in the United States [1] and may be powered either by direct electrical current or by battery. Manually powered breast pumps may also be called "hand pumps," which can be confused with hand expression.

For mothers who choose to use a pump, pumping for 15 minutes or until 2 minutes after milk flow ceases is often recommended, and this approach results in the highest volume of expressed milk, with higher fat content noted in milk removed at the end of a session of milk expression. However, studies have shown that 80% of the expressed milk is collected in the first 6 minutes, so mothers who have time constraints and are not pump dependent may wish to consider shorter durations of milk expression based on their own individual needs.[7] A vacuum range of 0 to −250 mm Hg and 47 to 55 cycles/min may result in optimal volumes.[8] A fundamental principle of pumping is that the level of vacuum chosen must be comfortable for the mother. Vacuum settings that are high enough to cause pain greatly increase the risk of tissue damage from pumping. One study of 21 mothers estimated that maximal comfortable vacuum is approximately −191 ± 9 mm Hg.[9] One option is to begin a pumping session with a stimulation pattern of 1 to −250 mm Hg at 105 to 120 cycles/min, which may initiate let-down more rapidly.[10] However, it is important for mothers to know that the initiation of let-down with a pump may be slower than with a breastfeeding infant. Let-down may occur earlier during pumping if a mother looks at a photograph of her baby or smells an item of her baby's clothes.

Simultaneous (as opposed to sequential) pumping of both breasts is generally preferred when using electric pumps.[11] In clinical trials, milk volumes expressed with simultaneous pumping was similar or increased compared with sequential pumping.[11–13] Simultaneous pumping also takes less time, which may be of value to many mothers.[12] Several other interventions have been shown to be effective at increasing pumped milk volume. Breast massage,[11] warm compresses before beginning milk expression,[14] and/or warm nipple shields[15] may increase milk volume and decrease the time required for milk expression. In addition, recorded music-based interventions improve the volume of milk expressed by pumping.[16]

Identifying the best type or brand of bilateral electric pump may depend more on personal preference than on an objective standard. A study comparing the Symphony breast pump (Medela, Inc, McHenry, IL, USA) with the Classic breast pump (Medela, Inc) found no differences in milk output.[17] In another study, the Pump In Style pump (Medela, Inc) had both a higher volume of milk extracted and a higher creamatocrit compared with the Embrace pump (Playtex, Westport, CT, USA).[18] Bernabe-Garcia and colleagues[19] compared 4 different types of hand pumps and reported no difference between them with respect to the volume of milk expressed or the duration of milk expression. Mothers must be reminded that the volume of milk extracted by pumping may be larger or smaller than the amount extracted during an infant's feeding.[20] This topic is discussed later, but it is important to recognize that some mothers worry about milk supply when they notice what they perceive as a "small" volume of expressed milk,[21–24] and such milk supply concern can be a major risk factor for breastfeeding discontinuation.[22,25–35]

Considering the high prevalence of pump use, the frequency of adverse events associated with breast pumping seems to be low. The US Food and Drug Administration (FDA) received 37 reports of adverse events as a result of the use of breast pumps between 1992 and 2003, of which 24 reports identified at least 1 patient problem, including pain, soreness, discomfort, tissue damage, erythema, and swelling.[36] Breast pumps have rarely been associated with infectious disease. In 1 reported case, contamination of breast pump equipment with *Pseudomonas aeruginosa* caused illness in a set of premature twins. In a separate case, a mother's breast pump tubing changed color and was found to be colonized by *Serratia marcescens*.[37] This mother discontinued breastfeeding, although neither she nor her twin infants had had signs or symptoms of illness.

Hands-on Pumping

Hands-on pumping was pioneered by Jane Morton and is an approach that combines hand expression with simultaneous bilateral electric breast pumping. This approach often produces more milk than either bilateral breast pumping or hand expression alone.[38] This technique may be especially useful for mothers of premature newborns (see later section), who may need to generate a high level of breast milk production without direct breastfeeding. These results also highlight the importance of continued research into optimal methods of milk expression.

Comparative Effectiveness of Methods of Milk Expression

There have been several studies comparing different methods of milk expression in a variety of settings (**Table 1**). Once a mature milk supply is well established, bilateral electric breast pumping expresses more milk in less time than unilateral pumping, hand pumping, or hand expression.[3,4,39–41] Because electric pumps may remove up to 50% more milk than hand expression with greater ease, mothers who are making mature milk often strongly prefer electric pumps.[42,43] However, individual mothers may prefer manual pumps or hand expression, and many mothers may be able to express adequate milk volumes using any of these approaches. In addition, although bilateral electric breast pumps have better efficacy than hand pumps and express milk more efficiently than hand pumps, these differences may not have an effect on breast-feeding duration. Hayes and colleagues[44] examined mothers enrolled in the Women, Infants and Children (WIC) branch of the Hawaii Department of Public Health and found no difference in breastfeeding duration between working mothers who used an electric breast pump and those who used a hand pump.

ANATOMY OF MILK EXPRESSION

The anatomy of breast pumping is different from the anatomy of hand expression. Hand expression uses positive pressure to release milk from the ducts, and with experience, may also generate let-down, which can assist in the removal of milk. A breast pump generates negative pressure, which works in 2 ways. First, the pump initiates let-down of milk an average of 4 times per pumping session. Second, the negative pressure generated in the phalange of the pump extracts milk from the ducts in a manner similar to the negative pressure generated in the posterior pharynx of the infant. The pump draws the mother's nipple and areola deep into the phalange. Therefore, when using a pump, it is of paramount importance to choose a size for the pump shield that matches the nipple and areola of the mother. Use of a shield that is too small can cause trauma to the nipple.

PHYSIOLOGY OF MILK EXPRESSION

During mature milk production, milk expression increases maternal levels of oxytocin and prolactin. Pumping has a much stronger effect on prolactin levels than does hand expression, and studies have shown that pumping increases prolactin levels even more than does direct breastfeeding.[39,45] However, higher levels of prolactin and oxytocin do not necessarily correlate with increased milk production; a study comparing 2 different pumps found that one yielded a higher milk volume and a higher creamatocrit (indicating more complete breast emptying), whereas the other pump

Table 1
Studies comparing types of milk expression for mothers after the onset of lactogenesis II

Type of Study	Author/Year	Country	Comparison Groups	Finding
Randomized controlled or crossover trials in mothers of premature infants or sick patients in the NICU	Fewtrell et al,[111] 2001	UK	Hand pump vs electric pump	Similar volumes with simultaneous electric pump/manual pump with greater volume when sequentially pumped
	Groh-Wargo et al,[12] 1995	US	Simultaneous (bilateral) electric pump vs single electric pump	No difference in milk volumes. Decreased time spent for simultaneous pump
	Hill et al,[112] 1999	US	Simultaneous vs single electric pump	No difference in milk volumes
	Jones et al,[11] 2001	UK	Simultaneous vs sequential electric pumping, with or without breast massage	Simultaneous pumping resulted in greater volume compared with sequential pumping; breast massage had additive effect on both
	Meier et al,[57] 2012	US	Different electric pump suction patterns (2 groups, both simultaneous electric pumping)	A regimen with an "initiation" pattern mimicking a term infant's rapid sucking rate and irregular sucking rhythm; when used before lactogenesis II, resulted in higher volume than a standard pattern
	Paul et al,[114] 1996	India	Manual expression vs hand pump	Hand pump resulted in greater expression
	Slusher et al,[4] 2007	Kenya and Nigeria	Electric pump, foot-operated pedal pump, and manual expression	Electric pump resulted in greater expression
Crossover design for mothers of term infants (mothers who may be returning to work or school)	Auerbach,[13] 1990	US	Simultaneous vs single electric pump	Simultaneous pumping resulted in greater volume
	Green et al,[43] 1982	US	Electric pump vs hand pump vs manual	Electric pumping resulted in greater volume than either hand pump or manual expression; the last two had similar results
Observational study of mothers of premature infants	Morton et al,[38] 2009	US	Pre/post design of teaching "hands-on pumping"	Hands-on pumping resulted in increased milk expression volumes

showed a much higher release in prolactin. The physiologic relationship between pumping, milk production, and hormonal regulation is clearly complex, and the current evidence base in this area often raises more questions than it answers. For example, a study found that hormonal responses to pumping are blunted among mothers with a family history of alcoholism.[46] The hormonal response to milk expression during lactogenesis I has not been reported and might differ from the response during later phases of lactation.

MOTHER'S EXPERIENCES OF MILK EXPRESSION

Women's experiences of milk expression are diverse. Some mothers find expressing milk to be a pleasant, comfortable, or relaxing activity, whereas others find milk expression painful, stressful, or embarrassing. Providers must note that their own personal experience with milk expression may not be reflective of the experience of individual mothers in their practice. In a qualitative study of milk expression experiences, one mother reported, "I feel like a cow," whereas another said, "I like to be able to do it."[47] One study found that 64% of mothers who expressed breast milk had expressed in the presence of family or friends, but 36% had not.[2] In the development of the Breast Milk Expression Experience Scale, mothers' learning experiences related to breast milk expression ranged from 1.5 to 5 on a scale of 1 to 5, and mothers' personal experiences ranged from 1 to 3.6 on a scale of 1 to 5.[48] Clearly, women differ in their experience and perception of milk expression. **Box 2** provides some suggested parent resources regarding milk expression.

INDICATIONS FOR MILK EXPRESSION

There are a variety of indications for milk expression, and the type and approach to milk expression may vary by indication. Return to work or school is the most common

---

Box 2
Resources for milk expression

Websites

Breastfeeding the High Risk Newborn (Lucile Packard Children's Hospital at Stanford) http://www.lpch.org/DiseaseHealthInfo/HealthLibrary/hrnewborn/bresthub.html

Office of Women's Health, US Department of Health and Human Services http://www.womenshealth.gov/breastfeeding/

La Leche League International http://www.lalecheleague.org/

Videos

Video of hand expression (Newborn Nursery at Lucile Packard Children's Hospital) http://newborns.stanford.edu/Breastfeeding/HandExpression.html

The Marmet Hand Expression Technique (about.com) http://video.about.com/breastfeeding/Hand-Expression-Technique.htm

A Premie Needs His Mother. First Steps to Breastfeeding Your Premature Baby. Jane Morton, MD http://www.breastmilksolutions.com/premie_needs.html

Books

The Womanly Art of Breastfeeding by the La Leche League

The Breastfeeding Mother's Guide to Making More Milk by Diana West

Nursing Mother, Working Mother, Revised Edition by Gale Pryor and Kathleen Huggins

reason for regular breast pumping, and working mothers should note that the time of day affects the volume of milk extracted by pumping, with the highest volumes expressed from 6 AM to noon and the lowest volumes expressed from 6 PM onward.[42] Some mothers have no trouble expressing enough milk while working, but for those who do, it may be advisable to breastfeed the baby just before leaving for work and just after returning from work and to use a bilateral electric breast pump every 3 hours while separated from the baby. After 6 months of age, babies begin to eat solid food, maternal milk supply becomes more stable, and mothers may not need to pump as frequently or at all during separations.[49]

Some mothers express milk as a substitute for direct breastfeeding. This situation may occur when an infant is born premature or critically ill (see later section) and may also be necessary for newborns with a cleft palate, who may not be able to generate adequate negative pressure to feed directly from their mothers' breast. Some mothers do not want to breastfeed directly, and some have infants who have difficulty establishing an effective latch. These women may choose to feed their baby pumped milk only, but it is difficult to maintain milk supply by expression alone. Among mothers of healthy term infants who were pumping only, without direct breastfeeding, none were able to provide breast milk through 6 months.[50] Mothers may also express milk because of casual, occasional mother–infant separation or because they want others to have the experience of feeding the baby. In some cases, mothers may express milk when they have consumed alcohol, drugs, or medication that is contraindicated with breastfeeding. In such situations, the milk must be discarded after expression.

Another common indication for milk expression is to encourage a larger milk supply. Because the use of a breast pump twice daily for 2 weeks in addition to ordinary breastfeeding increases milk production by an average of 175 mL/d for mothers who already have a good milk supply,[18] it may be thought that milk expression has a similar effect on mothers who are experiencing milk supply challenges. For example, mothers may often initiate milk expression because of delayed onset of lactation, high newborn weight loss, or other newborn signs of inadequate milk intake. Although such milk expression after breastfeeding may often be recommended for mothers with milk supply concern, the evidence base for it is limited, with 1 randomized trial finding a trend toward lower milk transfer from mother to infant for mothers who pumped in addition to breastfeeding.[51] Further research is needed to demonstrate the optimal approaches to milk expression for mothers having trouble establishing an adequate mature milk supply.

A globally important indication for milk expression is the use of flash pasteurization of breast milk. Much pediatric HIV infection worldwide is caused by breastfeeding, especially after complementary foods are introduced around 6 months of age. However, substituting other fluids for breast milk may result in even higher morbidity and mortality from gastroenteritis and other infectious diseases. Expressing breast milk could help reduce mother-to-infant transmission after 6 months if mothers are able to treat the expressed milk with flash pasteurization in their home kitchen. This technique has been demonstrated to be feasible and safe, with its effectiveness requiring further study.[5,52]

EARLY MILK EXPRESSION

Early milk expression, before the onset of lactogenesis II, differs from milk expression occurring after the onset of lactogenesis II in several important respects and is discussed separately in this section. In the United States, about half of breastfeeding mothers express milk during the first week after birth, and almost all who express milk in this early time do so using a mechanical pump.[53] The first few days after birth are a period of dramatic maternal hormonal changes, with rapidly increasing levels of prolactin and oxytocin initiating and maintaining lactation. The effect of milk expression on hormones during this early period is unknown, but it is possible that early expression may raise hormone levels and hasten the onset of lactogenesis II. However, it is also possible that early milk expression is not effective at hastening lactogenesis II. Milk volume is low during lactogenesis I, and at each feeding or expression, mothers produce about 0 to 5 mL of colostrum, a thick fluid rich in immunoglobulins. These small volumes are in stark contrast to the volumes produced once lactogenesis II begins, and mothers begin to make copious volumes of mature, white milk. The effect of the type of expression on the volume of milk expressed before the onset of mature milk production has not yet been determined, with some studies reporting that hand expression removes more milk than pumping and some studies reporting the opposite.[40,54–56] One study also found that a breast pump suction pattern that mimics the rapid suck rate and irregular suck rhythm of a breastfeeding newborn before the onset of lactogenesis II did not have a significant effect on the volume of colostrum or the timing of onset of lactogenesis II but was associated with a higher milk output beginning on day 6.[57]

A challenge associated with any method of early milk expression is that expression allows mothers to visualize the small volumes of milk. Mothers who are solely breastfeeding may not have a sense of how much milk they are producing, whereas milk expression makes mothers aware of the volume. Unfortunately, mothers who are not able to express significant volumes of milk may experience feelings of embarrassment and increased milk supply concern.[47] This situation is especially challenging because maternal concern regarding low milk supply can become a self-fulfilling prophecy. Mothers with concerns about low milk supply may begin formula supplementation, which may lead to decreased infant breastfeeding demand and increased milk stasis, which may in turn lead to truly insufficient milk supply. In addition, it is important to remember that mothers in the immediate postpartum period may have residual pain or fatigue from childbirth and may have less comfort with exposing and manipulating their breasts than mothers who have been breastfeeding for weeks or months. Therefore, a mother's reaction to milk expression before the onset of lactogenesis II may be unrelated to her reaction to milk expression once the onset of mature milk production has begun.

A recent Cochrane review found a "lack of data relating to how various methods and techniques of milk expression or pumping assist mothers to meet their own goals."[40] Indeed, the outcome studies have highly variable findings, and there is some evidence that the timing of initiating of pumping might have an influence. Pumping in the first month does not have a significant influence on breastfeeding duration.[58] Furthermore, one study found that expressing breast milk (defined as either use of a mechanical pump or hand expression) in the first 3 weeks was associated with breastfeeding discontinuation by 3 months of age.[28]

The method of expression taught in the immediate postpartum period may have a significant effect on breastfeeding and may even affect breastfeeding duration. A randomized controlled trial that compared breast pumping to hand expression reported that early hand expression increased breastfeeding rates at 2 months by 25% compared with early breast pumping.[59] The positive effect of learning hand expression instead of pumping might be attributable to 2 factors: first, normal colostrum volume might appear more appropriate when expressed by hand rather than by pump, and second, mothers who hand expressed initially reported greater comfort expressing in front of others than mothers who initially pumped.

The WHO and the Academy of Breastfeeding Medicine recommend teaching milk expression to mothers before discharge from birth hospitalization.[60,61] In addition, the Center for Disease Control has endorsed the WHO's Baby Friendly Hospital Initiative, which requires teaching of milk expression to all mothers during birth hospitalization.[62] These policies are based on research showing that frequent milk expression improves breastfeeding duration for mothers who have returned to paid employment[63–69] and the idea that mothers are available during the birth hospitalization to learn milk expression. However, Chen and colleagues[70] reported that receiving breast pump education from a physician or physician assistant was a risk factor for shorter breastfeeding duration, whereas receiving breast pump education from a class or support group was a protective factor associated with a longer breastfeeding duration. These associations could be attributable to differences in the quality of counseling received from these different sources, but the study's results might also be attributable to the fact that breast pump teaching by a physician is a marker of learning breast pumping as an inpatient, which, as discussed earlier, may not be the best time to learn pumping.

MILK STORAGE FOR HEALTHY TERM NEWBORN

Room temperature milk storage is safe for at least 3 to 4 hours and may be safe for up to 8 hours when it has been expressed in a clean manner and stored in cooler room temperatures. Milk may be stored for at least 72 hours refrigerated at 4°C or less, and may be stored for 6 to 12 months in a freezer at −17°C or less. New, warm milk should not be added to cooled, stored milk as this could increase bacterial contamination. Although several companies make cooler bags for the transport and storage of expressed breast milk, these cooler bags maintain a temperature of 15°C or less, and only one study has examined the safety of milk stored at this temperature.[71] Further research is needed in this area. The antibacterial activity in milk declines the longer it is stored, and some studies have noted a decline in the levels of vitamin C in milk frozen for more than 3 months.[72,73] Frozen milk should be thawed in the refrigerator overnight or by running under warm water or gentle agitation in a dish of warm water; refrigerated milk may be served cool or warmed as noted for thawing frozen milk.[74]

EXPRESSION OF MILK FOR PRETERM INFANTS IN THE NEONATAL INTENSIVE CARE UNIT

Mothers whose infants are admitted to the neonatal intensive care unit (NICU) face more challenges than other mothers in initiating and sustaining breast milk feeding.[75,76] These mothers are more likely to have experienced complications in pregnancy and childbirth, such as cesarean section delivery, and may be receiving medications that may interfere with breastfeeding or milk expression.[77,78] In addition, the physical environment of the NICU may not be conducive for breastfeeding or pumping, and the infant's illness may preclude oral feeding for some time. These challenges are most prominent for mothers of preterm infants, as such infants may not actually be able to breastfeed for up to several weeks until they transition from tube feedings to oral feedings.[79] Support in initiating milk expression early in the hospital course helps to increase the likelihood of achieving full breast milk feeding.

MATERNAL COUNSELING FOR THE PRETERM OR CRITICALLY ILL NEWBORN

Early counseling of mothers of preterm or critically ill newborns is a crucial component of ensuring sufficient breast milk for this population. Mothers who have given birth prematurely are more likely to have characteristics that make them less likely to breastfeed, including younger age; lower-income strata; having usage of tobacco, alcohol, and drugs; and having medical complications.[80–82] Because mothers with these risk factors may not have thought about breastfeeding before delivery, may have already made a decision to formula feed,[83–85] or may not have received much guidance on the topic of breast milk,[85–87] they may benefit greatly from education on the specific benefits of breast milk for preterm infants. Such counseling may motivate mothers to provide breast milk during their infants' hospitalization, even if they do not eventually make the commitment to breastfeeding after discharge.

Counseling on both the benefits of breast milk and techniques to initiate and maintain supply can be discussed early on, even before birth, if the mother is hospitalized with the likelihood of preterm birth. Although some hospitals may assign a lactation consultant to offer counseling on milk expression, repeated counseling by several members of the team including obstetricians, labor and delivery nurses, nutritionists, social workers, neonatologists, and NICU nurses may help to reinforce the importance of breast milk for preterm infants.[88] The benefit of breast milk for the premature population is well described,[89–91] and it can be suggested to the mother that breast milk and her task of milk expression is a medical therapy that cannot be replaced by pharmaceuticals and is something that only she can provide for her infant.[92]

Clinicians may wonder if early counseling on breast milk may cause more anxiety for a family in an already stressful and traumatic situation. In a study of a counseling intervention aimed at mothers of premature infants who were initially planning to formula feed, 69 of 81 (85%) mothers initiated breast milk expression, compared with 100% of a control group of mothers intending to breastfeed. Initiation rates did not differ by race or income status. Anxiety status and stress as measured by several scales did not increase with counseling for either group and actually declined during the hospital course.[93]

CREATING AN OPTIMAL ENVIRONMENT FOR NICU PATIENTS

Adequate resources including equipment, environment, and staff training are necessary to support clinicians and parents in the effort to provide breast milk for premature and critically ill neonates. The success of a mother in initiating and sustaining breast milk expression until discharge requires a multidisciplinary approach.[94] Education of staff on breast milk feeding should involve all health care professionals in the NICU, including nurses, nurse practitioners, therapists, neonatologists, and anyone who may have contact with parents.[95] The presence of a physician attitude that breast milk expression is the responsibility of nurses alone has been identified as a potential barrier to improving practice in nurseries.[96] Studies have shown that sociodemographic factors such as younger age, lower educational attainment, non-White race, and inadequate prenatal care are associated with decreased success in breast milk provision for preterm infants.[81,82,97] These high-risk groups should be considered as targets for implementation of the best practices and quality improvement efforts,[98] and it should not be assumed that these risk factors preclude successful establishment of milk expression.

The California Perinatal Quality Care Collaborative (CPQCC) has published a Nutritional Toolkit that outlines several aspects of supporting breast milk provision for premature infants.[94] Using this toolkit as a basis for the best practices, a multihospital collaborative project to improve quality in this area resulted in a 25% increase in breast milk provision for very-low-birthweight (VLBW) infants and a corresponding decrease in necrotizing enterocolitis.[99] Other examples of comprehensive nutrition plans that facilitate breast milk feeding and eventual transition to breastfeeding have been developed by individual NICUs.[98,100] Although the WHO's Baby Friendly Hospital Initiative is primarily designed for the healthy newborn population, implementation of the Ten Steps to Successful Breastfeeding may also lead to increased breast milk provision in the NICU.[101]

TIMING OF MILK EXPRESSION FOR THE PRETERM INFANT

An early start to pumping greatly increases the likelihood of sufficient breast milk supply for the preterm infant. An earlier start to milk expression is more likely to lead to success in lactation and sustained expression. Mothers of newborns who are not breastfeeding should begin milk expression in the first 6 hours after birth, and there may be benefit to starting sooner, within 1 hour of delivery if no contraindications exist.[97,102]

Earlier gestational age at birth is associated with delayed lactogenesis II, and mothers should be counseled about this expectation to avoid frustration in the first days of milk expression.[103] Informing mothers about the variation in milk production in the first few days may potentially prevent mothers from becoming discouraged, and this may be important because some mothers may stop pumping after a few days without milk production because of the perception that they are not being successful. It may also help some mothers to be aware that differences in milk volumes from the left and right breasts may occur, particularly for primiparous mothers, and do not have an impact on total milk output.[104,105]

Frequency of pumping is another important aspect of ensuring enough supply. Mothers should be encouraged to pump a minimum of 8 times a day and potentially up to 12 times a day during the first several weeks when breast milk supply is being established.[100] In the first few days before the onset of mature milk production, the mother should pump for 10 to 15 minutes each session. As the milk begins to come in, the mother should continue to pump for about 2 minutes after the final droplets of milk are released to ensure that the breasts are completely emptied.[106]

APPROACHES TO NICU MILK EXPRESSION

Although the equipment and techniques of milk expression are the same for mothers of healthy newborns as for those of newborns in the NICU, the approach to milk expression needs to be more intense for mothers who are expressing for premature or critically ill infants. There have been several trials comparing the effectiveness of various pumping regimens and pump types, but the importance of any particular method is probably less important than having a concerted approach.[4,96]

For premature babies, electric pumping may be the most efficient approach and is likely to produce more milk volume in the long run.[4] Simultaneous (as opposed to sequential) pumping is generally preferred.[11] In clinical trials of mothers who had given birth prematurely, milk volumes expressed with simultaneous pumping were similar or increased compared with sequential pumping.[11–13] Simultaneous pumping also provides some efficiency, thereby providing more free time for mothers to spend resting or visiting with their infant.[12] This extra time may be more important for mothers of premature babies, as it may be necessary to express milk for weeks or months. Pain and discomfort while pumping, which may be due to vacuum level or phalange size, should be addressed early to prevent a mother from giving up because of those reasons.

Other methods for increasing milk supply have been studied. Breast massage may help to increase expressed volumes,[11] as may combining hand expression with electric pumping.[38] A mechanical pumping pattern that was designed to closely mimic the pattern of a healthy term infant has been shown to increase efficiency and supply.[57] The pattern consisted of 2 phases, the first 2 minutes consisting of rapid suction events, which simulated a nonnutritive initiation phase, and a second slower phase mimicking nutritive sucking to facilitate regular milk flow. Relaxation at the bedside while pumping, skin-to-skin contact, and kangaroo care may also help to facilitate increased milk production.[96,107–109] Galactagogues may be another consideration when there is a concern about inadequate supply (see articles by Rowe and colleagues and Chantry and Howard elsewhere in this issue). In order to ensure establishment of an adequate milk supply, a mother needs access to breast pumps in the postpartum area, the NICU, and at home. Therefore, each NICU should have an adequate supply of equipment for use in the hospital in conjunction with an efficient program for providing equipment for home use. Hospital-grade pumps are approved by the FDA for multiple users, and providers must disinfect and clean the pump between users. Each user must have her own pump kit that she does not share. Women who receive health care coverage through Medicaid or those who qualify for WIC typically are covered through those programs for home use of a hospital-grade pump. Programs may vary by state. For mothers whose infants are hospitalized in the NICU, private insurance companies and health maintenance organizations should also cover pumps, but individual plans may vary. A sample letter to request insurance coverage for pump equipment is available in the CPQCC toolkit.[110]

In situations in which electric pumps are not available because of resource limitations, manual pumps may be just as efficient as electric pumps.[111,112] Manual pumps may also be preferable for mothers who feel intimidated or uncomfortable with electric pumps. Hand expression may be especially useful in the first days to initiate supply,[38,113] because the suction generated by pumps may not fully simulate the biologic action of breastfeeding. However, hand expression may not be as efficient as mechanical pumping in the long term and therefore may be considered an adjunct at various times during the hospital course.[114]

Hand expression may also be helpful in the first day or two to capture small amounts of colostrum for the premature infant. As even small drops are valuable for the preterm neonate, providing small volumes may also demonstrate to the mother her ability to contribute to her infant's care. Hand expression may be particularly useful in this situation to reduce loss to plastic tubing. Medela, Inc, produces a small, 35-mL milk collection container with a curved bottom that is designed to minimize loss of colostrum. The smaller size may also help by setting a reasonable expectation for mothers in the first few days of milk expression. Mothers of twins and higher-order multiples face the greater challenge of providing milk for more than 1 infant. Although having a goal of pumping for more than 1 infant may seem intimidating, observational studies of premature infants have shown that mothers of twins seem to be more successful in sustaining breast milk feeding for their premature infants.[81,115]

STORAGE AND COLLECTION IN THE NICU

Each NICU should have its own guidelines about milk collection and storage. If a baby is not receiving milk immediately after pumping, the milk should be refrigerated. If the baby will not receive the milk within the next 48 hours, it should be frozen. General hygiene techniques including washing of hands with soap and water should be followed. Milk collected at each session of breast milk expression should be held in a different container and labeled. The Human Milk Banking Association of North America (HMBANA) publishes a manual of the best practices for expressing, storing, and handling of human milk in hospital and at home.[116]

One consideration for premature infants is the possibility of cytomegalovirus (CMV) transmission through mother's breast milk.[117–121] The concern for premature infants is that postnatal CMV transmission through maternal breast milk may sometimes cause serious illness. Although freeze-thawing has been a recommended method for reducing transmission, it may not be effective for all cases.[121] General guidelines from the nutrition toolkit of the CPQCC suggest the following steps to reduce CMV transmission[94]: (1) Screen mothers of VLBW infants. (2) Screen infants of CMV-seropositive mothers for CMV if maternal breast milk will be provided. (3) Colostrum may be given fresh or frozen. (4) If the mother is CMV seropositive, freeze all maternal breast milk for at least 24 hours before feeding until the infant is greater than 32 weeks corrected age or feeding directly at the breast. Infants who exhibit symptoms consistent with CMV infection such as respiratory illness, hepatitis, leukopenia, or thrombocytopenia should be tested for CMV. The previous suggestions are not universally accepted, and each institution should review the literature and consider their own policies on handling of breast milk during the first few weeks for premature infants. This subject is a somewhat controversial area, and further research is needed to establish a strong evidence base.

MAINTENANCE AND MONITORING OF MILK SUPPLY

Expression of breast milk for preterm infants is often required for several weeks to even months, and even mothers who were initially motivated require continued support to sustain adequate supply. For mothers of VLBW infants, the challenges of having to express breast milk in the absence of actual breastfeeding can ultimately lead to low rates of expression by the time of hospital discharge.[75,76,81]

The first 2 weeks are a critical period for initiation and maintenance of lactation in this population but one in which other priorities of NICU care may overshadow the attention given to breast milk expression by both parents and clinicians.[122] Because preterm infants often do not receive full enteral feedings for at least 2 weeks, mothers may be falsely reassured that they have expressed "enough" milk during that period, which may lead eventually to an inadequate supply. The Rush Mothers' Milk Club program provides a milk volume record for pump-dependent mothers, which is monitored by staff to alert clinicians if intervention may be needed to increase supply.[122] The mother should be counseled to have an aim of increasing milk supply early on to build a reserve to at least 350 mL/d and ideally 750 to 1000 mL/d during the first 2 weeks.[55,122–124] This goal ensures an eventual adequate supply for VLBW infants.

SPECIAL CONSIDERATIONS FOR CRITICALLY ILL TERM INFANTS

For term infants who are in the NICU, there may be several considerations for feeding. Some infants are admitted for critical illnesses, requiring a prolonged period without enteral feeding. Others are relatively well but require admission for monitoring, phototherapy, or intravenous antibiotics. These latter infants may be able to feed orally for some or all their feedings. In some situations, infants may start to feed orally but may not have the full strength and capacity to take enough nutrition on their own. Even in situations in which the infant has the capacity to breastfeed for all feeding, circumstances may prevent the mother from being at the hospital for all feedings, necessitating milk expression during the times that she is away. In these cases, the mother should seek to either breastfeed or pump about 8 times a day to maintain her milk supply. If the mother is breastfeeding but the infant has not yet established an adequate latch and suck, the mother should express after each breastfeeding session.

For infants who have significant congenital anomalies and/or those requiring surgical management, breast milk feeding may not be considered a priority. However, because such infants are at higher risk of feeding intolerance, infections, and other morbidities, breast milk may be even more important for this population. The promotion of breast milk for surgical patients benefits from all the components of an effective approach as described earlier for premature infants, including adequate counseling, staff support, and early, frequent milk expression. The multidisciplinary team that provides counseling and monitoring may also include physicians, nurses, and nurse practitioners from the surgical team. A successful project to increase breast milk feeding in infants with complex surgical anomalies has been described.[125] Key components of this project were a multidisciplinary planning team, increased education, and bedside nurse involvement in monitoring of milk volumes.

SUMMARY

Breast milk expression, whether by hand, manual pump, or electric pump, is a useful tool for breastfeeding promotion and may be essential for the provision of milk to a baby who cannot breastfeed. The indications for breast milk expression are varied, ranging from maternal employment to extreme prematurity, and the approaches and techniques of milk expression should be tailored to the indication for expression. Milk expression is not necessarily an intuitive process for mothers, both in terms of technique and in terms of maternal experience, and adequate counseling and monitoring by the clinician are needed to help ensure that each mother's milk expression approach leads to the intended goals for her family's specific circumstances.

REFERENCES

1. Labiner-Wolfe J, Fein SB, Shealy KR, et al. Prevalence of breast milk expression and associated factors. Pediatrics 2008;122(Suppl 2):S63–8.
2. Clemons SN, Amir LH. Breastfeeding women's experience of expressing: a descriptive study. J Hum Lact 2010;26(3):258–65.
3. Slusher TM, Slusher IL, Keating EM, et al. Comparison of maternal milk (breastmilk) expression methods in an African nursery. Breastfeed Med 2012;7(2): 107–11.
4. Slusher T, Slusher IL, Biomdo M, et al. Electric breast pump use increases maternal milk volume in African nurseries. J Trop Pediatr 2007;53(2):125–30.
5. Chantry CJ, Young SL, Rennie W, et al. Feasibility of using flash-heated breastmilk as an infant feeding option for HIV-exposed, uninfected infants after 6 months of age in urban Tanzania. J Acquir Immune Defic Syndr 2012;60(1): 43–50.
6. Pittard WB 3rd, Geddes KM, Brown S, et al. Bacterial contamination of human milk: container type and method of expression. Am J Perinatol 1991; 8(1):25–7.
7. Prime DK, Kent JC, Hepworth AR, et al. Dynamics of milk removal during simultaneous breast expression in women. Breastfeed Med 2012;7(2):100–6.
8. Mitoulas LR, Lai CT, Gurrin LC, et al. Effect of vacuum profile on breast milk expression using an electric breast pump. J Hum Lact 2002;18(4):353–60.
9. Kent JC, Mitoulas LR, Cregan MD, et al. Importance of vacuum for breastmilk expression. Breastfeed Med 2008;3(1):11–9.
10. Kent JC, Ramsay DT, Doherty D, et al. Response of breasts to different stimulation patterns of an electric breast pump. J Hum Lact 2003;19(2):179–86 [quiz: 87–8, 218].

11. Jones E, Dimmock PW, Spencer SA. A randomised controlled trial to compare methods of milk expression after preterm delivery. Arch Dis Child Fetal Neonatal Ed 2001;85(2):F91–5.
12. Groh-Wargo S, Toth A, Mahoney K, et al. The utility of a bilateral breast pumping system for mothers of premature infants. Neonatal Netw 1995;14(8):31–6.
13. Auerbach KG. Sequential and simultaneous breast pumping: a comparison. Int J Nurs Stud 1990;27(3):257–65.
14. Yigit F, Cigdem Z, Temizsoy E, et al. Does warming the breasts affect the amount of breastmilk production? Breastfeed Med 2012. [Epub ahead of print].
15. Kent JC, Geddes DT, Hepworth AR, et al. Effect of warm breastshields on breast milk pumping. J Hum Lact 2011;27(4):331–8.
16. Keith DR, Weaver BS, Vogel RL. The effect of music-based listening interventions on the volume, fat content, and caloric content of breast milk produced by mothers of premature and critically ill infants. Adv Neonatal Care 2012; 12(2):112–9.
17. Meier PP, Engstrom JL, Hurst NM, et al. A comparison of the efficiency, efficacy, comfort, and convenience of two hospital-grade electric breast pumps for mothers of very low birthweight infants. Breastfeed Med 2008; 3(3):141–50.
18. Hopkinson J, Heird W. Maternal response to two electric breast pumps. Breastfeed Med 2009;4(1):17–23.
19. Bernabe-Garcia M, Lopez-Alarcon M, Villegas-Silva R, et al. Effectiveness of four manual breast pumps for mothers after preterm delivery in a developing country. J Am Coll Nutr 2012;31(1):63–9.
20. Mitoulas LR, Lai CT, Gurrin LC, et al. Efficacy of breast milk expression using an electric breast pump. J Hum Lact 2002;18(4):344–52.
21. Hill PD. Insufficient milk supply syndrome. NAACOGS Clin Issu Perinat Womens Health Nurs 1992;3(4):605–12.
22. Hill PD. The enigma of insufficient milk supply. MCN Am J Matern Child Nurs 1991;16(6):312–6.
23. Hill PD, Humenick SS. Development of the H & H Lactation Scale. Nurs Res 1996;45(3):136–40.
24. Flaherman VJ, Hicks KG, Cabana MD, et al. Maternal experience of interactions with providers among mothers with milk supply concern. Clin Pediatr 2012; 51(8):778–84.
25. Chan SM, Nelson EA, Leung SS, et al. Breastfeeding failure in a longitudinal post-partum maternal nutrition study in Hong Kong. J Paediatr Child Health 2000;36(5):466–71.
26. Lewallen LP, Dick MJ, Flowers J, et al. Breastfeeding support and early cessation. J Obstet Gynecol Neonatal Nurs 2006;35(2):166–72.
27. Amir LH, Cwikel J. Why do women stop breastfeeding? A closer look at 'not enough milk' among Israeli women in the Negev Region. Breastfeed Rev 2005;13(3):7–13.
28. Schwartz K, D'Arcy HJ, Gillespie B, et al. Factors associated with weaning in the first 3 months postpartum. J Fam Pract 2002;51(5):439–44.
29. Rempel LA. Factors influencing the breastfeeding decisions of long-term breastfeeders. J Hum Lact 2004;20(3):306–18.
30. Yang Q, Wen SW, Dubois L, et al. Determinants of breast-feeding and weaning in Alberta, Canada. J Obstet Gynaecol Can 2004;26(11):975–81.
31. Williams PL, Innis SM, Vogel AM, et al. Factors influencing infant feeding practices of mothers in Vancouver. Can J Public Health 1999;90(2):114–9.

32. Evans ML, Dick MJ, Lewallen LP, et al. Modified breastfeeding attrition pre-diction tool: prenatal and postpartum tests. J Perinat Educ 2004;13(1):1–8.

33. Colin WB, Scott JA. Breastfeeding: reasons for starting, reasons for stopping and problems along the way. Breastfeed Rev 2002;10(2):13–9.

34. Blyth R, Creedy DK, Dennis CL, et al. Effect of maternal confidence on breast-feeding duration: an application of breastfeeding self-efficacy theory. Birth 2002;29(4):278–84.

35. Forman MR, Lewando-Hundt G, Graubard BI, et al. Factors influencing milk insufficiency and its long-term health effects: the Bedouin Infant Feeding Study. Int J Epidemiol 1992;21(1):53–8.

36. Brown SL, Bright RA, Dwyer DE, et al. Breast pump adverse events: reports to the food and drug administration. J Hum Lact 2005;21(2):169–74.

37. Faro J, Katz A, Berens P, et al. Premature termination of nursing secondary to *Serratia marcescens* breast pump contamination. Obstet Gynecol 2011; 117(2 Pt 2):485–6.

38. Morton J, Hall JY, Wong RJ, et al. Combining hand techniques with electric pumping increases milk production in mothers of preterm infants. J Perinatol 2009;29(11):757–64.

39. Zinaman MJ, Hughes V, Queenan JT, et al. Acute prolactin and oxytocin responses and milk yield to infant suckling and artificial methods of expression in lactating women. Pediatrics 1992;89(3):437–40.

40. Becker GE, Cooney F, Smith HA. Methods of milk expression for lactating women. Cochrane Database Syst Rev 2011;(12):CD006170.

41. Garza C, Johnson CA, Harrist R, et al. Effects of methods of collection and storage on nutrients in human milk. Early Hum Dev 1982;6(3):295–303.

42. Boutte CA, Garza C, Fraley JK, et al. Comparison of hand- and electric-operated breast pumps. Hum Nutr Appl Nutr 1985;39(6):426–30.

43. Green D, Moye L, Schreiner RL, et al. The relative efficacy of four methods of human milk expression. Early Hum Dev 1982;6(2):153–9.

44. Hayes DK, Prince CB, Espinueva V, et al. Comparison of manual and electric breast pumps among WIC women returning to work or school in Hawaii. Breast-feed Med 2008;3(1):3–10.

45. Hill PD, Aldag JC, Demirtas H, et al. Association of serum prolactin and oxytocin with milk production in mothers of preterm and term infants. Biol Res Nurs 2009; 10(4):340–9.

46. Mennella JA, Pepino MY. Breastfeeding and prolactin levels in lactating women with a family history of alcoholism. Pediatrics 2010;125(5):e1162–70.

47. Morse JM, Bottorff JL. The emotional experience of breast expression. J Nurse Midwifery 1988;33(4):165–70.

48. Flaherman VJ, Gay B, Scott C, et al. Development of the breast milk expression experience measure. Matern Child Nutr 2012. [Epub ahead of print].

49. Morse JM, Harrison MJ, Prowse M. Minimal breastfeeding. J Obstet Gynecol Neonatal Nurs 1986;15(4):333–8.

50. Geraghty SR, Khoury JC, Kalkwarf HJ. Human milk pumping rates of mothers of singletons and mothers of multiples. J Hum Lact 2005;21(4):413–20.

51. Chapman DJ, Young S, Ferris AM, et al. Impact of breast pumping on lactogen-esis stage II after cesarean delivery: a randomized clinical trial. Pediatrics 2001; 107(6):E94.

52. Mbuya MN, Humphrey JH, Majo F, et al. Heat treatment of expressed breast milk is a feasible option for feeding HIV-exposed, uninfected children after 6 months of age in rural Zimbabwe. J Nutr 2010;140(8):1481–8.

53. Centers for Disease Control. Web Tables Report for the Infant Feeding Practices Study. Published 2011. Available at: http://cdc.gov/ifps/pdfs/data/IFPS2_tables_ch3.pdf. Accessed December 20, 2011.

54. Flaherman VJ, Aby J, Burgos AE, et al. Randomized trial of early limited formula to reduce formula use at 1 week and promote breast-feeding at 3 months in infants with high early weight loss. Abstract Presentation, Pediatric Academic Societies Annual Meeting. Boston, 2012.

55. Slusher T, Hampton R, Bode-Thomas F, et al. Promoting the exclusive feeding of own mother's milk through the use of hindmilk and increased maternal milk volume for hospitalized, low birth weight infants (<1800 grams) in Nigeria: a feasibility study. J Hum Lact 2003;19(2):191–8.

56. Ohyama M, Watabe H, Hayasaka Y. Manual expression and electric breast pumping in the first 48 h after delivery. Pediatr Int 2010;52(1):39–43.

57. Meier PP, Engstrom JL, Janes JE, et al. Breast pump suction patterns that mimic the human infant during breastfeeding: greater milk output in less time spent pumping for breast pump-dependent mothers with premature infants. J Perinatol 2012;32(2):103–10.

58. Geraghty S, Davidson B, Tabangin M, et al. Predictors of breastmilk expression by 1 month postpartum and influence on breastmilk feeding duration. Breastfeed Med 2012;7(2):112–7.

59. Flaherman VJ, Gay B, Scott C, et al. Randomised trial comparing hand expression with breast pumping for mothers of term newborns feeding poorly. Arch Dis Child Fetal Neonatal Ed 2012;97(1):F18–23.

60. UNICEF/WHO. Baby-Friendly Hospital Initiative: Revised, Updated and Expanded for Integrated Care, Section 1, Background and Implementation, Preliminary version. Published 2006. Available at: http://www.who.int/nutrition/topics/BFHI_Revised_Section1.pdf. Accessed January 17, 2008.

61. Academy of Breastfeeding Medicine Clinical Protocol Committee. ABM Clinical Protocol #2 (2007 revision): guidelines for hospital discharge of the breastfeeding term newborn and mother: "the going home protocol". Breastfeed Med 2007;2(3):158–65.

62. Centers for Disease Control. Vital signs: hospital support for breastfeeding. Published 2011. Available at: http://www.cdc.gov/VitalSigns/Breastfeeding/. Accessed February 1, 2012.

63. Auerbach KG, Guss E. Maternal employment and breast-feeding. A study of 567 women's experiences. Am J Dis Child 1984;138(10):958–60.

64. Hills-Bonczyk SG, Avery MD, Savik K, et al. Women's experiences with combining breast-feeding and employment. J Nurse Midwifery 1993;38(5):257–66.

65. Whaley SE, Meehan K, Lange L, et al. Predictors of breastfeeding duration for employees of the Special Supplemental Nutrition Program for Women, Infants, and Children (WIC). J Am Diet Assoc 2002;102(9):1290–3.

66. Forte A, Mayberry LJ, Ferketich S. Breast milk collection and storage practices among mothers of hospitalized neonates. J Perinatol 1987;7(1):35–9.

67. Auerbach KG, Walker M. When the mother of a premature infant uses a breast pump: what every NICU nurse needs to know. Neonatal Netw 1994;13(4):23–9.

68. Chamberlain LB, McMahon M, Philipp BL, et al. Breast pump access in the inner city: a hospital-based initiative to provide breast pumps for low-income women. J Hum Lact 2006;22(1):94–8.

69. Nyqvist KH, Sjoden PO, Ewald U. Mothers' advice about facilitating breastfeeding in a neonatal intensive care unit. J Hum Lact 1994;10(4):237–43.

70. Chen PG, Johnson LW, Rosenthal MS. Sources of education about breastfeeding and breast pump use: what effect do they have on breastfeeding duration? An analysis of the infant feeding practices survey II. Matern Child Health J 2012; 16(7):1421–30.

71. Hamosh M, Ellis LA, Pollock DR, et al. Breastfeeding and the working mother: effect of time and temperature of short-term storage on proteolysis, lipolysis, and bacterial growth in milk. Pediatrics 1996;97(4):492–8.

72. Buss IH, McGill F, Darlow BA, et al. Vitamin C is reduced in human milk after storage. Acta Paediatr 2001;90(7):813–5.

73. Bank MR, Kirksey A, West K, et al. Effect of storage time and temperature on folacin and vitamin C levels in term and preterm human milk. Am J Clin Nutr 1985;41(2):235–42.

74. Academy of Breastfeeding Medicine Protocol Committee. ABM clinical protocol #8: human milk storage information for home use for full-term infants (original protocol March 2004; revision #1 March 2010). Breastfeed Med 2010;5(3): 127–30.

75. Lefebvre F, Ducharme M. Incidence and duration of lactation and lactational performance among mothers of low-birth-weight and term infants. CMAJ 1989;140(10):1159–64.

76. Hill PD, Aldag JC, Chatterton RT, et al. Comparison of milk output between mothers of preterm and term infants: the first 6 weeks after birth. J Hum Lact 2005;21(1):22–30.

77. Garite TJ, Combs CA. Obstetric interventions beneficial to prematurely delivering newborn babies: antenatal corticostetroids, progesterone, magnesium sulfate. Clin Perinatol 2012;39(1):33–45.

78. Lee HC, Gould JB. Survival advantage associated with cesarean delivery in very low birth weight vertex neonates. Obstet Gynecol 2006;107(1):97–105.

79. Sridhar S, Arguello S, Lee HC. Transition to oral feeding in preterm infants. NeoReviews 2011;12(3):e141–7.

80. Alexander GR, Weiss J, Hulsey TC, et al. Preterm birth prevention: an evaluation of programs in the United States. Birth 1991;18(3):160–9.

81. Lee HC, Gould JB. Factors influencing breast milk versus formula feeding at discharge for very low birth weight infants in California. J Pediatr 2009;155(5): 657–662.e1–2.

82. Flacking R, Wallin L, Ewald U. Perinatal and socioeconomic determinants of breastfeeding duration in very preterm infants. Acta Paediatr 2007;96(8): 1126–30.

83. Wiemann CM, DuBois JC, Berenson AB. Racial/ethnic differences in the decision to breastfeed among adolescent mothers. Pediatrics 1998;101(6):e11.

84. Maehr JC, Lizarraga JL, Wingard DL, et al. A comparative study of adolescent and adult mothers who intend to breastfeed. J Adolesc Health 1993;14(6):453–7.

85. Hill GJ, Arnett DB, Mauk E. Breast-feeding intentions among low-income pregnant and lactating women. Am J Health Behav 2008;32(2):125–36.

86. Lu MC, Prentice J, Yu SM, et al. Childbirth education classes: sociodemographic disparities in attendance and the association of attendance with breastfeeding initiation. Matern Child Health J 2003;7(2):87–93.

87. Bailey JM, Crane P, Nugent CE. Childbirth education and birth plans. Obstet Gynecol Clin North Am 2008;35(3):497–509, ix.

88. Rice SJ, Craig D, McCormick F, et al. Economic evaluation of enhanced staff contact for the promotion of breastfeeding for low birth weight infants. Int J Technol Assess Health Care 2010;26(2):133–40.

89. Patel AL, Meier PP, Engstrom JL. The evidence for use of human milk in very low-birthweight preterm infants. NeoReviews 2007;8:e459–66.

90. Schanler RJ. The use of human milk for premature infants. Pediatr Clin North Am 2001;48(1):207–19.

91. Sisk PM, Lovelady CA, Dillard RG, et al. Early human milk feeding is associated with a lower risk of necrotizing enterocolitis in very low birth weight infants. J Perinatol 2007;27(7):428–33.

92. Merewood A. Breastfeeding: promotion of a low-tech lifesaver. NeoReviews 2007;8(7):e296–300.

93. Sisk PM, Lovelady CA, Dillard RG, et al. Lactation counseling for mothers of very low birth weight infants: effect on maternal anxiety and infant intake of human milk. Pediatrics 2006;117(1):e67–75.

94. California Perinatal Quality Care Collaborative. Nutritional support of the very low birth weight infant. Stanford (CA): California Perinatal Quality Care Collaborative; 2008.

95. Pineda RG, Foss J, Richards L, et al. Breastfeeding changes for VLBW infants in the NICU following staff education. Neonatal Netw 2009;28(5):311–9.

96. Renfrew MJ, Craig D, Dyson L, et al. Breastfeeding promotion for infants in neonatal units: a systematic review and economic analysis. Health Technol Assess 2009;13(40):1–146, iii–iv.

97. Furman L, Minich N, Hack M. Correlates of lactation in mothers of very low birth weight infants. Pediatrics 2002;109(4):e57.

98. Meier PP, Engstrom JL, Mingolelli SS, et al. The Rush Mothers' Milk Club: breastfeeding interventions for mothers with very-low-birth-weight infants. J Obstet Gynecol Neonatal Nurs 2004;33(2):164–74.

99. Lee HC, Kurtin PS, Wight NE, et al. A quality improvement project to increase breastmilk use in very low birth weight infants. Pediatrics, in press.

100. Dougherty D, Luther M. Birth to breast–a feeding care map for the NICU: helping the extremely low birth weight infant navigate the course. Neonatal Netw 2008;27(6):371–7.

101. Merewood A, Philipp BL, Chawla N, et al. The baby-friendly hospital initiative increases breastfeeding rates in a US neonatal intensive care unit. J Hum Lact 2003;19(2):166–71.

102. Parker LA, Sullivan S, Krueger C, et al. Effect of early breast milk expression on milk volume and timing of lactogenesis stage II among mothers of very low birth weight infants: a pilot study. J Perinatol 2012;32(3):205–9.

103. Henderson JJ, Hartmann PE, Newnham JP, et al. Effect of preterm birth and antenatal corticosteroid treatment on lactogenesis II in women. Pediatrics 2008;121(1):e92–100.

104. Engstrom JL, Meier PP, Jegier B, et al. Comparison of milk output from the right and left breasts during simultaneous pumping in mothers of very low birthweight infants. Breastfeed Med 2007;2(2):83–91.

105. Hill PD, Aldag JC, Zinaman M, et al. Comparison of milk output between breasts in pump-dependent mothers. J Hum Lact 2007;23(4):333–7.

106. Meier PP, Brown LP, Hurst NM. Breastfeeding the preterm infant. In: Riordan J, Auerbach KG, editors. Breastfeeding and human lactation. 2nd edition. Boston: Jones & Bartlett; 1998. p. 449–73.

107. Meier PP. Breastfeeding in the special care nursery. Prematures and infants with medical problems. Pediatr Clin North Am 2001;48(2):425–42.

108. Feher SD, Berger LR, Johnson JD, et al. Increasing breast milk production for premature infants with a relaxation/imagery audiotape. Pediatrics 1989;83(1):57–60.

109. Spatz DL. Ten steps for promoting and protecting breastfeeding for vulnerable infants. J Perinat Neonatal Nurs 2004;18(4):385–96.

110. Appendix 4-L1. #1 Sample letter: explanation of medical need for breast pump. In: California Perinatal Quality Care Collaborative. Nutritional support of the very low birth weight Infant. 2008. p. 100–1.

111. Fewtrell MS, Lucas P, Collier S, et al. Randomized trial comparing the efficacy of a novel manual breast pump with a standard electric breast pump in mothers who delivered preterm infants. Pediatrics 2001;107(6):1291–7.

112. Hill PD, Aldag JC, Chatterton RT. Effects of pumping style on milk production in mothers of non-nursing preterm infants. J Hum Lact 1999;15(3):209–16.

113. Morton J, Wong RJ, Hall JY, et al. Combining hand techniques with electric pumping increases the caloric content of milk in mothers of preterm infants. J Perinatol 2012;32(10):791–6.

114. Paul VK, Singh M, Deorari AK, et al. Manual and pump methods of expression of breast milk. Indian J Pediatr 1996;63(1):87–92.

115. Killersreiter B, Grimmer I, Buhrer C, et al. Early cessation of breast milk feeding in very low birthweight infants. Early Hum Dev 2001;60(3):193–205.

116. 2011 Best practice for expressing, storing and handling human milk in hospitals, homes, and child care settings. 3rd editon. Fort Worth (TX): HMBANA; 2011.

117. Bryant P, Morley C, Garland S, et al. Cytomegalovirus transmission from breast milk in premature babies: does it matter? Arch Dis Child Fetal Neonatal Ed 2002; 87(2):F75–7.

118. Hamprecht K, Goelz R, Maschmann J. Breast milk and cytomegalovirus infection in preterm infants. Early Hum Dev 2005;81(12):989–96.

119. Hamprecht K, Maschmann J, Muller D, et al. Cytomegalovirus (CMV) inactivation in breast milk: reassessment of pasteurization and freeze-thawing. Pediatr Res 2004;56(4):529–35.

120. Lee HC, Enright A, Benitz WE, et al. Postnatal cytomegalovirus infection from frozen breast milk in preterm, low birth weight infants. Pediatr Infect Dis J 2007;26(3):276.

121. Maschmann J, Hamprecht K, Weissbrich B, et al. Freeze-thawing of breast milk does not prevent cytomegalovirus transmission to a preterm infant. Arch Dis Child Fetal Neonatal Ed 2006;91(4):F288–90.

122. Meier PP, Engstrom JL. Evidence-based practices to promote exclusive feeding of human milk in very low-birthweight infants. NeoReviews 2007;8(11):e467–77.

123. Wight NE, Morton JA, Kim JH. Managing breastfeeding in the NICU. In: Wight NE, Morton JA, Kim J, editors. Best medicine: human milk in the NICU. Amarillo (TX): Hale Publishing; 2008. p. 97–135.

124. Hurst NM, Meier PP. Breastfeeding the preterm infant. In: Riordan J, Sudbury M, editors. Breastfeeding and human lactation. London: Jones & Bartlett; 2005. p. 367–408.

125. Edwards TM, Spatz DL. An innovative model for achieving breast-feeding success in infants with complex surgical anomalies. J Perinat Neonatal Nurs 2010;24(3):246–53 [quiz: 254–5].

Donor Human Milk Banking and the Emergence of Milk Sharing

Susan Landers, MD[a,b,*], Ben T. Hartmann, PhD[c,d]

KEYWORDS

- Donor human milk banking • Premature infant • Necrotizing enterocolitis
- Risk management • Milk sharing

KEY POINTS

- Provide evidence for the safety and efficacy of feeding donor human milk to premature babies.
- Review current milk banking practices in North America.
- Review the effects of long-term storage, handling, and heat treatment methods on various components of donor human milk.
- Describe risk management and quality control methods in donor human milk banking.

INTRODUCTION

Today in North America, there are 13 donor milk banks that make up the Human Milk Banking Association of North America (HMBANA). These banks are located in San Jose, CA; Denver, CO; Indianapolis, IN; Coralville, IA; Kalamazoo, MI; Raleigh, NC; Columbus, OH; Austin, TX; Fort Worth, TX; Kansas City, MO; Newtonville, MA; Calgary, Alberta; and Vancouver, BC, Canada (https://www.hmbana.org). Four more milk banks scattered throughout North America are currently in development and scheduled to open in 2013. These banks are not-for-profit entities. In 2006, Prolacta Bioscience, Inc (Monrovia, CA, USA), was founded as a for-profit entity to provide a commercial alternative to human milk banking, specifically, formulations of human

Disclosures: Dr Ben Hartmann has accepted Sponsored Travel from Medela AG, a manufacturer of breast pumping equipment. Dr Susan Landers currently serves on the Medical Advisory Board for Medela, Inc (Breastfeeding US, 1101 Corporate Drive, McHenry, IL, USA).
[a] Pediatrix Medical Group, 1301 Concord Terrace, Sunrise, FL 33323, USA; [b] Seton Family of Hospitals, Department of Neonatology, 1201 West 38th Street, Austin, TX 78705, USA; [c] Neonatology Clinical Care Unit, Perron Rotary Express Milk Bank, King Edward Memorial Hospital, 1st Floor Block A, Bagot Road, Subiaco 6008, Western Australia; [d] Centre for Neonatal Research and Education, The University of Western Australia, M550, 35 Stirling Highway Crawley, Perth 6009, Western Australia
* Corresponding author. Seton Medical Center, Department of Neonatology, 1201 West 38th Street, Austin, TX 78705.
E-mail address: susan_landers@pediatrix.com

milk designed for premature and critically ill infants (http://www.prolacta.com). Donor human milk is now being provided to patients throughout North America from both sources. Since the 1990s, with evidence of safety and increased amount of research on the clinical benefits of feeding donor human milk, milk banking has proliferated globally. Milk banking now exists in many countries, including Australia, Brazil, France, Germany, Italy, Switzerland, Norway, Finland, United Kingdom, Bulgaria, Slovakia, and South Africa.

In the United States, HMBANA is responsible for human milk banking practices and procedures, but there is currently no official federal oversight or regulation of milk banking. The original HMBANA guidelines were written in 1985, with input from the Centers for Disease Control (CDC) and the Food and Drug Administration (FDA). All HMBANA milk banks function under the supervision of medical advisory boards. Prolacta Bioscience, Inc, reports following FDA regulations for both food and pharmaceuticals for their milk products. However, the FDA reviewed the practice of milk donor banking in the United States and decided against federal regulation of human milk banking (http://www.fda.gov/AdvisoryCommittees/CommitteesMeetingMaterials/PediatricAdvisoryCommittee/ucm201871.htm). Only a few states (eg, Texas) have regulations and state laws specifying guidelines related to procurement, processing, and distribution of human milk. New York and California have laws requiring milk banks to be licensed with the state before distributing milk, and California regulates milk banks in a manner similar to tissue banks.

In North America, not-for-profit milk banks (HMBANA) are generally community based or hospital based, function independently, and are operated with hospital or grant funding. Each bank charges a processing fee for dispensed donor milk, ranging from $3 to $5 per ounce. The milk banks serve not only hospitalized inpatients but also outpatients. Milk banks typically prioritize hospitals and neonatal intensive care units (NICUs) within their state but reach out to serve other states as well. For example, in the first decade of its existence the Mother's Milk Bank of Austin served 56 hospitals and NICUs throughout Texas, 11 in Florida, 10 in Midwestern states, and 8 in South Atlantic states.

The greatest barrier to the use of donor human milk in NICUs is the lack of consensus among neonatologists regarding the efficacy of donor human milk feedings for all preterm babies. The cost borne by hospitals for purchasing the milk is another significant barrier, as whether or not private and/or Medicaid insurance coverage exists for donor milk varies from state to state. In addition, hospitals continue to express concerns about the availability of donor milk (especially preterm donor milk), the need for small aliquot volumes, the lack of uniform NICU-based milk preparation and fortification protocols, and the additional burden to the hospital, such as the necessity of tracking recipients and documentation of informed consent.

MANAGEMENT OF DONOR MILK BANKS

Within North America, milk banking guidelines and procedures are largely standardized and evidence-based. Donor selection occurs after careful characterization of the potential donor's health history. Donors must be in good health, taking no medications or herbals and nursing an infant less than 1 year old. Lactating women who have extra milk after feeding their own infant or who have experienced perinatal loss donate to milk banks. Donor screening is rigorous and involves verbal and written questionnaires and laboratory serologic blood testing (cost, $150–$300 per donor) for human immunodeficiency virus (HIV)-1, HIV-2, human T-lymphotropic virus (HTLV)-I and II, hepatitis B virus (HBV), hepatitis C virus (HCV), syphilis, and tuberculosis. Donors with positive test results are excluded. Other donor exclusion criteria include high-risk behaviors for HIV, use of illegal drugs, smoking or use of tobacco products, drinking more than 2 alcoholic drinks per day, a history of organ or tissue transplant, any blood transfusion in the prior 12 months, tattoo or body piercing within the last 12 months, and past travel to UK for more than 3 months or to Europe for more than 5 months, from 1980 to 1996. These are the same donor exclusion criteria used by American Association of Blood Banks (AABB; www.aabb.org). Prolacta Bioscience, Inc, uses some additional techniques for donor screening and quality control, including donor milk drug testing, DNA fingerprinting to ensure that the donor milk belongs to the screened donor, a cold chain delivery system and data logging technology, and polymerase chain reaction (PCR) testing for infectious agents in milk pools both before and after pasteurization.

Donor education for proper collection, storage, and transport of milk is paramount. In North America, donors are given instructions and specific protocols for expressing milk, proper hygiene, handling, and labeling. The milk is stored at $-20°C$ in polyethylene containers and transported on dry ice, and long-term freezing at $-20°C$ occurs at each milk bank. Frozen milk is later defrosted, pooled, and mixed, using universal precautions. Some milk banks conduct prepasteurization bacteriologic screening, which screens for donor technique and possible trends in colonization of pathogens. HMBANA milk banks perform heat processing with the Holder method using a commercial pasteurizer ($62.5°C$ for 30 minutes). Prolacta Bioscience uses the high-temperature, short-time (HTST) pasteurization method ($72°C$ for 16 seconds). All milk banks perform postpasteurization bacteriologic testing, which verifies pasteurization. No milk with any positive culture results after pasteurization is dispensed from HMBANA banks. Pasteurized milk is then chilled and stored for later use and dispensed with a physician's prescription.

FACTORS AFFECTING THE SAFETY OF DONOR MILK

Many factors influence the current safety of donor human milk. These include the nature of donor screening, donor honesty (about unknown medications or herbal exposure), potential infectious agents, milk changes from storage and preservation, milk component changes from heat treatment methods, and quality control of milk banking techniques. Infection risks associated with donor human milk feedings are thought to be negligible. There have been no reported cases of viral transmission or infection from the feeding of pasteurized donor human milk. However, many hospitals and neonatologists prefer to obtain informed consent for the remote possibility of infection and for the possibility of unknown drug or herbal exposure. Others assume donor milk feeding is the standard of care and obtain consent for its use only as part of the general consent for medical treatment.

Concerns remain regarding donor milk, as neonatologists aim to safeguard infants against the potential for exposure to pathogens, such as gram-negative organisms, methicillin-resistant *Staphylococcus aureus*, and group B beta-hemolytic *Streptococcus*. Neonatologists do not uniformly understand that mother's own milk is frequently colonized with bacteria, nor do most know that pasteurized donor milk is dispensed as a sterile product.[1] In fact, prepasteurization bacteriologic screening studies have shown that a wide variety of bacteria are present in donor human milk.[2] However, Holder pasteurization is an effective means to remove any detectable bacteria from donor milk.[2,3] In addition, pasteurized donor milk (without fortifiers or other additives) remains culture-negative for 24 hours after thawing and routine handling in the NICU.[4] The HTST treatment method has also shown to be effective in eradicating pathogenic bacteria within the first 12 seconds of heating.[5]

Physicians commonly express concern about possible viral transmission, especially cytomegalovirus (CMV) and HIV. Hamprecht and colleagues[6] have compared the effects of 2 heat treatment methods (Holder vs HTST, in this study 72°C for only 5 seconds) on CMV infectivity and on milk components. Both heat treatment methods effectively inhibited CMV, as measured by PCR, CMV-RNA assay, and microculture assay for infectivity.[6] Another study also found the HTST process to be highly effective in eradicating HIV and marker viruses for HBV and HCV.[5]

Concerns have been raised about the adverse effects of milk storage and processing on the antiinfective properties of donor milk. Concentrations of immunomodulatory proteins (lysozyme, lactoferrin, lactoperoxidase, and secretory IgA) are reduced 50% to 80% by pasteurization, and to a lesser extent by frozen storage, when compared with fresh milk.[7,8] The levels of other immunoactive cytokines (interferon, tumor necrosis factor, and interleukin) and many important growth factors (granulocyte colony-stimulating factor, hepatocyte growth factor, heparin-binding epidermal-like growth factor, transforming growth factor, and erythropoietin) are significantly reduced by Holder pasteurization.[9,10] In addition, antioxidants are measurably altered by heat treatment.[11] HTST pasteurization, when compared with Holder pasteurization, has been shown to be less harmful in reducing enzymes that mark the immunologic quality of the milk.[6] Studies comparing heat treatment methods (Holder vs HTST) in their alteration of bactericidal and antioxidant capacities of human milk have shown that only short heating methods, 62°C to 72°C for 5 seconds, preserve the concentrations of growth factors in human milk.[12]

RECOMMENDATIONS AND CURRENT CLINICAL USES OF DONOR HUMAN MILK

In 2003, the World Health Organization and United Nations Children's Fund (UNICEF) recommended that for health situations where infants cannot or should not be breast-fed, the best alternative to expressed breast milk from an infant's own mother is breast milk from a healthy wet nurse or human milk bank. American Academy of Pediatrics (AAP) policy supports the use of pasteurized donor milk when mother's own milk is not available (**Box 1**).[13] Human milk banks in North America adhere to guidelines for quality control of screening and testing donors and pasteurize all milk before distribution. The AAP, CDC, and FDA do not recommend feeding fresh human milk from unscreened donors because of the risk of transmitting infectious agents.

Box 1
Recently updated AAP policy recommendations (Pediatr 2012;129:e827–41)

1. "The potent benefits of human milk are such that all preterm infants should receive human milk. Mother's own milk, fresh or frozen, should be the primary diet for preterm infants, and it should be fortified appropriately for the infant born weighing less than 1,500 grams."

2. "If mother's own milk is unavailable despite significant lactation support, pasteurized donor milk should be used."

3. "Quality control of pasteurized donor milk is important and should be monitored."

Donor milk is most often used for the nutritional support of very premature infants and infants with malabsorption syndromes and/or severe feeding intolerance. Preventative uses include necrotizing enterocolitis (NEC) and inflammatory bowel disease. In North America, other common clinical therapeutic uses for donor milk include short gut syndrome (post-NEC), infectious diseases (acute gastroenteritis, sepsis, and pneumonia), postsurgical gut healing (omphalocele, gastroschisis, bowel obstruction, and intestinal fistulas), immunologic diseases (severe allergies and IgA deficiency), chronic renal failure, congenital heart disease, inborn errors of metabolism, and failure to thrive.

CLINICAL STUDIES OF DONOR MILK USE

A recent Cochrane Database systematic review of 8 randomized controlled trials found that feeding very preterm infants (<32 weeks gestation and <1800 g birth weight) formula compared with donor milk resulted in higher rates of growth in the short term. Weight gain, linear growth, and head growth were improved in infants fed formula compared with infants who received donor milk. There was no evidence of an effect on long-term growth rates or on neurodevelopmental outcomes.[14]

Most compelling is the finding of this Cochrane review, as well as 2 other systematic reviews indicating a 4-fold increased risk of NEC in preterm or low birth weight infants fed formula compared with those fed donor human milk (**Table 1**).[15,16] Some of these older studies, however, did not include a large proportion of extremely premature infants, and nutritional protocols did not evaluate human milk fortifiers (HMFs) or contemporary preterm formula.

Studies have not proved conclusively that donor milk feeding reduces infection in preterm babies. Although a large national cohort of extremely low-birth-weight preterm babies found that early feedings with either donor or mother's own milk were associated with decreased rates of late-onset sepsis,[17] a randomized controlled trial found that infants fed donor milk, supplementing their mother's own milk, had similar rates of late-onset sepsis, compared with infants fed preterm formula and mother's own milk,[18] and a systematic review did not find that donor milk reduces sepsis in preterm infants.[19]

There are few recent trials of donor milk in preterm infants. One such trial in extremely preterm infants assigned infants to supplementation of mother's own milk feeding to either donor milk or formula. This study showed no significant difference in the rates of NEC and/or late-onset sepsis, measured together.[18] Further, it showed poor growth in infants who were supplemented with donor human milk compared with the formula-fed babies. However, limitations of this trial, including lack of measurement of the protein content of the donor milk used, were of concern.[20] Later studies have shown better growth in premature infants managed with adjustable, individualized fortification of donor human milk.[21]

The most recent trial of donor milk was a large multicenter randomized controlled trial conducted to examine the occurrence of NEC in extremely preterm infants fed an exclusively human milk–based diet.[22] Study infants were fed predominantly their

Table 1
Risk of necrotizing enterocolitis in preterm or low birth weight infants fed formula milk versus donor breast milk. (Reference # 14)

Study Author, Year	Formula Milk	Donor Breastmilk	Weight	Risk Ratio (95% CI)
Gross,[47] 1983	3/26	1/41	8.1%	4.73 (0.52,43.09)
Tyson et al,[48] 1983	1/44	0/37	5.7%	2.53 (0.11,60.39)
Lucas et al,[49] 1984	4/76	1/83	10.0%	4.37 (0.50,38.23)
Lucas et al,[49] 1984	5/173	2/170	21.0%	2.46 (0.48,12.49)
Schanler et al,[18] 2005	10/88	5/78	55.3%	1.77 (0.63,4.96)
Total	23/407	9/409	100%	2.46 (1.19,5.08)

Data from Quigley MA, Henderson G, Anthony MT, et al. Formula milk versus donor breast milk for feeding preterm or low birth weight infants. Cochrane Database Syst Rev 2007;(4):CD002971.

mother's own milk (70%–80%) and were randomly assigned to supplementation with bovine fortifier or with Prolact+H2MF (Prolacta Bioscience). Two groups received pasteurized donor human milk–based HMF when the enteral intake was approximately 25% (40 mL/kg/d) and approximately 65% (100 mL/kg/d) of full feedings. Both groups received pasteurized donor human milk when mother's milk was unavailable. The third group received bovine milk–based HMF when the enteral intake reached 100 mL/kg/d and preterm formula if no mother's milk was available. A remarkable 50% reduction in the rate of NEC and a 90% reduction in the rate of surgical NEC were seen among babies fed the human milk–based fortifier, donor human milk, and mother's milk. In this trial, rates of late-onset sepsis and bronchopulmonary dysplasia did not differ by study groups.[22]

As hospitals in the United States remain concerned about the cost of donor human milk, especially the high cost of the Prolacta human milk–based fortifier ($6.25/ml), the findings from the trial described earlier were used to determine the adjusted incremental costs of donor human milk, HMF, and preterm formula for extremely low-birth-weight infants.[23] Those fed human milk–based fortifier were found to have lower expected NICU length of stay and costs of hospitalization, resulting in net savings of almost 4 NICU days and $8167 (95% confidence interval, $4405–$11,930) per infant. Compared with feeding mother's milk fortified with bovine milk–based supplements, a completely human milk–based diet that includes mother's milk fortified with donor human milk–based HMF was predicted to result in potential net savings in the total cost of care. This study predicted the economic value of NEC risk reduction, which seems to justify the current cost of human milk–based fortifier.[23]

As a result, many neonatologists now confidently provide donor human milk to preterm babies when mother's own milk is unavailable. Hospitals often use specific criteria as indications for use of donor human milk, for example, all infants under a certain birth weight or gestational age, and for a specified period of hospital stay. Most NICUs routinely practice nutritional and growth monitoring and use individualized nutrient fortification when feeding donor human milk to extremely preterm babies.[24]

However, unless additional studies address concerns about growth and development of preterm babies fed donor human milk, some remain unconvinced of the cost-effectiveness of donor milk feedings for all preterm or extremely preterm infants.[25]

RECIPIENTS OF DONOR MILK

In the United States, most patients who receive donor human milk are very premature infants; however, large volumes of donor milk are consumed also by outpatients. From 1999 to 2010, the Mother's Milk Bank of Austin dispensed donor milk for use by outpatients for certain diseases, including feeding intolerance, failure to thrive, gastroesophageal reflux, postsurgical NEC, other postsurgical bowel abnormalities, congenital malformations, milk protein allergies, and chronic renal failure. These outpatients often received donor milk for 4 to 6 months. In addition, donor milk was distributed to 73 healthy, full-term adopted infants whose parents chose to purchase and feed donor milk. Thus, some have raised questions about the use of donor milk, a scarce commodity, for outpatients, as well as for older infants and children.[26]

THE NUTRITIONAL CONTENT OF DONOR MILK

Neonatologists remain concerned about the lack of standardization of donor milk and its effects on managing the growth of very premature patients and have thus urged HMBANA milk banks to label the macronutrient and mineral content of the donor milk. Several recent publications document that there is considerable variation in macronutrient content in donor milk (**Table 2**).[27,28] The variability of composition in donor milk is largely due to natural biologic variability, but some concern exists regarding the effects of heat treatment on nutritional composition. Valentine and colleagues[29] showed that pasteurization did not substantially alter the levels of donor milk fatty acids and amino acids, whereas others have reported an effect of pasteurization on milk macronutrient composition.[3,30] Further studies are needed to elucidate which nutritional components of donor milk may be altered by pasteurization.

INTERNET-BASED MILK SHARING

The emergence of donor human milk sharing via the Internet has become problematic. Internet-based and community sharing of donor human milk is now commonplace. In 1990, the first Internet-based milk-sharing network was called "Eats On Feets." At present, this network has chapters in almost every state throughout the United States. The Eats on Feets Web site (http://www.eatsonfeets.org) describes its mission as supporting the safe sharing of breast milk by facilitating (1) informed choice—mothers must understand the options, including risks and benefits, of all infant- and child-feeding methods; (2) donor screening—mothers must question donors about their health and lifestyle and may request blood screening test results; (3) safe handling—mothers are expected to handle their milk with clean hands and equipment and use proper storage methods; (4) home pasteurization—mothers may want to "pasteurize" milk at home, heating the milk using their stovetop to inactivate HIV or by using a single bottle pasteurizer that performs the Holder method of pasteurization.

Other Web sites, such as MilkShare (http://milkshare.birthingforlife.com), offer access to milk donors. Similarly, the Human Milk for Human Babies (HM4HB) global network (http://www.hm4hb.net) has online chapters that facilitate access to human milk and indicate that their purpose is to provide a "commerce-free space where women can share milk in a safe, ethical manner." This approach to donor milk distribution relies solely on the recipients and donors, for whom they list roles and responsibilities. The Web site provides a review of safety issues, recommendations for storage, and some educational videos that describe flash heating, a method of pasteurization that was developed in the context of HIV prevention in Africa and validated for home use by a mother using her own milk.[31] The safety of this process in the context of Internet milk sharing is unknown.

In 2011, the US FDA addressed this issue of Internet-based milk sharing and made recommendations that potential users first consult with a health care provider about using a source other than the baby's mother and consider the possible health and safety risks for the baby from exposure to infectious diseases or chemical contaminants, and advised against feeding infants breast milk acquired directly from

Table 2				
Reported donor human milk composition				
Macronutrients	**Fat (g/dL)**	**Protein (g/dL)**	**Lactose (g/dL)**	**Calories (kcal/dL)**
Preterm milk, Australia PREM, $N = 47$	4.16 ± 0.9	1.35 ± 0.3	6.7 ± 0.6	69.7 ± 8.7
Coefficient of variation (%)	21.5	24.5	8.9	—
Term milk, US, Prolacta, $N = 273$	3.22 ± 1.0	1.16 ± 0.25	7.8 ± 0.88	65 ± 11
Ranges	0.71–7.06	0.7–2.1	4.86–12.67	38–110

individuals or through the Internet. The FDA further advised that if parents decide to feed a baby with donor human milk, they should use milk only from a source that has screened its donors and taken other precautions to ensure milk safety. Parents were referred to human milk banks that screen donors, collect, process, handle, test, and store the milk, and to the HMBANA Web site. FDA has not been involved in establishing these voluntary guidelines or state standards.

MILK BANK MANAGEMENT: RESPONSE TO CLINICAL CONCERNS
Protecting Donor Milk Recipients from Risk

The reemergence of informal milk sharing and ongoing concerns expressed by clinicians regarding the safety of donor milk provide an opportunity to reexamine the way that contemporary human milk banks operate, providing an opportunity for milk banks to respond to these issues and consider approaches that may alleviate these concerns to provide greater consistency in the practice and management of milk banking.

Human milk provides multiple levels of protection from infection that are important for the newborn human infant,[32] including secretory immunoglobulin A (sIgA) and, in lower concentrations, IgG and IgM,[33] which protect against infections caused by viruses, bacteria, or parasites.[32] Fatty acids and monoglycerides released from milk fat by the action of lipase[32] have antibacterial, antifungal, and antiviral activities.[32] Glycosylated proteins and oligosaccharides provide specific protection against infectious agents or bacterial toxins. Many other breast milk components act as antiinflammatory agents and immunomodulators,[32] including cytokines, growth factors, hormones, leukocytes, macrophages, neutrophils, and lymphocytes.[33] However, breast milk also commonly contains bacteria, occasionally fungi and viruses, and rarely other infectious agents (eg, prions). There may also be pharmacologically active chemicals (medicines and environmental toxins) that may present a risk to breast milk–fed infants. Apart from significant viruses such as HIV and some medications, these biologic or chemical contaminants are rarely of concern for a mother of a breastfeeding infant. However, a donor milk bank must consider the risk presented to its recipient population by the potential presence of these factors in donated milk. In most circumstances, milk banks screen the donor population in a manner that minimizes the introduction of risk. However, as the milk is expressed, it comes in contact with a pump and storage bottles and is pooled, stored (refrigerated and frozen), thawed, and usually pasteurized before being fed to preterm infants. Each of these steps may introduce new risks to the product and has the potential to alter or destroy components that provide the levels of immunologic protection. Thus, milk banks must define a process that balances both product quality and safety for the intended recipient.

The requirements of HMBANA milk banks have been described here and elsewhere.[34] Published descriptions of international milk banking practices are also available, for example, those from Sweden,[35] Italy,[36] United Kingdom,[37] Norway,[38] and Australia.[27] Brazil has the largest network of breast milk banks in the world; their operations are regulated by city, state, and national agencies and supported by public systems of milk donation, storage, and transportation (http://www.brasil.gov.br/sobre/health/programs-and-campaigns/milk-banks). Many developed countries around the world have established donor milk banks; some dispense raw milk, and others pasteurize the donor milk. The new Human Milk Banking Association of South Africa (http://hmbasa.org.za) provides online resources for milk banks in low resource areas and instructions on a modified version of the flash-heating technique. Most international milk banks routinely pasteurize the milk,[27,35–37] but some provide raw unpasteurized donor milk,[38] whereas others do both.[35] All the milk banks screen donors for antibodies HIV-1 and HIV-2, HCV, and HBV surface antigen. Some also screen for HTLV-I, HTLV-II,[27,34,35,37,38] and syphilis[27,34,37]; one requires a chest radiograph for active tuberculosis[35]; and those not pasteurizing may screen for CMV.[38]

Thus, the practice of milk banking varies internationally, as does the risk environment with respect to the donor population, for example, the prevalence of infectious diseases. These potential risks may have different significance where the recipient population varies (eg, extremely preterm, late preterm, full-term newborns, or older individuals). Therefore, it is impossible to propose a single model of milk banking that is appropriate in all international settings. It is therefore interesting to consider how milk banks can respond to develop practices that maintain quality and safety in different contexts. It would be beneficial to define a methodology for the ongoing assessment of quality and safety in human milk banking.

Toward Standard Practice in Donor Human Milk Banking

An increasingly common approach by milk banks is to assess the hazards during processing using risk management tools developed by the food industry.[27,36,37] Thus, there has been increasing application of Hazard Analysis Critical Control Point (HACCP) in milk banking, a methodology described in the food industry (www. codexalimentarius.org) and also in the milk banking literature.[27,36,37] HACCP is a system that identifies, evaluates, and controls hazards that are significant for food safety in a systematic manner, defining 5 preliminary steps and 7 principles that must be undertaken.[27,36] HACCP also provides a systematic way to document this approach allowing transparency. This transparency provides a great benefit to human milk banking, which has maintained a long history of safe operation but has failed to communicate how this safety record has been achieved.

An underlying "quality principle" for donor screening is that milk banks must ensure that infectious agents, medicines, and/or chemicals, if present in donor human milk, do not present an unacceptable clinical risk to the intended recipient population. To ensure that this principle is achieved, a milk bank could apply a modified HACCP methodology. Considering the first 3 preliminary steps of a HACCP, a milk bank could assemble a multidisciplinary team, including a milk bank medical director, microbiologist, and a milk bank quality manager who would then identify the product (donor milk), the producer (the donor population), any intended or existing control methods (donor screening, pasteurization), and the intended use (define the clinical acuity of the intended recipient population). Next, the milk bank could undertake a formal risk assessment on the potential risks in donated milk. Considering the first part of our quality principle, milk banks could prepare a list of potential infectious agents, including viruses (enveloped and nonenveloped, known and unknown), bacteria (pathogenic), prions, vaccines (live attenuated virus).

The milk bank HACCP team could then prepare a list of all hazards that may be expected to occur in donated human milk from the point of production to the point of consumption. For example, the viral risks of transmission in donor milk may be summarized as shown in **Table 3**.[5,6,36,39–45] The next step would be to conduct a formal risk assessment using specifically developed consequence and likelihood tables for each identified hazard to quantify (rank) them, identify any that are not appropriately controlled, and document the milk bank's management of these risks. The milk bank HACCP team would be responsible for a consensus decision regarding consequences and likelihood descriptors. The judgment should be made bearing in mind the existing or proposed control measures and their effectiveness. For each hazard, a numerical Consequence Severity Level and the Likelihood Level is applied

Table 3
Potential viral hazards in human milk

Hazard	Identified in Breast Milk	Cause of Illness in Infant	Comment	References
HIV-1 and 2	Yes (HIV1)	Yes	Serologic screening available, Holder and HTST pasteurization inactivate HIV-1	5,39–41
HTLV-I and II	Yes (HTLV-I)	Yes (HTLV-I) Inconclusive (HTLV-II)	Serologic screening available Holder pasteurization inactivates HTLV-I[a]	39,42
Hepatitis B and C	Yes (HBsAg)	Unlikely	Serologic screening available No evidence that Holder pasteurization inactivates HBV or HCV	39,40,43
Cytomegalovirus	Yes	Yes	Serologic screening available Holder and HTST pasteurization inactivate the virus	6,39
Rubella (wild type and vaccine)	Yes (both)	No evidence	—	40,43
Herpes simplex virus	Yes (with active breast lesions)	Unlikely	—	43
Varicella zoster virus (VZV) and vaccine	Yes (VZV DNA) Unknown (vaccine)	Unlikely	—	43
Yellow fever virus and vaccine	Not confirmed	Yes (vaccine)	—	44
Other nonenveloped viruses[b]	Unknown	Unknown	Transmitted by respiratory droplets or fecal–oral route. Could be transmitted by contaminated pump equipment Survive low pH, drying, and thermal disinfection	45
Other enveloped viruses[b]	Unknown	Unknown	Require an intact lipid envelope for infectivity and most are labile in response to acids, detergent, and heat.	45

a Experiments not conducted with human milk.
b Milk banks may choose to consider generic risks as a way to manage the potential transmission of currently unknown or emergent viral risks—a comparison would be the emergence of HIV in the 1980s, which resulted in the closure of many milk banks.

to provide a Level of Risk, which corresponds to a Risk Score and defines a management response to this risk.

The process described earlier should be undertaken for each identified potential hazard in donor human milk (eg, each viral hazard described in **Table 3**). Any risks rated "unacceptable" should be clearly identified and require additional control measures to ensure patient safety. If this method is applied in conjunction with a traditional HACCP assessment of hazards during the actual processing of product, the milk bank will have a sound and transparent assessment of the potential risks of their product to recipients. This procedure will give clinicians more confidence in the safety of the product, ensure that appropriate precautions have been taken to protect recipients, and give regulators confidence that the milk bank has delivered these outcomes.

Future Developments in Donor Milk Banking

The major process step related to quality and safety of donor milk is clearly thermal pasteurization (Holder or HTST). The negative effect of heat on product quality is unavoidable at temperatures and exposure times required to kill common bacteria, and researchers are examining alternative pasteurization technologies used by the food industry for microbiological control. Most alternative methods either directly or indirectly result in thermal damage of protein. However, short-wave ultraviolet light (UVC), particularly that in the narrow wavelength of 250 to 260 nm, is lethal to most microorganisms, including bacteria, viruses, protozoa, mycelial fungi, and yeasts, at ambient temperatures.[46] The UVC damage directly alters microbial DNA such that the microorganism can no longer reproduce and the risk of disease is eliminated.[46] A barrier to its use in human milk is the lack of penetration through opaque fluids; however, research is ongoing to examine the use of turbulent flows to combat this issue.[46]

If and when future research demonstrates that an alternate method of processing is effective at bacterial and viral inactivation and that there are no detrimental effects of the method itself, there will be a challenge to milk banks to introduce an alternative to the established thermal processing methods. The previously described risk assessment methodology can be applied to any new technology. A milk bank will have a thorough risk assessment of its current processing method and a quantitative score for this process. Should a similar risk assessment with the alternative technology in place be conducted and it resulted in an equivalent or lower level of risk score (using the modified HACCP approach), it should be reasonable for the milk bank to introduce this new technology. The formalization of this process ensures transparency in this decision for the recipients of donor milk and the clinicians ordering the milk.

SUMMARY

This response to clinical perspectives and concerns in donor milk banking has focused on examining the potential for standardization of management practices. In taking this risk assessment approach, it is relevant to consider the risk of not providing donor human milk when a mother's own milk is not available. Where the potential risks of donor milk banking are well managed, the risk of formula feeding is quantifiably greater than that of donor milk feeding. The potential to further increase product quality with the introduction of new technology may provide an even greater benefit to recipients where mother's own milk is unavailable. This response should also illustrate the significant difference between donor milk banking and informal milk sharing. Individuals engaging in informal milk sharing must understand and accept the potential risks involved with this process. However, where a donor milk bank operates, it is the responsibility of the bank to appropriately manage these issues for their recipient population.

REFERENCES

1. Wight ME, Morton JA, Kim JH. Best medicine: human milk in the NICU. Amarillo (TX): Hale Publishing; 2008.
2. Landers S, Updegrove K. Bacteriological screening of donor human milk before and after Holder pasteurization. Breastfeed Med 2012;5:117–21.
3. deSegura AF, Escuder D, Montilla A, et al. Heating-induced bacteriological and biochemical modifications in human donor milk after Holder pasteurization. J Pediatr Gastroenterol Nutr 2012;54:197–203.
4. Cohen RS, Huang CFR, Xiong SC, et al. Cultures of Holder pasteurized donor human milk after use in a neonatal intensive care unit. Breastfeed Med 2012;7: 282–4.
5. Terpstra FG, Rechtman DJ, Lee ML, et al. Antimicrobial and antiviral effect of high temperature short-time (HTST) pasteurization applied to human milk. Breastfeed Med 2007;2:27–33.
6. Hamprecht K, Maschmann J, Müller D, et al. Cytomegalovirus (CMV) inactivation in breast milk: reassessment of pasteurization and freeze-thawing. Pediatr Res 2004;56(4):529–35.
7. Akinbi H, Meinzen-Derr J, Auer C, et al. Alterations in the host defense properties of human milk following prolonged storage or pasteurization. J Pediatr Gastroenterol Nutr 2010;51:347–52.
8. Czank D, Prime DK, Hartmann B, et al. Retention of the immunological proteins of pasteurized human milk in relation to pasteurizer design and practice. Pediatr Res 2009;66(4):374–9.
9. Ultalan PB, Keeney SE, Palkowetz KH, et al. Heat susceptibility of interleukin-10 and other cytokines in donor human milk. Breastfeed Med 2009;4(3):137–44.
10. Ewaschuk JB, Unger S, O'Connor DL, et al. Effect of pasteurization on selected immune components of donated human breast milk. J Perinatol 2011;31:593–8.
11. Silvestre D, Miranda M, Muriach M, et al. Antioxidant capacity of human milk: effect of thermal conditions for the pasteurization. Acta Paediatr 2008;97:1070–4.
12. Goelz R, Hihn E, Hamprecht K, et al. Effects of different CMV heat-inactivation-methods on growth factors in human breast milk. Pediatr Res 2009;65(4):458–61.
13. Section on Breastfeeding. American Academy of Pediatrics. Breastfeeding and the use of human milk. Pediatrics 2012;129:e827–41.
14. Quigley MA, Henderson G, Anthony MT, et al. Formula milk versus donor breast milk for feeding preterm or low birth weight infants. Cochrane Database Syst Rev 2007;(4):CD002971.
15. Boyd CA, Quigley MA, Brocklehurst P. Donor breast milk versus infant formula for preterm infants: systematic review and meta-analysis. Arch Dis Child Fetal Neonatal Ed 2007;92:F169–75.
16. McGuire W, Anthony MY. Donor human milk versus formula for preventing necrotizing enterocolitis in preterm infants: systematic review. Arch Dis Child Fetal Neonatal Ed 2003;88:F11–4.
17. Ronnestad A, Abrahamsen TG, Medbo S, et al. Late onset septicemia in Norwegian national cohort of extremely premature infants receiving very early full human milk feeding. Pediatrics 2005;115(3):269–76.
18. Schanler RJ, Lau C, Hurst NM, et al. Randomized trial of donor human milk versus preterm formula as substitutes for mothers' own milk in the feeding of extremely premature infants. Pediatrics 2005;116(2):400–6.
19. DeSilva A, Jones PW, Spencer SA. Does human milk reduce infection rates in preterm infants? A systematic review. Arch Dis Child Fetal Neonatal Ed 2004;89:F509.

20. Wight NE. Donor milk: down but not out. Pediatrics 2005;116:1610.
21. Arslanoglu S, Moro GE, Ziegler EE. Adjustable fortification of human milk to preterm infants: does it make a difference? J Perinatol 2006;26:614–21.
22. Sullivan S, Schanler RJ, Kim JH, et al. An exclusively human milk-based diet is associated with a lower rate of necrotizing enterocolitis than a diet of human milk and bovine milk-based products. J Pediatr 2010;156(4):562–7.
23. Vaidyanathan G, Hay JW, Kim JH. Costs of necrotizing enterocolitis and cost-effectiveness of exclusively human milk-based products in feeding extremely premature infants. Breastfeed Med 2012;7:29–37.
24. Landers S. Maximizing the benefits of human milk feeding for the preterm infant. Pediatr Ann 2003;32(5):298–306.
25. McGuire W. Donor human milk for preterm infants [letter]. Pediatrics 2012;130(2): e462.
26. Miracle DJ, Szucs KA, Torke AM, et al. Contemporary ethical issues in human milk banking in the United States. Pediatrics 2011;128:1–6.
27. Hartmann BT, Pang WW, Keil AD, et al. Best practice guidelines for the operation of a donor human milk bank in an Australian NICU. Early Hum Dev 2007;83: 667–73.
28. Wojcik KY, Rechtman DJ, Lee ML, et al. Macronutrient analysis of a nationwide sample of donor breast milk. J Am Diet Assoc 2009;109:137–40.
29. Valentine CJ, Morrow G, Fernandez S, et al. Docosahexaenoic acid and amino acid contents in pasteurized donor milk are low for preterm infants. J Pediatr 2010;157:906–10.
30. Vieira AA, Soares FV, Pimenta HP, et al. Analysis of the influence of pasteurization, freezing/thawing, and other processes on human milk's macronutrient concentration. Early Hum Dev 2011;87(8):577–80.
31. Israel-Ballard K, Chantry C, Dewey K, et al. Viral, nutritional, and bacterial safety of flash-heated and pretoria-pasteurized breast milk to prevent mother-to-child transmission of HIV in resource-poor countries: a pilot study. J Acquir Immune Defic Syndr 2005;40(2):175–81.
32. May JT. Breastmilk and infection - a brief overview. Breastfeed Rev 1999;7(3): 25–7.
33. Hanson LA. Immunobiology of human milk - how breastfeeding protects babies. Amarillo (TX): Pharmasoft; 2004. p. 241.
34. HMBANA. Guidelines for the establishment and operation of a human milk bank; 2011.
35. Omarsdottir S, Casper C, Åkerman A, et al. Breast milk handling routines for preterm infants in Sweden: a national cross-sectional study. Breastfeed Med 2008;3(3):165–70.
36. Arslanoglu S, Bertino E, Tonetto P, et al. Guidelines for the establishment and operation of a donor human milk bank. J Matern Fetal Neonatal Med 2010; 23(Suppl 2):1–20.
37. National Institute for Health and Clinical Excellence. Donor breast milk banks: the operation of donor milk bank services, vol. Clinical guideline (CG) 93. National Institute for Health and Clinical Excellence; 2010. p. 1–132.
38. Grøvslien AH, Grønn M. Donor milk banking and breastfeeding in Norway. J Hum Lact 2009;25(2):206–10.
39. Ruff AJ. Breastmilk, breastfeeding, and transmission of viruses to the neonate. Semin Perinatol 1994;18(6):510–6.
40. Buescher ES. Human milk and infectious diseases. In: Hale TW, Hartmann PE, editors. Textbook of human lactation. Amarillo (TX): Hale Publishing; 2007. p. 193–214.

41. Orloff S, Wallingford J, McDougal J. Inactivation of human immunodeficiency virus type I in human milk: effects of intrinsic factors in human milk and of pasteurisation. J Hum Lact 1993;9:13–7.
42. Yamato K, Taguchi H, Yoshimoto S, et al. Inactivation of lymphocyte-transforming activity of human T-cell leukemia virus type 1 by heat. Jpn J Cancer Res 1986;77: 13–5.
43. Jones CA. Neonatology for the generalist: maternal transmission of infectious pathogens in breast milk. J Paediatr Child Health 2001;37:576–82.
44. Kuhn S, Twele-Montecinos L, MacDonald J, et al. Case report: probable transmission of vaccine strain of yellow fever virus to an infant via breast milk. CMAJ 2011; 183(4):E243–5.
45. Murray PR, Rosenthal KS, Pfaller MA, editors. Medical microbiology. 5th edition. Philadelphia: Elsevier Mosby; 2005. p. 963.
46. Bintsis T, Litopoulou-Tzanetaki E, Robinson R. Existing and potential applications of ultraviolet light in the food industry: a critical review. J Sci Food Agric 2000;80: 637–45.
47. Gross SJ. Growth and biochemical response of preterm infants fed human milk or modified infant formula. N Engl J Med 1983;308(5):237–41.
48. Tyson JE, Lasky RE, Mize CE, et al. Growth, metabolic response, and development in very-low-birth-weight infants fed banked human milk or enriched formula. I. Neonatal findings. J Pediatr 1983;103(1):95–104.
49. Lucas A, Gore SM, Cole TJ, et al. Multicentre trial on feeding low birth weight infants: effects of dieton early growth. Archives of Disease in Childhood 1984; 59:722–30.

Nutritional Management of the Breastfeeding Dyad

Christina J. Valentine, MD, MS, RD[a],*, Carol L. Wagner, MD[b]

KEYWORDS

- Maternal-infant nutrition • Exclusive breastfeeding • Lactation • Macronutrients
- Micronutrients

KEY POINTS

- Maternal nutrient requirements are heightened during lactation.
- Some nutrients including vitamins A, D, B1, B2, B6, and B12, fatty acids, and iodine are required in the maternal diet to ensure optimal levels in breast milk and, thus, the goal for infant dietary intake.
- Complementary foods should begin by 6 months of age in exclusively breastfed infants with a focus on zinc-rich and iron-rich food sources.

INTRODUCTION

Nutritional management of the breastfeeding dyad begins with focus on a varied and balanced diet for the mother. Exclusive breastfeeding is recommended for the first 6 months of life, and provides preferred nutrition to support optimal growth and development in infancy.[1,2] The mammary gland is a unique organ, designed to support infant survival, and is capable of providing adequate milk volume to the infant even under dire nutritional circumstances in the mother.[3] Specific attention should be paid to maternal food sources that contain vitamins A, B1, B2, B3, B6, B12, C, and D, fatty acids, and iodine, as the concentration of these nutrients in human milk are at least partially dependent on maternal diet and body stores. Conversely calories, protein, folate, minerals, and trace elements in human milk are not dependent on maternal diet. Nevertheless, to avoid depletion of maternal nutrient stores, the recommended dietary intakes of these nutrients are greater for lactating women than for an average adult.

Vitamin supplementation of breastfed infants is recommended for only vitamins D and K. Even among mothers taking recommended dietary supplements, vitamin D is typically found at low concentrations in human milk, insufficient to meet the daily requirements of 400 IU/d for the exclusively breastfeeding infant.[4,5] Therefore, 400 IU/d of vitamin D is recommended by the American Academy of Pediatrics (AAP)

[a] Perinatal Institute, Division of Neonatology, Cincinnati Children's Hospital Medical Center, Cincinnati, OH 45229, USA; [b] Department of Neonatology, Medical University of South Carolina, Charleston, SC, USA
* Corresponding author.
E-mail address: Christina.Valentine@nationwidechildrens.org

Pediatr Clin N Am 60 (2013) 261–274
http://dx.doi.org/10.1016/j.pcl.2012.10.008
0031-3955/13/$ – see front matter © 2013 Published by Elsevier Inc.
pediatric.theclinics.com

for all breastfeeding infants, beginning within the first few days after birth until weaning.[5] Regardless of maternal diet or supplementation, vitamin K concentration is also extremely low in human milk.[6] Since 1961 the AAP has recommended an injection of vitamin K in the newborn period to prevent hemorrhagic disease of the newborn.[7,8]

This article reviews the suggested nutrient intakes for the nursing mother and her infant as well as the physiologic basis for these recommendations.

HUMAN MILK NUTRIENTS
Nutrients Affected by Maternal Diet

Experimental studies indicate that vitamins A, B1 (riboflavin), B2 (thiamin), B3 (niacin) or the precursor tryptophan, B6 (pyridoxine), B12 (cobalamin), and D are necessary in the maternal diet to ensure adequate concentrations in breast milk.[9,10] These nutrients do not affect lactogenesis per se but are transferred into milk by transport from the peripheral blood of the mother across the mammary epithelium.[11]

Vitamin A

Colostrum is particularly rich in vitamin A.[12] The content of vitamin A in human milk depends on maternal stores and is transported in the lipid fraction of human milk primarily as retinyl ester.[13] It has been estimated that over the first 6 months of lactation, infants receive 60 times the amount of vitamin A that they received during the 9 months of pregnancy.[14] However, women lacking food sources of vitamin A demonstrate low concentrations in both plasma and milk.[12] Milk concentrations correlate with plasma concentrations and can be useful as a biomarker of maternal vitamin A status. In populations with low levels of vitamin A, breastfeeding is associated with significant protection of infants against xerophthalmia.[14,15] Postnatal supplementation of mothers may improve maternal nutritional status[16] and infant stores of vitamin A.[17]

The B vitamins except for folate

Vitamins B1, B2, B3, B6, and B12[9] are not stored and are therefore necessary in the diet. These vitamins are readily transported across the mammary gland, but grain diets that are not fortified with B vitamins, diets low in animal products and thus in B12 intake,[18] or disease conditions that influence a mother's B12 status[19] may result in low concentrations of these B vitamins in human milk.[20] Likewise, the use of oral contraceptives before pregnancy and lactation can adversely affect vitamin B6 concentrations in mother's milk.[21] Women living in areas of the world that lack food fortification strategies are particularly vulnerable. In developed nations, mothers consuming specialty diets or fad diets, mothers who have had an intestinal injury or gastric bypass, or mothers who are consuming gluten-free diets that are not replacing the vitamin B usually obtained from wheat products could also be at risk.

Vitamin C

Maternal dietary vitamin C has been correlated with maternal milk concentrations in some studies.[22,23] In a study of 200 women a significant seasonal variability in concentrations of vitamin C was noted, with the higher concentration evident in summer months.[23] In supplementation studies, however, the supplement in the maternal diet did not correspond to maternal milk concentrations, implying a regulatory mechanism for vitamin C in milk.[24] Nevertheless, mothers should be encouraged to consume a healthy diet that is replete with vitamin C.

Vitamin D

This vitamin is a precursor hormone, and unlike other nutrients that can only be obtained from diet, the vast majority of vitamin D is derived from its synthesis within the skin following ultraviolet B exposure. Only a small portion of the daily requirement comes from the diet, mainly from fatty fish, organ meats such as liver, eggs (in the form of vitamin D3 or cholecalciferol), and mushrooms (in the form of vitamin D2 or ergocalciferol). In a recent vitamin D supplementation trial conducted during pregnancy (sponsored by the National Institute of Child Health and Human Development [NICHD]), the average daily intake of women was approximately 200 IU/d compared with the 10,000 to 20,000 IU that are generated within 24 hours of whole-body sunlight exposure (without sunscreen).[25] It was thought for decades that the sole purpose of vitamin D was for calcium homeostasis and to prevent rickets in children.[26] However, advances made in the past decade using molecular techniques demonstrate the significant role that vitamin D plays in immune function, both innate and adaptive.[27–29] Given this recently expanded view of vitamin D, it is clear that its role in immune modulation during lactation and in the breastfeeding infant is just beginning to be understood.[30,31]

The content of vitamin D in human milk itself has also been a source of controversy. Studies of the vitamin D or antirachitic content of human milk showed that on average there was approximately 70 IU/L and that this amount was barely able to provide for the breastfeeding infant who had no sunlight exposure.[4,32] The AAP revised their recommendations in 2008 to include vitamin D supplementation of 400 IU/d within the first few days after delivery in all breastfeeding infants and in any infant who consumes less than 1 L of formula per day (which contains $\sim$400 IU/L).[5] Such a recommendation provides adequate vitamin D to the breastfeeding infant but does not address the needs of the mother, nor does it address the issue of why breast milk has marginal sufficiency of vitamin D.

Recent studies have demonstrated that vitamin D supplementation in the mother improves her vitamin D status, thereby improving her milk antirachitic activity and, thus, the transfer of vitamin D to her infant.[33–35] In an initial pilot study, vitamin D2, 2000 IU/d versus 4000 IU/d, was given to mothers and the transfer to their fully breastfeeding infants was tracked. There was an increase in maternal total circulating 25(OH)D, a concomitant increase in milk antirachitic activity, and improved infant vitamin D status that significantly correlated with maternal vitamin D status.[34] A second pilot study performed by this group compared maternal supplementation vitamin of 400 IU/d (the amount found in most prenatal vitamins) with 6400 IU/d.[33] The infants whose mothers were randomized to 400 IU/d also received 400 IU/d, and those infants whose mothers were randomized to 6400 IU/d received placebo (0 IU/d). Mothers who received the 6400 IU/d dose had improved vitamin D status that resulted in 25(OH)D levels in their infants comparable with levels of those infants who were receiving 400 IU/d. There was no toxicity associated with the higher dosing regimen; however, the sample size for this pilot study was small. A larger, 2-site NICHD trial initiated in 2006 was recently completed. Although the results of this larger study are not yet fully available, there was no reported toxicity in either the mother or the infant, and the preliminary analyses are consistent with the findings of the earlier pilot study.[36] These studies clearly indicate that breast milk is only deficient or "minimally sufficient" in vitamin D if the mother is deficient or "minimally sufficient" herself. There is a strong correlation between maternal vitamin D status, milk antirachitic activity, and infant vitamin D status.

The current recommendation of the AAP,[5] reiterated by the Institute of Medicine (IOM),[37] is to supplement the infant with 400 IU/d to achieve vitamin D sufficiency in the breastfeeding infant. It is suggested that the mother continues to take her prenatal vitamin containing between 400 and 600 IU. Data from recent vitamin D supplementation trials that have the potential to shift the paradigm of care are awaited. In the meantime, it is essential to educate women who choose to breastfeed about the various options to improve their vitamin D status and that of their breastfeeding infant.

Fatty acids are made by the mammary gland[38] but the content of fatty acids in human milk largely depends on maternal diet and body stores.[39–42] The essential fatty acids, including the ω-6 linoleic acid series and ω-3 linolenic acid series, are required in the diet to avoid essential fatty-acid deficiency in both mother and infant.[43] Over the last century dietary habits have changed in North America and elsewhere, increasing the ratio of ω-6 to ω-3 long-chain polyunsaturated fatty acids (LCPUFAs).[44] These LCPUFAs exert unique biological effects, and thus should not be grouped together to examine their effects. Immune homeostasis is affected in the mother and infant as the different fatty acids modulate a very different prostaglandin[45] and cytokine expression.[46,47] Perhaps the most potent of the ω-3 fatty acids is docosahexaenoic acid (DHA), which has beneficial anti-inflammatory activity. Another important biological effect of DHA pertains to brain development and cognition. A provocative study by Jensen and colleagues[48] examined supplementation with a modest 200 mg/d of DHA in the nursing mother's diet for the first 4 months postpartum, and demonstrated that sustained attention scores at 5 years of age improved in the intervention offspring compared with controls.[48]

Careful attention to reading the label on dietary supplements is necessary, as it has been observed that DHA supplements can consist of a mere 23 mg/d in some fish-oil products. In the Midwest, motivated nursing women taking a varied diet and their prenatal vitamins have a low concentration of DHA in their milk at 0.1%,[49] similar to women in developing countries on meager food sources.[50] Supplementing these breastfeeding mothers with 1 g DHA in comparison with placebo increased milk concentrations significantly for the nursing infant.[51] Most expert panels suggest that adult women ingest 3 ω-3–rich fish sources per week or a minimum of 300 to 1000 mg of DHA per day[52–54] while pregnant or breastfeeding.

Finally, the forms of fats consumed by the mother are also consumed by the breastfed infant. That is, as for unsaturated fats, if saturated or *trans* fats predominate in the mother's diet, these fats are also transferred to the infant through breast milk. The murine model of obesity demonstrates a direct relationship between saturated fats in the mouse pup and fat deposition,[55] thus prompting careful examination of the mother's diet and recommendations for a healthy balance of dietary sources of ω-6 and ω-3 fatty acids.

Iodine

Iodine concentration in breast milk is strongly influenced by the mother's iodine status.[56] Iodine is essential for thyroid and developmental function.[57] Fortunately, the mammary gland is able to concentrate iodine and often provides adequate iodine to the infant even in mothers of insufficient status.[56] Iodine status is measured by median urinary iodine concentration in response to salt iodization.[56] The current World Health Organization (WHO) recommendation is a daily maternal intake of 250 µg/d during lactation to ensure that deficiency does not occur.[58,59] Women who live where iodized salt programs exist appear to have reasonable iodine status.

Fig. 1 describes the targets for both maternal and infant diets during lactation.

Nutrients Not Evidently Dependent on Maternal Diet

Energy and protein

These components are provided to the breastfed infant through human milk almost regardless of the mother's diet.[3,60,61] Energy restriction or exercise during lactation that is modest (deficits of 500 kcal/d or exercise 45 minutes 4–5 times per week) does not affect milk volume, lactose, or protein concentrations.[62,63] Rather, if the energy costs of milk production are not met by maternal diet, maternal stores will

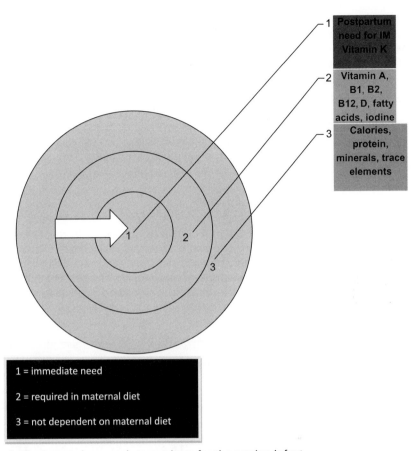

1 = immediate need

2 = required in maternal diet

3 = not dependent on maternal diet

Fig. 1. The targeted approach to nutrients for the nursing infant.

be depleted to ensure adequate milk production. It appears that maternal plasma prolactin increases with negative energy balance and may protect lactogenesis.[64]

Calcium

Calcium homeostasis in the mother is another good example of maternal use of stores to protect lactation. The calcium found in milk is regulated in the mammary gland by citrate and casein unrelated to maternal dietary intake of calcium or vitamin D.[65] Based on stable isotope studies, Mohammad and colleagues[62] demonstrated that calcium stores from bone are used during lactation to assure availability to milk production. Overall, the bone loss during lactation is transient, and does not increase the risk of osteoporosis or bone fractures in later life.[66] However, women may experience bone loss if their calcium intake is less than 500 mg/d[63] and should therefore include good sources of calcium in their diet.

Vitamin E

This vitamin is present in 3 forms: α-tocopherol, β-tocopherol, and γ-tocopherol, with α-tocopherol the most active form.[67] The level of α-tocopherol is significantly higher in early milk and correlates with lipid concentrations,[67,68] but does not appear to be affected by maternal diet or smoking.[69]

Folate and the minerals zinc, copper, iron, and zinc

These nutrients are similarly regulated, so that their concentrations in milk do not depend on maternal diet. Thus, for these nutrients the quality the mother's diet does not affect the quality of her milk but is important for maintaining her own health.[70]

NUTRIENT REQUIREMENTS DURING LACTATION

Nutritional demands are higher for the mother while nursing. These metabolic demands translate into the requirements for an additional 300 calories and a total of 71 g of protein per day.[60] **Table 1** shows the recommendations for nutrients during lactation. Nutrient intakes for the average woman are best achieved by a diet consisting of a variety of foods.

Minimum Daily Food Intakes Suggested to Meet Maternal Nutrient Requirements

Box 1 summarizes the minimum daily food intakes suggested to meet nutritional needs during lactation. Vegetarians, women with dietary restrictions, or those with a history of intestinal or gastric surgery should consult with a registered dietitian to critically evaluate their intake and receive a specialized dietary plan to ensure that vitamin B12, iron, and zinc intakes are adequate. In addition, consumers can design their own individual menu plans on www.myplate.gov.

Table 1
Maternal daily recommended intakes of micronutrients during lactation[a]

Nutrients (Unit)	Maternal Age	
	14–18 y	19–50 y
Water-Soluble Vitamins		
B1 (mg)	1.4	1.4
B2 (mg)	1.6	1.6
B3 (mg)	17	17
B6 (mg)	2	2
B12 (μg)	2.8	2.8
Pantothenic acid (mg)	7	7
Biotin (μg)	35	35
Vitamin C (mg)	115	120
Folate (μg)	500	500
Fat-Soluble Vitamins		
A (μg)	1200	1300
D (IU)[b]	600	600
E (mg)	19	19
K (μg)	75	90
Minerals		
Calcium[b] (mg)	1300	1000
Phosphorus (mg)	1250	700
Zinc (mg)	13	12
Iron (mg)	10	9

[a] Dietary reference intakes as recommended by the Institute of Medicine, 2005.
[b] Calcium and vitamin D intake as recommended by the Institute of Medicine, 2010.

Box 1
Suggested minimum food sources for the lactating mother
Dairy Group: 3 one-cup servings: High in vitamins A and D: milk, yogurt
Protein: 6.5 oz (184 g): Iron, zinc, potassium: lean meats, chicken, beans, peas, nuts, seeds
ω-3–Rich fish sources: salmon, trout, herring, sardines; ω-3 rich eggs
(do not eat shark, swordfish, kingfish, which can be high in mercury)
Grains: 8 half-cup or 1-slice servings: Make sure grains fortified with folic acid and iron
Vegetables: 3 one-cup raw servings: High in vitamins A and K: carrots, pumpkin, squash, sweet potatoes, cooked greens, tomatoes, red sweet peppers
Fruits: 2 one-cup servings: Cantaloupe, mango, apricots, bananas, honeydew melon, oranges

Dietary Supplements for the Mother

Food sources should provide the majority of nutrients for the nursing mother, but for some nutrients supplementation is important. The IOM recommends supplementation with 600 IU/d of vitamin D if sun exposure and baseline vitamin D concentrations are low in the mother.[37] Often North American dietary intake of salmon or fatty fish is low,[39,41] requiring some source of supplementation. Additional DHA/ω-3 may be achieved by dietary supplements or by consumption of 4 ω-3–enriched eggs per week.[71] In women unable to eat fish or egg sources, a dietary supplement may be needed to achieve a daily intake of 300 mg to 1 g per day.

INFANT NUTRIENT REQUIREMENTS
Exclusive Breastfeeding

The WHO recommends exclusive feeding on human milk for the first 6 months of life.[2] With this recommendation comes the responsibility to also ensure that the mother's diet is adequate, as described earlier. The assumed intake of 750 mL of breast milk per day at an average energy and protein content of approximately 67 kcal and 1 g of protein per deciliter[60] provides breastfed infants with adequate intake for growth and development (**Table 2**).[60]

Iron Deficiency

Approximately 50% of the anemia diagnosed in the latter half of infancy is due to iron deficiency.[72] To avoid iron deficiency, the AAP Committee on Nutrition, citing concern for infants born with low iron stores such as low birth weight infants and infants of diabetic mothers, recommends that exclusively breastfed infants receive supplemental iron at 1 mg/kg/d beginning at 4 months and continuing until appropriate iron-containing complementary foods have been introduced.[73] Previously ill or preterm infants may have special requirements for iron supplementation[74] before 4 to 6 months of life[75] and complementary foods around 13 weeks corrected age[76,77] to improve iron status and linear growth.[77] Concern regarding iron status in infancy pertains to the role of iron nutriture on brain development and function.[78]

Iron status in infants depends not only on their nutrient intake but also on cord-clamping practices after delivery. If infants have a delay in cord clamping longer than 180 seconds, their iron status is improved.[79] In a randomized controlled trial with 400 term infants, delayed cord clamping resulted in a 45% higher serum ferritin concentration and significantly lower prevalence of iron-deficiency anemia at 4 months

Table 2
Nutrient requirements of infants by age[a]

Nutrient (Unit)	Age of Infant	
	0–6 mo	7–12 mo
Water-Soluble Vitamins		
B1 (mg)	0.2	0.3
B2 (mg)	0.3	0.4
B3 (mg)	2	4
Pantothenic acid (mg)	1.7	1.8
Biotin (μg)	5	6
B6 (mg)	0.1	0.3
B12 (μg)	0.4	0.5
Vitamin C (mg)	40	50
Folate (μg)	65	80
Fat-Soluble Vitamins		
A (μg)	400	500
D (IU)[b]	400	400
E (mg)	4	5
K (μg)	2	2.5
Minerals		
Calcium[b] (mg)	200	260
Phosphorus (mg)	100	275
Zinc (mg)	2	3
Iron (mg)	0.27	11

[a] Dietary reference intakes as recommended by the Institute of Medicine, 2005.
[b] Vitamin D and calcium Intake as recommended by the Institute of Medicine, 2010.

compared with the early clamping group.[79] A study testing cord clamping at 2 minutes in comparison with a control group demonstrated adequate iron status extending to 6 months.[80] A meta-analysis of 15 controlled trials determined that cord clamping for 2 minutes would indeed maximize infant iron status throughout the first 6 months of infancy.[81]

The recommendation to supplement all exclusively breastfed infants with iron at 4 months, rather than target infants at greater risk for iron deficiency for early screening and/or supplementation, is controversial.[82–84] Although a full discussion of the pros and cons of universal iron supplementation at 4 months is beyond the scope of this article, concerns focus primarily on the potential harm of universal iron supplementation[82–84] and lack of acknowledgment of the alternative method to enhance iron nutriture, which is to delay umbilical cord clamping.[82] Until further data are available, at least close attention to iron status is merited by 4 months in infants at greater risk for iron deficiency[84] and at 6 months in term infants of normal birth weight without other risk factors.

Complementary foods that begin with strained/pureed meats[85] or use of egg yolk as described by the Makrides and colleagues[86] will boost iron status. Zinc status can also be low for exclusively breastfed infants at 6 months. A recent randomized trial conducted by Krebs[87] described enhanced balance of zinc in infants who were started on a meat source at 6 months. The current WHO commentary on complementary foods for the breastfed infant corroborates introductions of meat and egg yolk as

---

Box 2
Introducing complementary foods in the exclusively breastfed infant

First foods: strained/pureed meats, egg yolks, iron/zinc fortified cereals

- 6 months to 1 year
- 1 to 2 tablespoons at a time, 3 to 4 times per day

Second foods: yellow/orange and dark green vegetables, fruits

- 6 months to 1 year
- 1 to 2 tablespoons at a time, 3 to 4 times per day

Third foods: foods with thick texture, seeds, nuts, other milk sources

- After 1 year

---

a good source of iron and zinc. However, women who are practicing vegetarians, without intake of meat or egg yolk in the diet, should seek out an infant cereal fortified with iron and zinc.[87] The bioavailability of iron can be an issue depending on the iron additive, so attention should be paid to the specific form of supplement used in the cereal.[88] A complementary feeding schedule is shown in **Box 2**.

Complementary Foods for Infants

It is recommended that provision of complementary foods be started at 6 months, along with continued breastfeeding, to ensure adequate iron and zinc[60] when the infant's nutrient needs cannot be met exclusively by breastfeeding. Human milk concentrations of many nutrients decline rapidly during the 6- to 12-month lactational stage.[70,89,90] Thus, providing adequate complementary foods to the infant is imperative in avoiding iron deficiency and/or growth failure.

Nutrient Supplements Needed by the Breastfed Infant

As with the maternal diet, meeting infant nutritional needs by means of food intake is preferred. However, meeting this goal is not always possible in modern life. For example, given the limitation of sunshine, and the link between marginal vitamin D status in the mother and low concentrations of vitamin D in human milk, the AAP in 2008[5] and the IOM in 2010[37] recommended that all breastfed infants and all infants consuming less than 1 liter of formula per day (which contains 400 IU/L) receive 400 IU vitamin D per day as a dietary supplement starting within a few days of birth. If iron sources are not adequate in complementary foods, additional supplementation is necessary.[91]

SUMMARY

Lactation is adequately sustained almost regardless of maternal nutrition, but attention to maternal nutrition during lactation can improve human milk composition in relation to some vitamins, fatty-acid constituents, and iodine. A varied and healthy diet can satisfy most nutritional needs of a nursing mother, and provide adequate milk for her infant. However, as maternal diet may not always be adequate, continued use of multivitamins is recommended. Vitamin K is needed for the breastfed infant immediately after delivery and a vitamin D supplement is recommended for the breastfed infant within the first few days of life. At-risk infants may benefit from iron supplementation at 4 months of age. After the infant reaches 6 months, consumption of complementary foods should begin with food sources rich in iron and zinc.

REFERENCES

1. Section on Breastfeeding. Breastfeeding and the use of human milk. Pediatrics 2012;129(3):e827–41.
2. Pan American Health Organization; World Health Organization. Guiding principles for complementary feeding of the breastfed child. Washington, DC/Geneva: PAHO/WHO (Pan American Health Organization/World Health Organization); 2003.
3. Butte NF, Garza C, Stuff JE, et al. Effect of maternal diet and body composition on lactational performance. Am J Clin Nutr 1984;39(2):296–306.
4. Greer FR, Marshall S. Bone mineral content, serum vitamin D metabolite concentrations, and ultraviolet B light exposure in infants fed human milk with and without vitamin D2 supplements. J Pediatr 1989;114(2):204–12.
5. Wagner CL, Greer FR. Prevention of rickets and vitamin D deficiency in infants, children, and adolescents. Pediatrics 2008;122(5):1142–52.
6. Pietschnig B, Haschke F, Vanura H, et al. Vitamin K in breast milk: no influence of maternal dietary intake. Eur J Clin Nutr 1993;47(3):209–15.
7. Greer FR, Marshall S, Cherry J, et al. Vitamin K status of lactating mothers, human milk, and breast-feeding infants. Pediatrics 1991;88(4):751–6.
8. Greer FR, Mummah-Schendel LL, Marshall S, et al. Vitamin K1 (phylloquinone) and vitamin K2 (menaquinone) status in newborns during the first week of life. Pediatrics 1988;81(1):137–40.
9. Allen LH. B vitamins in breast milk: relative importance of maternal status and intake, and effects on infant status and function. Adv Nutr 2012;3(3):362–9.
10. Kang-Yoon SA, Kirksey A, Giacoia G, et al. Vitamin B-6 status of breast-fed neonates: influence of pyridoxine supplementation on mothers and neonates. Am J Clin Nutr 1992;56(3):548–58.
11. Rasmussen KM. The influence of maternal nutrition on lactation. Annu Rev Nutr 1992;12:103–17.
12. Strobel M, Tinz J, Biesalski HK. The importance of beta-carotene as a source of vitamin A with special regard to pregnant and breastfeeding women. Eur J Nutr 2007;46(Suppl 1):I1–20.
13. Stoltzfus RJ, Underwood BA. Breast-milk vitamin A as an indicator of the vitamin A status of women and infants. Bull World Health Organ 1995;73(5):703–11.
14. Bahl R, Bhandari N, Wahed MA, et al. Vitamin A supplementation of women postpartum and of their infants at immunization alters breast milk retinol and infant vitamin A status. J Nutr 2002;132(11):3243–8.
15. Mahalanabis D. Breast feeding and vitamin A deficiency among children attending a diarrhoea treatment centre in Bangladesh: a case-control study. BMJ 1991;303(6801):493–6.
16. Oliveira-Menegozzo JM, Bergamaschi DP, Middleton P, et al. Vitamin A supplementation for postpartum women. Cochrane Database Syst Rev 2010;(10):CD005944.
17. Agne-Djigo A, Idohou-Dossou N, Kwadjode KM, et al. High prevalence of Vitamin A deficiency is detected by the modified relative dose-response test in six-month-old Senegalese breast-fed infants. J Nutr 2012;142(11):1991–6.
18. Specker BL, Miller D, Norman EJ, et al. Increased urinary methylmalonic acid excretion in breast-fed infants of vegetarian mothers and identification of an acceptable dietary source of vitamin B-12. Am J Clin Nutr 1988;47(1):89–92.

19. Grange DK, Finlay JL. Nutritional vitamin B12 deficiency in a breastfed infant following maternal gastric bypass. Pediatr Hematol Oncol 1994;11(3):311–8.
20. Deegan KL, Jones KM, Zuleta C, et al. Breast milk vitamin B-12 concentrations in Guatemalan women are correlated with maternal but not infant vitamin B-12 status at 12 months postpartum. J Nutr 2012;142(1):112–6.
21. Kirksey A, Ernst JA, Roepke JL, et al. Influence of mineral intake and use of oral contraceptives before pregnancy on the mineral content of human colostrum and of more mature milk. Am J Clin Nutr 1979;32(1):30–9.
22. Ortega RM, Quintas ME, Andres P, et al. Ascorbic acid levels in maternal milk: differences with respect to ascorbic acid status during the third trimester of pregnancy. Br J Nutr 1998;79(5):431–7.
23. Tawfeek HI, Muhyaddin OM, al-Sanwi HI, et al. Effect of maternal dietary vitamin C intake on the level of vitamin C in breastmilk among nursing mothers in Baghdad, Iraq. Food Nutr Bull 2002;23(3):244–7.
24. Byerley LO, Kirksey A. Effects of different levels of vitamin C intake on the vitamin C concentration in human milk and the vitamin C intakes of breast-fed infants. Am J Clin Nutr 1985;41(4):665–71.
25. Hollis BW, Johnson D, Hulsey TC, et al. Vitamin D supplementation during pregnancy: double-blind, randomized clinical trial of safety and effectiveness. J Bone Miner Res 2011;26(10):2341–57.
26. Nutrition Co. Committee on Nutrition. The prophylactic requirement and the toxicity of vitamin D. Pediatrics 1963;31(3):512–25.
27. Walker VP, Zhang X, Rastegar I, et al. Cord blood Vitamin D status impacts innate immune responses. J Clin Endocrinol Metab 2011;96(6):1835–43.
28. Liu PT, Stenger S, Li H, et al. Toll-like receptor triggering of a vitamin D-mediated human antimicrobial response. Science 2006;311(5768):1770–3.
29. Hewison M. Vitamin D and the immune system: new perspectives on an old theme. Endocrinol Metab Clin North Am 2010;39(2):365–79.
30. Hollis BW, Wagner CL. Vitamin D and pregnancy: skeletal effects, nonskeletal effects, and birth outcomes. Calcif Tissue Int 2012. [Epub ahead of print].
31. Wagner CL, Taylor SN, Johnson DD, et al. The role of vitamin D in pregnancy and lactation: emerging concepts. Womens Health (Lond Engl) 2012;8(3):323–40.
32. Gartner L, Greer F, American Academy of Pediatrics, Section on Breastfeeding Medicine and Committee on Nutrition. Prevention of rickets and vitamin D deficiency: new guidelines for vitamin D intake. Pediatrics 2003;111(4):908–10.
33. Wagner CL, Hulsey TC, Fanning D, et al. High-dose vitamin D3 supplementation in a cohort of breastfeeding mothers and their infants: a 6-month follow-up pilot study. Breastfeed Med 2006;1(2):59–70.
34. Hollis B, Wagner C. Vitamin D requirements during lactation: high-dose maternal supplementation as therapy to prevent hypovitaminosis D in both mother and nursing infant. Am J Clin Nutr 2004;80(Suppl 6):1752–8.
35. Basile L, Taylor S, Wagner CL, et al. The effect of high-dose vitamin D supplementation on serum vitamin D levels and milk calcium concentration in lactating women and their infants. Breastfeed Med 2006;1(1):32–5.
36. Wagner C, Howard C, Hulsey T, et al. Preliminary results of a randomized controlled trial of maternal supplementation with 6400 IU vitamin D/day compared with maternal, & infant supplementation of 400 IU/day in achieving sufficiency in the breastfeeding mother-infant dyad. [abstract]. Trieste (Italy): ISRHML Conference; Int Soc Res Human Milk Lactation, 2012.

37. Food and Nutrition Board. Standing Committee on the Scientific Evaluation of Dietary Reference Intakes. Dietary reference intakes for Vitamin D and calcium. Washington, DC: National Academy Press; 2010.
38. Shennan DB, Peaker M. Transport of milk constituents by the mammary gland. Physiol Rev 2000;80(3):925–51.
39. Innis SM. Polyunsaturated fatty acids in human milk: an essential role in infant development. Adv Exp Med Biol 2004;554:27–43.
40. Jensen CL, Voigt RG, Prager TC, et al. Effects of maternal docosahexaenoic acid intake on visual function and neurodevelopment in breastfed term infants. Am J Clin Nutr 2005;82(1):125–32.
41. Brenna JT, Diau GY. The influence of dietary docosahexaenoic acid and arachidonic acid on central nervous system polyunsaturated fatty acid composition. Prostaglandins Leukot Essent Fatty Acids 2007;77(5–6):247–50.
42. Makrides M, Neumann MA, Gibson RA. Effect of maternal docosahexaenoic acid (DHA) supplementation on breast milk composition. Eur J Clin Nutr 1996;50(6):352–7.
43. Friedman Z, Danon A, Stahlman MT, et al. Rapid onset of essential fatty acid deficiency in the newborn. Pediatrics 1976;58(5):640–9.
44. Brenna JT, Varamini B, Jensen RG, et al. Docosahexaenoic and arachidonic acid concentrations in human breast milk worldwide. Am J Clin Nutr 2007;85(6):1457–64.
45. Ratnayake WM, Galli C. Fat and fatty acid terminology, methods of analysis and fat digestion and metabolism: a background review paper. Ann Nutr Metab 2009; 55(1–3):8–43.
46. Lu J, Jilling T, Li D, et al. Polyunsaturated fatty acid supplementation alters proinflammatory gene expression and reduces the incidence of necrotizing enterocolitis in a neonatal rat model. Pediatr Res 2007;61(4):427–32.
47. Cotogni P, Muzio G, Trombetta A, et al. Impact of the omega-3 to omega-6 polyunsaturated fatty acid ratio on cytokine release in human alveolar cells. JPEN J Parenter Enteral Nutr 2011;35(1):114–21.
48. Jensen CL, Voigt RG, Llorente AM, et al. Effects of early maternal docosahexaenoic acid intake on neuropsychological status and visual acuity at five years of age of breast-fed term infants. J Pediatr 2010;157(6):900–5.
49. Valentine CJ, Morrow G, Fernandez S, et al. Docosahexaenoic acid and amino acid contents in pasteurized donor milk are low for preterm infants. J Pediatr 2010;157(6):906–10.
50. Jensen RG. Lipids in human milk. Lipids 1999;34(12):1243–71.
51. Valentine CJ, Morrow G, Pennell M, et al. Randomized controlled trial of docosahexaenoic acid supplementation in Midwestern U.S. human milk donors. Breastfeed Med 2012. [Epub ahead of print].
52. Carlson SE. Docosahexaenoic acid supplementation in pregnancy and lactation. Am J Clin Nutr 2009;89(2):678S–84S.
53. Koletzko B, Cetin I, Brenna JT. Dietary fat intakes for pregnant and lactating women. Br J Nutr 2007;98(5):873–7.
54. Simopoulos AP, Leaf A, Salem N Jr. Workshop on the essentiality of and recommended dietary intakes for omega-6 and omega-3 fatty acids. J Am Coll Nutr 1999;18(5):487–9.
55. Rolls BA, Gurr MI, van Duijvenvoorde PM, et al. Lactation in lean and obese rats: effect of cafeteria feeding and of dietary obesity on milk composition. Physiol Behav 1986;38(2):185–90.
56. Zimmermann MB. The impact of iodised salt or iodine supplements on iodine status during pregnancy, lactation and infancy. Public Health Nutr 2007; 10(12A):1584–95.

57. Heidemann PH, Stubbe P, Thal H, et al. Influence of iodine prophylaxis on thyroid function and iodine excretion in newborn infants and their mothers: comparison between Sweden and Germany. Acta Endocrinol 1986;113(Suppl 1):S47–8.

58. Andersson M, de Benoist B, Delange F, et al. Prevention and control of iodine deficiency in pregnant and lactating women and in children less than 2-years-old: conclusions and recommendations of the Technical Consultation. Public Health Nutr 2007;10(12A):1606–11.

59. Azizi F, Smyth P. Breastfeeding and maternal and infant iodine nutrition. Clin Endocrinol (Oxf) 2009;70(5):803–9.

60. Dewey KG. Energy and protein requirements during lactation. Annu Rev Nutr 1997;17:19–36.

61. Lonnerdal B. Effects of milk and milk components on calcium, magnesium, and trace element absorption during infancy. Physiol Rev 1997;77(3):643–69.

62. Mohammad MA, Sunehag AL, Haymond MW. Effect of dietary macronutrient composition under moderate hypocaloric intake on maternal adaptation during lactation. Am J Clin Nutr 2009;89(6):1821–7.

63. Dewey KG, Lovelady CA, Nommsen-Rivers LA, et al. A randomized study of the effects of aerobic exercise by lactating women on breast-milk volume and composition. N Engl J Med 1994;330(7):449–53.

64. Dewey KG. Effects of maternal caloric restriction and exercise during lactation. J Nutr 1998;128(Suppl 2):386S–9S.

65. Kent G, Gay S, Inouye T, et al. Vitamin A-containing lipocytes and formation of type III collagen in liver injury. Proc Natl Acad Sci U S A 1976;73(10): 3719–22.

66. Kalkwarf HJ. Lactation and maternal bone health. Adv Exp Med Biol 2004;554: 101–14.

67. Jansson L, Akesson B, Holmberg L. Vitamin E and fatty acid composition of human milk. Am J Clin Nutr 1981;34(1):8–13.

68. Chappell JE, Francis T, Clandinin MT. Vitamin A and E content of human milk at early stages of lactation. Early Hum Dev 1985;11(2):157–67.

69. Szlagatys-Sidorkiewicz A, Zagierski M, Luczak G, et al. Maternal smoking does not influence vitamin A and E concentrations in mature breastmilk. Breastfeed Med 2012;7:285–9.

70. Lonnerdal B, Keen CL, Hurley LS. Iron, copper, zinc, and manganese in milk. Annu Rev Nutr 1981;1:149–74.

71. Lewis NM, Seburg S, Flanagan NL. Enriched eggs as a source of N-3 polyunsaturated fatty acids for humans. Poult Sci 2000;79(7):971–4.

72. Tawia S. Iron and exclusive breastfeeding. Breastfeed Rev 2012;20(1):35–47.

73. Baker RD, Greer FR. Diagnosis and prevention of iron deficiency and iron-deficiency anemia in infants and young children (0-3 years of age). Pediatrics 2010;126(5):1040–50.

74. Griffin I, Cooke RJ. Iron retention in preterm infants fed low iron intakes: a metabolic balance study. Early Hum Dev 2010;86(Suppl 1):49–53.

75. Long H, Yi JM, Hu PL, et al. Benefits of Iron supplementation for low birth weight infants: a systematic review. BMC Pediatr 2012;12:99.

76. Palmer DJ, Makrides M. Introducing solid foods to preterm infants in developed countries. Ann Nutr Metab 2012;60(Suppl 2):31–8.

77. Marriott LD, Foote KD, Bishop JA, et al. Weaning preterm infants: a randomised controlled trial. Arch Dis Child Fetal Neonatal Ed 2003;88(4):F302–7.

78. Fretham SJ, Carlson ES, Georgieff MK. The role of iron in learning and memory. Adv Nutr 2011;2(2):112–21.

79. Andersson O, Hellstrom-Westas L, Andersson D, et al. Effect of delayed versus early umbilical cord clamping on neonatal outcomes and iron status at 4 months: a randomised controlled trial. BMJ 2011;343:d7157.

80. Chaparro CM, Neufeld LM, Tena Alavez G, et al. Effect of timing of umbilical cord clamping on iron status in Mexican infants: a randomised controlled trial. Lancet 2006;367(9527):1997–2004.

81. Hutton EK, Hassan ES. Late vs early clamping of the umbilical cord in full-term neonates: systematic review and meta-analysis of controlled trials. JAMA 2007; 297(11):1241–52.

82. Schanler RJ, Feldman-Winter L, Landers S, et al. Concerns with early universal iron supplementation of breastfeeding infants. Pediatrics 2011;127(4):e1097 [author reply: e1101–4].

83. Furman LM. Exclusively breastfed infants: iron recommendations are premature. Pediatrics 2011;127(4):e1098–9 [author reply: e1101–4].

84. Dewey KG, Domellof M, Cohen RJ, et al. Iron supplementation affects growth and morbidity of breast-fed infants: results of a randomized trial in Sweden and Honduras. J Nutr 2002;132(11):3249–55.

85. Fomon SJ, Nelson SE, Ziegler EE. Retention of iron by infants. Annu Rev Nutr 2000;20:273–90.

86. Makrides M, Hawkes JS, Neumann MA, et al. Nutritional effect of including egg yolk in the weaning diet of breast-fed and formula-fed infants: a randomized controlled trial. Am J Clin Nutr 2002;75(6):1084–92.

87. Krebs NF. Dietary zinc and iron sources, physical growth and cognitive development of breastfed infants. J Nutr 2000;130(Suppl 2S):358S–60S.

88. Fomon SJ. Nutrition of normal infants. St Louis (MO): Mosby-Year Book; 1993.

89. Schanler RJ, Oh W. Composition of breast milk obtained from mothers of premature infants as compared to breast milk obtained from donors. J Pediatr 1980; 96(4):679–81.

90. Krebs NF, Hambidge KM. Zinc requirements and zinc intakes of breast-fed infants. Am J Clin Nutr 1986;43(2):288–92.

91. Dee DL, Sharma AJ, Cogswell ME, et al. Sources of supplemental iron among breastfed infants during the first year of life. Pediatrics 2008;122(Suppl 2): S98–104.

Maternal Medication, Drug Use, and Breastfeeding

Hilary Rowe, BSc(Pharm), PharmD, ACPR[a], Teresa Baker, MD[b],
Thomas W. Hale, PhD[c],*

KEYWORDS

- Breastfeeding • Medications • Infant exposure • Antidepressants • Antibiotics

KEY POINTS

- Drugs transfer into milk as a function of molecular weight. The higher the molecular weight, the less the drug transfers into human milk.
- Drugs transfer into human milk as a function of the maternal plasma level. The higher the plasma level, the higher the transfer into human milk.
- Drugs with poor oral bioavailability seldom produce significant clinical levels in human milk, and are generally poorly absorbed by the infant.
- Drugs that transfer into the brain compartment also likely transfer into human milk but this does not mean that the levels in milk are clinically high or even clinically relevant.
- The transfer of drugs into human milk is one of the purest forms of compartment pharmacokinetics. Good knowledge of the kinetics and chemistry of a medication aids in predicting levels in human milk but nothing is better than a well-done clinical trial in a human model.

INTRODUCTION

While rates of breastfeeding early postpartum are greater than 74.6%, the US Centers for Disease Control and Prevention's 2012 breastfeeding report card found breastfeeding at 6 months was 47.2%, and breastfeeding at 12 months was 25.5%.[1] Although there are many social factors that lead to this high rate of discontinuation, the use of medications must be considered. The average number of different medications (excluding iron, minerals, folic acid, vitamins) taken per mother in a small American study was 4 throughout lactation (0.9 medications per month).[2]

[a] Maternal Fetal Medicine, Fraser Health, Surrey, British Columbia, Canada; [b] Obstetrics and Gynecology, Texas Tech University School of Medicine, Amarillo, TX 79106, USA; [c] Pharmacy Department, Surrey Memorial Hospital, 13750- 96th Avenue, Surrey, British Columbia V3V 1Z2, Canada
* Corresponding author. Department of Pediatrics, Texas Tech University School of Medicine, 1400 Coulter, Amarillo, TX 79106.
E-mail address: thomas.hale@ttuhsc.edu

Pediatr Clin N Am 60 (2013) 275–294
http://dx.doi.org/10.1016/j.pcl.2012.10.009
0031-3955/13/$ – see front matter © 2013 Elsevier Inc. All rights reserved.

With so many women using drug therapy during lactation, pediatricians and obstetricians are faced with the challenge of determining which medications are suitable for breastfeeding mothers. Although there is more literature available about the transfer of medications into breast milk, this is often not communicated to students and clinicians; therefore, many women are advised to stop breastfeeding or avoid drug therapy based on information obtained from product monographs.

Even without specific medication data from human studies, a good understanding of the kinetic principles and mechanisms of medication entry into breast milk can help a clinician make an informed decision that often allows the mother to continue breastfeeding while treating her medical condition. This article discusses the most important concepts needed to understand how medications enter breast milk to aid in clinical decisions and highlights suitable medications for breastfeeding mothers.

KEY CONCEPTS OF MEDICATION ENTRY INTO BREAST MILK

Although all medications enter milk to some degree, clinically relevant levels are seldom attained. Most drugs simply transfer in and out of the milk compartment by passive diffusion from a region of high concentration to a region of low concentration. Some active transport systems exist for immunoglobulins, electrolytes, and particularly iodine, but facilitated transport systems are limited. Fewer than 10 drugs are known to be selectively transported into human milk.

Medications that enter breast milk often have certain physicochemical characteristics.[3] They are generally low in molecular weight (less than 500 Da), they often attain higher maternal plasma levels, they are generally poorly bound to plasma proteins, and they have a higher pK_a (pH at which a drug is equally ionic and nonionic; polar or ionic medications are less likely to leave the breast milk compartment). Human milk has a low pH (7–7.2) which causes some medications with a higher pK_a (>7.2) to become ionized and trapped in milk.

In addition, clinicians also need to consider the oral bioavailability of the drug in the infant's gastrointestinal tract. Many drugs are simply not absorbed in the gastrointestinal tract of infants. The stage of lactation is important. More medication can enter breast milk in the colostral phase, but only minimal doses are transferred to the infant during this phase because of the limited volume of colostrum. With mature milk, there is a larger volume but less medication enters breast milk because of tight cell to cell junctions.

CALCULATING INFANT EXPOSURE

Perhaps the most useful tool in clinical practice is to calculate the actual dose received by the infant. To do this, the actual concentration of medication in the milk and the volume of milk transferred must be known. Although not always available, data on milk levels are available for many drugs. More recent studies now calculate the average area under the curve (AUC) value for the medication (C_{ave}).[4] This methodology accurately estimates the average daily level of the drug in milk, and hence the average intake by the infant. Although the actual volume of milk ingested is highly variable and depends on the age of the infant and the extent to which the infant is exclusively breastfed, many clinicians use a value of 150 mL/kg/d to estimate the amount of milk ingested by the infant. The most useful and accurate measure of exposure is to calculate the relative infant dose (RID) as shown in **Fig. 1**.

The RID is generally expressed as a percentage of the mother's dose, and it provides a standardized method of relating the infant's dose in milk to the maternal dose. Bennett[5] was the first to recommend that an RID of more than 10% should

Relative Infant Dose

$$RID = \frac{Dose.infant \left(\dfrac{mg/kg}{day} \right)}{Dose.mother \left(\dfrac{mg/kg}{day} \right)}$$

Dose.infant = dose in infant/day

Dose.mother = dose in mother/day

Fig. 1. Calculating the RID.

be the theoretical level of concern for most medications. However, the 10% level of concern is relative and each situation should be evaluated individually according to the overall toxicity of the medication.

UNIQUE INFANT FACTORS

To evaluate the risk of the medication, infants should be categorized as low, moderate, or high risk. Infants at low risk are generally older (6–18 months), receive lower volumes of breast milk, and are able to metabolize and handle drugs more efficiently. Mothers in the terminal stage of lactation (>1 year) often produce relatively lower quantities of milk. Thus, the absolute clinical dose transferred is often low.

Infants at moderate risk are term infants who are aged between 2 weeks and 6 months. Those at higher risk are premature, newborns, or infants with acute or chronic medical conditions that may be affected by the medication or may impair the clearance of medications in the infant (eg, renal dysfunction).

PSYCHIATRIC CONDITIONS

Recent data from 17 American states indicate that postpartum depression affects 12% to 20% of women.[6] Fortunately for practitioners, there is increasing information available about the use of antidepressants during lactation that support the treatment of the condition while breastfeeding (**Table 1**). The selective serotonin reuptake inhibitors (SSRIs) are presently the mainstay of antidepressant therapy in women who are breastfeeding. **Table 1** provides the RID for common SSRIs. Clinical studies in breastfeeding patients consuming sertraline, fluvoxamine, and paroxetine clearly suggest that the transfer of these medications into human milk is low and uptake by the infant is even lower.[7–9] Thus far, no or minimal untoward effects have been reported following the use of these 3 agents in breastfeeding mothers. Sertraline is overwhelmingly favored because more than 50 mother-infant pairs have been evaluated in numerous studies, and milk and infant plasma levels are low to undetectable.

Fluoxetine has also been studied in more than 50 mother-infant pairs, and transfers into human milk at concentrations as high as 9% of the maternal dose.[10] Because of its long half-life and active metabolite, clinically relevant plasma levels in infants have been reported, but without major complications. Long-term studies, however, are not yet available. Because of a higher RID, fluoxetine is perhaps less preferred unless lower doses are used during pregnancy and early postpartum. However, in reality, the incidences of untoward effects are probably remote, and mothers who cannot tolerate other SSRIs should be maintained on the product that works best for them.

Table 1
Antidepressants and reported levels in breast milk

Antidepressant	RID (%)	Comments
Selective Serotonin Reuptake Inhibitors (SSRIs)		
Citalopram	3.6[87]	Compatible: SSRIs are recommended first-line agents for depression and anxiety and are suitable when breastfeeding. There have been 2 cases of excessive somnolence, decreased feeding, and weight loss with citalopram; however, most new data suggest these side effects are rare.[88,89] Fluoxetine has been reported to cause colic, fussiness, and crying[90,91]
Escitalopram	5.3[92]	
Fluvoxamine	1.6[8]	
Fluoxetine	5–9[90,91]	
Sertraline	0.54[7]	
Paroxetine	1.4[9]	
Serotonin Norepinephrine Reuptake Inhibitors (SNRIs)		
Venlafaxine	8.1[93]	Compatible: No adverse events reported in breastfed infants with these 3 medications
Desvenlafaxine	6.8[94]	
Duloxetine	0.1[95]	

In essence, if a product works, it is not advisable to change breastfeeding mothers to another product. Although almost all tricyclic antidepressants produce low RIDs and are well tolerated by the infant, they are seldom used due to intolerable anticholinergic side effects in the mother.

Benzodiazepines are often used with antidepressants to help with anxiety or can be used as sleep aids for short periods (when non-drug measures have failed). Kelly and colleagues[11] conducted a study to determine adverse event rates in infants exposed to benzodiazepines via breast milk. The 3 most commonly used benzodiazepines in this study were lorazepam (52%), clonazepam (18%), and midazolam (15%).[11] Of 124 women taking benzodiazepines only, 1.6% (2 of 124) of their infants (2–24 months old) had depression of the central nervous system.[11] There was no correlation between sedation and the benzodiazepine dose or duration of breastfeeding.[11] Of the 2 mothers who reported sedation, 1 was taking alprazolam occasionally and the other was taking 2 benzodiazepines (clonazepam and flurazepam) chronically.[11] If these agents are used, choose a product with a short half-life and use the lowest effective dose for the shortest duration to minimize exposure.[12]

Other medications used for sedation include first-generation antihistamines; the most commonly used medications are diphenhydramine, dimenhydrinate, and doxylamine. Dimenhydrinate's active ingredient is diphenhydramine and doxylamine has a similar structure to diphenhydramine; therefore, the RID for diphenhydramine (0.7%–1.5%) is often extrapolated to all 3 of these drugs and it is believed that none of them readily enter breast milk.[13]

There are 2 medications that are not part of the benzodiazepine family but are indicated for insomnia: zopiclone and zolpidem. A study of 12 mothers who took zopiclone 7.5 mg orally, 2 to 6 days postpartum for sleep, found that the RID was about 1.4% of the maternal dose and no adverse effects were reported in the infants.[14] Monitoring the infant for sedation and the ability to breastfeed is recommended with all sedating medications.

Atypical antipsychotics are another class of medications that are being used more commonly for many disorders such as psychosis, bipolar disorder, depression, and so forth. Three of the most commonly used atypical antipsychotics are risperidone (RID 4.3%), quetiapine (RID 0.09%), and olanzapine (1.6%). These medications have low

RIDs and are believed to be more suitable during breastfeeding than the older antipsychotics (phenothiazines), which have been associated with drowsiness and lethargy.[15–18]

Methylphenidate (RID 0.2%) and dextroamphetamine (RID 5.7%) have relatively low penetration into breast milk and no history of causing adverse effects in breastfed infants. However, the infants of all breastfeeding mothers on stimulants require monitoring for irritability, weight loss, or poor weight gain.[19,20]

Clinicians are often faced with the decision of whether or not antiepileptic or mood stabilizer medications are suitable while breastfeeding. If a mother is stable on a drug, vigilant monitoring of the infant can be done to evaluate safety, such as monitoring drug levels or signs of sedation. **Table 2** provides the RIDs of most antiepileptic and mood stabilizer drugs.

Valproic acid levels in milk are low with an RID of approximately 1.4% to 1.7%.[21] In a study of 16 patients receiving 300 to 2400 mg/d, valproic acid concentrations in milk ranged from 0.4 to 3.9 mg/L (mean = 1.9 mg/L).[21] Although it is generally agreed that the amount of valproic acid transferring to the infant via milk is low, given the high risk of teratology of valproic acid, this drug should probably be avoided in women in the early postpartum period, and certainly in women at high risk of pregnancy.

Lamotrigine has been studied in at least 26 breastfeeding mothers. Levels in milk seem significant with RIDs ranging from 9.2% to 18.3%.[22,23] The use of lamotrigine in breastfeeding mothers produces significant plasma levels in some breastfed infants, although they are apparently not high enough to produce side effects. Some investigators suggest it is advisable to monitor a symptomatic infant's plasma levels to ensure safety.[22] Premature infants should be closely monitored for apnea, sedation, and weakness. The maternal use of lamotrigine is probably compatible with breastfeeding of premature and full-term breastfeeding infants as long as the infant is closely observed for untoward symptoms.

The transfer of topiramate into human milk is significant. In a study of 3 women who received topiramate (150–200 mg/d) at 3 weeks postpartum, the RID ranged from 3% to 23% of the maternal daily dose.[24] Plasma levels were detectable in 2 of the 3 infants and were low, 10% to 20% of the maternal plasma level. At 4 weeks, the milk/plasma ratio dropped to 0.69 and infant plasma levels were less than 0.9 μM and 2.1 μM, respectively. The breast milk and plasma levels were drawn 10 to 15 hours after the last dose of topiramate, which gives an underestimate of the amount found in breast milk. Because the plasma levels found in breastfeeding infants were significantly less than in maternal plasma, the risk of topiramate in breastfeeding mothers is probably acceptable. Close observation including monitoring plasma levels in symptomatic infants is advised.

RECREATIONAL DRUGS

Alcohol readily transfers into human milk, with an average milk/plasma ratio of about 1.0. Yet the clinical dose of alcohol in human milk is not necessarily high. In a well-controlled study of 12 women who ingested 0.3 g/kg of ethanol, the mean maximum concentration of ethanol in milk was only 320 mg/L.[25] In an interesting study of the effect of alcohol on milk ingestion by infants, the rate of milk consumption by infants during the 4 hours immediately after exposure to alcohol (0.3 g/kg) in 12 mothers was significantly less.[26] Reduction of letdown is apparently dose dependent and requires alcohol consumption of 1.5 to 1.9 g/kg.[27] Other studies have suggested psychomotor delay in infants of moderate drinkers (2+ drinks daily). These reports also suggest that alcohol suppresses milk production significantly, which is secondary to alcohol suppression of

Table 2
Seizure and mood stabilizer medications and reported levels in breast milk

Drug	RID (%)	Comments
Valproic acid	1.4–1.7[21]	Probably compatible: In a study of 16 patients receiving 300–2400 mg/d of valproic acid, breast milk concentrations ranged from 0.4 to 3.9 mg/L (mean = 1.9 mg/L)[21] One case report of a 3-mo-old breastfed infant who developed thrombocytopenia, petechiae, a minor hematoma, and anemia 6 wk after his mother's valproic acid dose was doubled. The investigators report that the onset of symptoms occurred around the time of a minor cold but believe the adverse events were not related to a viral illness[96] Neurodevelopmental Effects of Antiepileptic Drugs study demonstrated adverse cognitive effects from valproic acid exposure in utero. In a 3-y follow-up study, 42% of children were breastfed; IQs for breastfed children did not differ from children who were not breastfed. Although this study did not show adverse effects, there are many confounding variables; until further trials are published, the long-term effects on cognitive development are unknown[97]
Carbamazepine	5.9[98]	Compatible: Levels in milk are reported to be low (2.8–4.5 mg/L); the estimated infant dose is less than 0.68 mg/kg/d. One report of increased liver function tests occurred in a 9-d-old infant[98]
Lithium	30.1[99]	Compatible with close observation: Because the RID for lithium is variable, this medication should only be used if found to be the most suitable mood stabilizer for the mother and the infant is full term and healthy. Studies suggest monitoring serum creatinine and blood urea nitrogen levels and thyroid function in the infant[99,100]
Lamotrigine	9.2%[23]	Compatible: Reports of significant plasma levels have occurred in some breastfed infants, although none have been high enough to produce side effects. It may be helpful to monitor the infant's plasma levels[23,101]
Topiramate	24.5[24]	Compatible: Levels in infants are 10%–20% of mothers; no adverse effects have been reported in breastfed infants[24]
Phenytoin	7.7[102]	Compatible: Low amounts enter breast milk; monitoring for sedation and infant levels should be done if symptoms occur

oxytocin release. Metabolism of alcohol in adults is approximately 28 g in 3 hours, so mothers who ingest alcohol in moderate amounts may return to breastfeeding after waiting for approximately 2 hours for each drink consumed.[28] Thus, mothers should avoid consuming alcohol or avoid breastfeeding during and for at least 2 hours per drink after consuming alcohol. Chronic or heavy consumers of alcohol should not breastfeed.

Studies on the use of cannabis in pregnant women seem to be somewhat inconsistent. Commonly called marijuana, the active component tetrahydrocannabinol (delta-9-THC) is rapidly distributed to the brain and adipose tissue. It is stored in fat tissues for long periods (weeks to months). Small to moderate secretion into breast milk has been documented.[29] In 1 mother who consumed marijuana 7 to 8 times daily, milk levels of THC were reported to be 340 μg/L.[29]

In 1 mother who consumed marijuana once daily, milk levels were reported to be 105 μg/L.[29] Analysis of breast milk in a chronic heavy user revealed an 8-fold accumulation in breast milk compared with plasma, although the dose received is apparently insufficient to produce significant side effects in the infant. Studies have shown significant absorption and metabolism in infants although long-term sequelae are conflicting. In 1 study of 27 women who smoked marijuana routinely during breastfeeding, no differences were noted in outcomes on growth, mental, and motor development.[30] In another study, maternal use of marijuana was shown to be associated with a slight decrease in the motor development in infants at 1 year of age, especially when used during the first month of lactation.[31] The data from this study were conflicted by the use of marijuana during the first trimester of pregnancy. Maternal use of marijuana during pregnancy and lactation had no detectable effect on the mental development of the infant at 1 year of age.

There are few documented hazards reported following the limited use of marijuana while breastfeeding. Recent data suggest significant changes in the endocannabinoid system after fetal exposure to marijuana.[32] This system has a major role in the development of the central nervous system (CNS) and is involved in mood, cognition, and reward and goal-directed behavior. Both animal and human data strongly suggest that marijuana exposure in pregnancy, and potentially lactation, may lead to neurobehavioral complications. Until further data can confirm these studies, use of this drug should be strongly discouraged.

Cigarette smoking not only exposes breastfed infants to nicotine and its metabolite cotinine but it also exposes the infant to toxic xenobiotics in the cigarette and environmental cigarette smoke. A study by Ilett and colleagues[33] assessed the difference in nicotine and cotinine exposure from smoking cigarettes or using nicotine patches in breastfeeding mothers. This study enrolled 15 women who smoked an average of 17 cigarettes a day into an 11-week smoking cessation program using nicotine patches (21 mg/d in weeks 1 to 6, 14 mg/d in weeks 7 and 8, 7 mg/d patch in weeks 9 and 10, weaning around week 11). This study found that the absolute infant dose (in nicotine equivalents) decreased by about 70% by the time the mother was using the 7-mg patch compared with the dose generated by smoking. In addition, the breast milk concentrations of nicotine and cotinine also decreased by 50% and 66%. The average nicotine equivalents for infants exposed via breast milk was 25.2 μg/kg/d for smoking, 23 μg/kg/d for the 21-mg patch, 15.8 μg/kg/d for the 14-mg patch, and 7.5 μg/kg/d for the 7-mg patch. Therefore, as the mother progresses through the patch strengths, the transfer of nicotine equivalents to the infant via breast milk is significantly decreased and the exposure to other toxins from cigarettes is eliminated.

It is not recommended that women smoke near their infants, in the home or before breastfeeding; therefore, should a mother who smokes wish to breastfeed, it would be suitable to recommend nicotine replacement therapy to help her quit while continuing to breastfeed.

Caffeine is a naturally occurring CNS stimulant present in many foods and drinks. The half-life in adults is 4.9 hours, but the half-life in neonates is as high as 97.5 hours. The half-life decreases with age to 14 hours at 3 to 5 months and 2.6 hours at 6 months and older. The average cup of coffee contains 100 to 150 mg of caffeine depending on preparation and country of origin.

Peak levels of caffeine are found in breast milk 60 to 120 minutes after ingestion. In a study of 5 patients after ingestion of 150 mg of caffeine, peak concentrations of caffeine in serum ranged from 2.39 to 4.05 μg/mL and peak concentrations in milk ranged from 1.4 to 2.41 mg/L, with a milk/serum ratio of 0.52.[34] The average concentration of caffeine in milk at 30, 60, and 120 minutes after ingestion was 1.58, 1.49, and 0.926 mg/L, respectively. Another study included 7 breastfeeding mothers who consumed 750 mg of caffeine per day for 5 days, and were 11 to 22 days postpartum. The average concentration of caffeine in the milk was 4.3 mg/L,[35] and the mean concentration of caffeine in the serum of the infants on day 5 was 1.4 μg/mL.

The occasional use of coffee or tea is not contraindicated, but persistent chronic use of caffeine may lead to high plasma levels of caffeine in the infant, particularly during the neonatal period.

PAIN/ANALGESIA

Analgesics are one of the most commonly used medications while breastfeeding. Options for pain control include acetaminophen, nonsteroidal antiinflammatory drugs (NSAIDs), and opioids. Most NSAIDs are used to reduce pain and inflammation and are generally a suitable choice in breastfeeding women. Ibuprofen, acetaminophen, and naproxen are probably the most commonly used analgesics in North America. Their RID in milk ranges from 0.65% for ibuprofen,[36] 8.81% for acetaminophen,[37] to 3.3% for naproxen.[38]

Opioids are often used for acute pain after cesarean delivery or for other procedures in breastfeeding mothers. Morphine is generally the preferred opioid used in breastfeeding mothers because of its poor oral bioavailability (26%) in the infant and low RID of 9.1%.[39] Hydrocodone is a suitable alternative, its active metabolite is hydromorphone, and its RID ranges from 0.2% to 9% (average 2.4%).[40] There have been 2 reports of adverse events with infants exposed to hydrocodone via breast milk.[41,42] In the first case, both mother and infant were sedated after the mother took 2 hydrocodone 10 mg/acetaminophen 650 mg tablets every 4 hours for mastitis. Once the dose was reduced to 1 tablet every 3 hours, the sedation resolved.[41] The second infant required intubation after exposure to a combination of opioids his mother had taken for a migraine (hydrocodone and methadone).[42]

The use of codeine has started to decline since the death of an infant whose mother was taking codeine while breastfeeding in 2005.[43] Both codeine and oxycodone are less favorable opioids because their metabolism is unpredictable (CYP 2D6 enzyme) producing active metabolites and data showing CNS depression in infants.[44] In a cohort of mothers using oxycodone, codeine, and acetaminophen for pain during lactation, infant sedation was reported in 20.1%, 16.7%, and 0.5% for each drug, respectively.[44] All opioids should be used with caution in breastfeeding mothers, using low doses and short courses, avoiding combinations with other opioids, monitoring the mother and child continuously for sedation/side effects, and constantly reevaluating the need for the opioid. Although methadone is not given as a pain medication and a full discussion of methadone is beyond the scope of this review, maternal use of methadone is not a contraindication to breastfeeding.

When possible, treating the cause of the underlying pain and using acetaminophen/NSAIDs are recommended.

HYPERTENSION

Several medications are used to treat hypertension, including diuretics, β-adrenergic blockers, calcium channel blockers, angiotensin-converting enzyme inhibitors

(ACEIs), and angiotensin receptor blockers (ARBs). Many of these medications are suitable during breastfeeding; however, some in the β-blocker family are known to cause problems for breastfed infants. The β-blockers of choice are metoprolol (RID 1.4%) and propranolol (RID 0.3%); neither medication has been associated with any adverse events in infants.[45,46] In addition, labetalol has not been associated with any adverse effects in infants and has a low RID of 0.6%.[47] Although rare, atenolol and acebutolol have both been associated with adverse effects in infants, such as cyanosis, tachypnea, bradycardia, hypotension, and low body temperature, and are not preferred agents.[48,49] There is presently no information about the transfer of carvedilol or bisoprolol into breast milk. In summary, monitoring the infant for hypotension, bradycardia, and lethargy is suggested when using β-blockers during lactation.

The most common calcium channel blockers are amlodipine, felodipine, nifedipine, verapamil, and diltiazem. Studies on nifedipine suggest a low RID of 2.3%, 1 hour after a 30-mg dose.[50] In a patient who took verapamil 80 mg 3 times a day, the average steady-state milk concentration of verapamil was 25.8 μg/L; no drug was found in the infant's plasma and the RID was estimated to be 0.15%.[51] There is 1 report of a patient who received diltiazem 60 mg 4 times a day; in this case, the RID was low (0.9%).[52] There have been no reports of adverse events in breastfed infants exposed to nifedipine, verapamil, or diltiazem.[50–52]

ACEIs are not only used for hypertension; they have numerous other indications such as heart failure, myocardial infarction, diabetes, kidney disease, and so forth. The 2 ACEIs with the most breastfeeding data are captopril and enalapril. In a study of 12 women who took captopril 100 mg 3 times a day, breast milk levels were about 4.7 μg/L 4 hours after the dose, the estimated RID was 0.002%, and no adverse effects were found.[53] In a study in which 5 mothers were given a single 20-mg dose of enalapril, the average maximum milk concentrations of enalapril and its active metabolite enalaprilat were 1.74 μg/L and 1.72 μg/L, respectively; the RID was estimated to be about 0.175%.[54] There are many ACEIs on the market, but captopril and enalapril are preferred until there are sufficient data available to confirm their safety in breastfed infants.

There are no data available on the use of ARBs in breastfeeding mothers. Until this information becomes available, ACEIs should be used instead of ARBs (candesartan, irbesartan, losartan, and so forth).

Diuretics are often used to help lower blood pressure and decrease edema. There are no published data on the amount of furosemide that enters breast milk. There is 1 case report of a woman who received hydrochlorothiazide 50 mg daily.[55] On day 28, the mean milk concentration of hydrochlorothiazide was 80 ng/mL, resulting in a total infant daily dose of 0.05 mg of hydrochlorothiazide.[55] Plasma levels of hydrochlorothiazide in this infant were undetectable and no adverse events were reported.[55]

Despite suggestions in the past that diuretics may suppress milk production,[56] no further details of this study or other studies have been published that confirm this controversy; at this time, there is no substantial evidence to suggest that diuretics reduce milk volume and or that diuretics are contraindicated in breastfeeding.

LIVER/GASTROINTESTINAL TRACT

The use of histamine-2 (H2) antagonists and proton pump inhibitors (PPIs) for gastroesophageal reflux disease (GERD) and nausea/vomiting in pregnancy is increasing. Famotidine is a preferred H2 antagonist. In a study of 8 women who were given famotidine 40 mg/d, the RID was estimated to be the lowest of the H2 antagonists at

1.9%.[57] Although ranitidine has a high milk/plasma ratio, it is also a preferred agent because the amount of ranitidine that enters breast milk is low; the RID ranges between 1.3% and 4.6% and the total daily infant dose is about 0.4 mg/kg/d.[58] Cimetidine has a high milk/plasma ratio and RID between 9.8% and 32.6%, with a total daily infant dose of about 5.58 mg/kg/d. Although this dose is lower than the pediatric therapeutic dose, the other 2 drugs are more suitable than cimetidine during breastfeeding.[57] The use of PPIs poses little risk to the infant because all of the current PPIs are unstable at low pH and thus little is absorbed by the infant orally. In addition, the RIDs of these medications are low, demonstrating minimal drug transfer into breast milk (omeprazole RID 1.1%, pantoprazole RID 0.95%).[59,60]

NAUSEA

The 3 medications that are considered most suitable for short-term treatment of nausea and vomiting during lactation are dimenhydrinate (see section on psychiatric conditions for more information), ondansetron, and metoclopramide. Although the milk levels of ondansetron are unknown, it is a preferred agent because it is commonly used during pregnancy and in young infants without any major reports of safety concerns.[61,62] Metoclopramide is an alternative for short-term use (due to maternal side effects) with a low RID of 4.7%.

INFECTIOUS DISEASE

Most antibiotics, such as penicillins and cephalosporins, have been well studied and are compatible with breastfeeding because of poor entry into breast milk (**Table 3**).[63] Although side effects are uncommon, those reported in infants exposed to antibiotics in breast milk are usually selflimiting, such as diarrhea and rash.[64] Two classes of antibiotics that have known complications in children and are generally perceived by clinicians and patients as contraindicated in breastfeeding mothers, are tetracyclines and fluoroquinolones.[65–67] Tetracyclines cause permanent dental staining that is dose and time dependent and reduced bone growth in children following deposition of the drug in the epiphyseal plate.[68] Although patients and some clinicians perceive doxycycline and tetracycline to be contraindicated, their short-term use (<3 weeks) is considered suitable in breastfeeding mothers as the transfer of these medications into milk is low.[65,69] Tetracycline enters milk poorly because it binds with calcium in breast milk and cannot be absorbed (absolute infant dose 0.17 mg/kg/d, RID 0.6%).[69] Absorption of doxycycline is delayed but more complete and it too has a low RID of 4.2% (absolute infant dose 0.12 mg/kg/d).[65]

Although fluoroquinolones have caused arthrotoxicity (blisters, fissures, and erosions in cartilage) in animal studies using beagle dogs aged 13 to 16 weeks and have been associated with reversible musculoskeletal adverse effects in children and adults, there have been few reports of arthropathy in human infants; therefore, these medications are generally not contraindicated in breastfeeding mothers.[66,70] Although metronidazole has been associated with mutagenicity and carcinogenicity in rodents, this risk has remained theoretic and has not been reported in humans.[71] Topical and vaginal forms are suitable in breastfeeding mothers because systemic absorption is limited.[71] The use of oral metronidazole produces a relatively high RID of 9% to 13% when 1200 mg/d is taken by the mother. No adverse effects have been reported other than a metallic taste to the milk, which may not be palatable to some infants.[72] If larger single doses of metronidazole are used (2 g), then breastfeeding should be delayed for 12 to 24 hours to reduce the infant's exposure to this medication.[73]

Table 3
Antibiotics and reported levels in breast milk

Antibiotics	RID (%)	Comments
Penicillins		
Amoxicillin	1[63]	Compatible: The penicillins are a class of medication that minimally transfer into human milk. They have been used for years in lactating mothers and no serious adverse events have been reported in infants
Ampicillin	0.3[103]	
Ampicillin + sulbactam	0.5[104]	
		There is no specific information about the quantity of clavulanate that enters breast milk[64]
Aminoglycosides		
Gentamicin	2.1[105]	Compatible: Gentamicin produced measurable blood levels (0.41 μg/mL) in 5 of 10 infants in a study in which women were given gentamicin 80 mg intramuscularly every 8 h.[105] The expected intake for an infant was negligible at 307 μg/d.[105] Oral absorption is believed to be low (<1%) except in premature neonates, however, this study showed that oral absorption did occur in half of their population of full-term infants[105]
Tobramycin	0–2.6[106,107]	
Cephalosporins		
Cefazolin	0.8[108]	Compatible: The cephalosporins are also suitable during lactation as they have low RIDs and no major adverse effects in infants have been reported after many years of use. In a case report in which cephalothin and then cephalexin + probenecid were administered to the mother, the infant had green liquid stools; this resolved without dehydration when the infant was supplemented (15% of intake) with goats milk[109]
Cephalexin	0.5[109]	
Cefuroxime	0.6[110]	
Ceftriaxone	4.1[111]	
Cefotaxime	0.3[112]	
Ceftazidime	0.9[113]	
Carbapenems		
Meropenem	0.18[114]	Compatible: Currently there is little information about the use of carbapenems in breastfeeding mothers. One published case report found the average and maximum concentrations of meropenem in milk were 0.48 μg/mL and 0.64 μg/mL, respectively; this gave an estimated infant daily dose of 97 μg/kg/d[114]

HEMATOLOGY

The use of antiplatelet and anticoagulant medications is increasing in women for prevention of cardiovascular disease, treatment of venous thrombosis during pregnancy, prevention of procedure-related thrombosis, and numerous other indications (**Table 4**). Older studies of aspirin are poor and were done using relatively high doses as opposed to the doses of 81 to 325 mg used today. In the older studies and using

Table 4
Hematologic medications and reported levels in breast milk

Coagulation Medications	RID (%)	Comments
Aspirin	10.8[115]	Compatible: Use of low-dose aspirin 81 mg is probably safe; however, little information is known about the relationship between the dose and risk of Reye syndrome in infants. Watch for thrombocytopenia and petechiae in infants[115]
Warfarin		Compatible: In a study of 13 mothers, none of them had detectable levels in breast milk and no adverse events were reported in breastfed infants[116]
Heparin		Compatible: Large molecular weight 12,000–15,000 Da; unlikely to enter breast milk and most likely destroyed in the infant's gastrointestinal tract[117]
Dalteparin sodium (low molecular weight heparin)		Compatible: In a study of 15 patients at a mean of 5.7 d after cesarean delivery, dalteparin levels in breast milk were <0.005–0.037 IU/mL. Oral absorption is unlikely and its levels in mature milk could be lower[118]
Clopidogrel		Probably compatible: To date there are no data on human breast milk. The plasma half-life is 6–8 h; its metabolite (thiol derivative) covalently bonds to platelet receptors with a half-life of 11 d. Because it produces an irreversible inhibition of platelet aggregation, any drug in milk could inhibit an infant's platelet function for a prolonged period. Based on the moderate molecular weight of 420 Da, low protein binding, and 50% oral bioavailability, this drug would not be the drug of choice while breastfeeding, but if required, should not be a contraindication[119]

a 1-g oral dose, the RID was reported as 9.4%.[74] Thus, the risk in using daily doses of 81 mg or even 325 mg is probably low. At present there are no data available on the use of clopidogrel, one of the most commonly used drugs in this field.

ENDOCRINE MEDICATIONS

The rate of diabetes is increasing and more mothers require insulin and oral hypoglycemics in pregnancy and throughout lactation. One of the first-line medications used for type 2 diabetes mellitus is metformin; this medication is part of the biguanide class of antidiabetic medications and has been studied in 5 lactating women and 3 infants.[75] The average peak and trough concentrations in breast milk for metformin were 0.42 µg/mL and 0.39 µg/mL, resulting in an RID of 0.65%.[75] In this study, 3 infants had their blood glucose monitored and no hypoglycemia occurred; therefore, metformin should be compatible with breastfeeding.[75]

Glyburide is a second-generation sulfonylurea and is one of the first-line therapies used for type 2 diabetes mellitus. In a study of 6 mothers given a single dose of glyburide 5 mg, and 2 mothers given a single dose of glyburide 10 mg, the drug was undetectable in breast milk at both doses (limit of detection 0.005 µg/mL).[76] In a group of 5 mothers who received daily doses of glyburide 5 mg or glipizide 5 mg, the same results were found; both medications were undetectable in breast milk.[76] In this study, the plasma glucose levels in the infants were normal, which would be expected if no medication had been consumed by the infant.

Insulin is used in the management of multiple endocrine diseases such as type 1 and type 2 diabetes mellitus, gestational diabetes, and diabetic ketoacidosis. Insulin is a large peptide molecule that is not believed to be secreted into human milk in clinically significant amounts; however, should it enter breast milk, no or very little absorption would occur because the infant's gastrointestinal tract would destroy it.[77] Thus, there is no contraindication with using insulin while breastfeeding.

CONTRACEPTIVES

It is hypothesized that the withdrawal of progesterone in the early postpartum period initiates lactogenesis.[78] Consequently, it has been suggested that if a mother begins progesterone or combined oral contraceptives (COCs) early postpartum (the first few days), it may interrupt the establishment of lactation.[78]

A recently published, double-blind, randomized trial compared the effect of initiating progesterone-only contraceptives (0.35 mg norethindrone) with COCs (0.035 mg ethinyl estradiol + 1 mg norethindrone) at 2 weeks postpartum.[79] This study found that there was no difference in continuation of breastfeeding between the 2 groups at 8 weeks (64.1% combined pills vs 63.5% progestin only) or 6 months.[79] In both groups, women who supplemented their infants with formula or had concerns about inadequate milk supply were more likely to stop breastfeeding.[79] There was no comparison of discontinuation rates of breastfeeding with a placebo group, so it is unknown if progesterone itself increased the rate of discontinuation, and only the mother's perception of changes in milk volume was analyzed, not actual volume measurements.[79]

Although this new study is interesting, an older study of 330 women who used non-hormonal contraceptives (NHC), COCs, and copper intrauterine devices (Cu IUD) found more infants were weaned at 6 and 8 months in the oral contraceptive group (16.3% COC, 9% NHC, 4.7% Cu IUD at 6 months).[80] However, by the end of 1 year, an equivalent number of women (about 40%) in each of the 3 groups were no longer breastfeeding.[80]

Therefore, any hormonal product, estrogen or progestin, may suppress lactation at any time (early postpartum or after establishment). NHCs should always be discussed with breastfeeding mothers as an alternative and the potential risk of a hormonal contraceptive should be understood before choosing such a product. If mothers prefer to use hormonal contraception, they should be advised to avoid contraceptive products for at least the first 4 weeks postpartum to allow the establishment of lactation and avoid increasing their risk of thrombosis during this period.[78,79,81]

DRUGS THAT STIMULATE MILK PRODUCTION

During gestation, prolactin levels can be as high as 400 ng/mL. After delivery and in the first 6 months postpartum, maternal prolactin levels decrease steadily to approximately 75 ng/mL at 6 months, even though milk production is unchanged.[82] In many mothers who are unable to produce an adequate supply of breast milk, prolactin levels are believed to have decreased to inadequate levels (<75 ng/mL). Therefore, in some cases, milk production may be restored with the use of dopamine antagonists (galactagogues), which stimulate the release of prolactin.

The 2 most common dopamine antagonists used for this purpose are metoclopramide (Reglan) and domperidone (Motilium). Metoclopramide is prescribed most frequently in the United States because domperidone is not approved by the US Food and Drug Administration (FDA). Prolactin release as stimulated by metoclopramide is clearly dose related. Ten to fifteen milligrams administered 3 times daily has been demonstrated to be most beneficial.[83] The dose of metoclopramide present in human milk is small: 6 to 24 μg/kg/d for children studied in the early postpartum period and 1 to 13 μg/kg/d for those studied after 8 to 12 weeks postpartum.[84] Side effects of this medication are severe, and include depression, extrapyramidal symptoms, gastric cramping, and tardive dyskinesia. However, no side effects were reported in this study when mothers were given metoclopramide 10 mg 3 times a day for a limited duration.[84]

Domperidone (Motilium) is another dopamine antagonist used to stimulate prolactin levels. It is only available in the United States via compounding pharmacies, because it has never been approved for use in the United States. Although the FDA has issued a black box warning, domperidone still remains the primary galactagogue used around the world.

A study of domperidone used a dose of 10 mg 3 times a day for 7 days in mothers of premature infants, and found an increase in mean milk volume of 44.5%. Levels of domperidone in milk were low in this study (1.2 ng/mL), consequently the infant dose was also low (<0.2 μg/kg/d) and no adverse effects were reported in the infant.[85]

Because breast milk production is dependent on persistent and increased prolactin levels produced by the dopamine antagonist, a slow withdrawal of either domperidone or metoclopramide over several weeks to a month is suggested to prevent loss of milk supply.

Fenugreek is the most commonly used herbal product for increasing breast milk production. There are numerous studies with conflicting data. The most recent placebo-controlled study published as an abstract in 2011 suggested that fenugreek had no effect on either prolactin levels or volume of breast milk.[86] This study included 26 mothers of premature infants who took fenugreek 1725 mg 3 times a day for 3 weeks. Although no adverse effects were noted in the study, herbal products are not controlled by the FDA so the quality and consistency of the product chosen would be unknown and may put the mother and/or infant at risk of unknown adverse effects. Fenugreek is not recommended to improve breast milk production.

SUMMARY

The number of new medications that are available to breastfeeding mothers requiring drug therapy is expanding daily. This makes it difficult for clinicians to assess the safety of medications in breast milk; however, knowing how to assess the key factors that influence a medication's suitability while breastfeeding allows clinicians to make collaborative clinical decisions with their patients to encourage breastfeeding. In reality, women can breastfeed safely while ingesting most medications, but not all. Clinicians who are aware of this field are better able to care for breastfeeding mothers and support breastfeeding.

REFERENCES

1. Centers for Disease Control and Prevention. Breastfeeding Report Card-United States, 2012. Available at: http://www.cdc.gov/breastfeeding/pdf/2012Breast feedingReportCard.pdf.
2. Stultz EE, Stokes JL, Shaffer ML, et al. Extent of medication use in breastfeeding women. Breastfeed Med 2007;2(3):145–51.
3. Hale TW. Medication and mothers' milk. 15th edition. Amarillo (TX): Hale Publishing; 2012.
4. Hale TW, Hartmann PE. Textbook of human lactation. Amarillo (TX): Hale Publishing; 2007.
5. Bennett PN. Drugs and human lactation. Amsterdam: Elsevier; 1996.
6. Centers for Disease Control and Prevention (CDC). Prevalence of self-reported postpartum depressive symptoms–17 states, 2004-2005. MMWR Morb Mortal Wkly Rep 2008;57(14):361–6.
7. Stowe ZN, Hostetter AL, Owens MJ, et al. The pharmacokinetics of sertraline excretion into human breast milk: determinants of infant serum concentrations. J Clin Psychiatry 2003;64(1):73–80.
8. Hagg S, Granberg K, Carleborg L. Excretion of fluvoxamine into breast milk. Br J Clin Pharmacol 2000;49(3):286–8.
9. Ohman R, Hagg S, Carleborg L, et al. Excretion of paroxetine into breast milk. J Clin Psychiatry 1999;60(8):519–23.
10. Kristensen JH, Ilett KF, Hackett LP, et al. Distribution and excretion of fluoxetine and norfluoxetine in human milk. Br J Clin Pharmacol 1999;48(4):521–7.
11. Kelly LE, Poon S, Madadi P, et al. Neonatal benzodiazepines exposure during breastfeeding. J Pediatr 2012;161(3):448–51.
12. Kanto JH. Use of benzodiazepines during pregnancy, labour and lactation, with particular reference to pharmacokinetic considerations. Drugs 1982;23(5): 354–80.
13. Rindi V. La eliminazione degli antistaminici di sintesi con il latte e l'azione latto-goga de questi. Riv Ital Ginecol 1951;34:147–57 [in Italian].
14. Matheson I, Sande HA, Gaillot J. The excretion of zopiclone into breast milk. Br J Clin Pharmacol 1990;30(2):267–71.
15. Hill RC, McIvor RJ, Wojnar-Horton RE, et al. Risperidone distribution and excretion into human milk: case report and estimated infant exposure during breast-feeding. J Clin Psychopharmacol 2000;20(2):285–6.
16. Croke S, Buist A, Hackett LP, et al. Olanzapine excretion in human breast milk: estimation of infant exposure. Int J Neuropsychopharmacol 2002;5(3):243–7.
17. Rampono J, Kristensen JH, Ilett KF, et al. Quetiapine and breast feeding. Ann Pharmacother 2007;41:711–4.
18. Wiles DH, Orr MW, Kolakowska T. Chlorpromazine levels in plasma and milk of nursing mothers. Br J Clin Pharmacol 1978;5(3):272–3.
19. Hackett LP, Kristensen JH, Hale TW, et al. Methylphenidate and breast-feeding. Ann Pharmacother 2006;40(10):1890–1.
20. Ilett KF, Hackett LP, Kristensen JH, et al. Transfer of dexamphetamine into breast milk during treatment for attention deficit hyperactivity disorder. Br J Clin Pharmacol 2006;63(3):371–5.
21. von Unruh GE, Froescher W, Hoffmann F, et al. Valproic acid in breast milk: how much is really there? Ther Drug Monit 1984;6(3):272–6.
22. Tomson T, Ohman I, Vitols S. Lamotrigine in pregnancy and lactation: a case report. Epilepsia 1997;38(9):1039–41.

23. Newport DJ, Pennell PB, Calamaras MR, et al. Lamotrigine in breast milk and nursing infants: determination of exposure. Pediatrics 2008;122(1):e223–31.

24. Ohman I, Vitols S, Luef G, et al. Topiramate kinetics during delivery, lactation, and in the neonate: preliminary observations. Epilepsia 2002;43(10):1157–60.

25. Mennella JA, Beauchamp GK. The transfer of alcohol to human milk. Effects on flavor and the infant's behavior [see comments]. N Engl J Med 1991;325(14):981–5.

26. Mennella JA. Regulation of milk intake after exposure to alcohol in mothers' milk. Alcohol Clin Exp Res 2001;25(4):590–3.

27. Cobo E. Effect of different doses of ethanol on the milk-ejecting reflex in lactating women. Am J Obstet Gynecol 1973;115(6):817–21.

28. Ho E, Collantes A, Kapur BM, et al. Alcohol and breast feeding: calculation of time to zero level in milk. Biol Neonate 2001;80(3):219–22.

29. Perez-Reyes M, Wall ME. Presence of delta9-tetrahydrocannabinol in human milk [letter]. N Engl J Med 1982;307(13):819–20.

30. Tennes K, Avitable N, Blackard C, et al. Marijuana: prenatal and postnatal exposure in the human. NIDA Res Monogr 1985;59:48–60.

31. Astley SJ, Little RE. Maternal marijuana use during lactation and infant development at one year. Neurotoxicol Teratol 1990;12(2):161–8.

32. Jutras-Aswad D, DiNieri J, Harkany T, et al. Neurobiological consequences of maternal cannabis on human fetal development and its neuropsychiatric outcome. Eur Arch Psychiatry Clin Neurosci 2009;259:395–412.

33. Ilett KF, Hale TW, Page-Sharp M, et al. Use of nicotine patches in breast-feeding mothers: transfer of nicotine and cotinine into human milk. Clin Pharmacol Ther 2003;74(6):516–24.

34. Tyrala EE, Dodson WE. Caffeine secretion into breast milk. Arch Dis Child 1979;54(10):787–800.

35. Ryu JE. Caffeine in human milk and in serum of breast-fed infants. Dev Pharmacol Ther 1985;8(6):329–37.

36. Weibert RT, Townsend RJ, Kaiser DG, et al. Lack of ibuprofen secretion into human milk. Clin Pharm 1982;1(5):457–8.

37. Bitzen PO, Gustafsson B, Jostell KG, et al. Excretion of paracetamol in human breast milk. Eur J Clin Pharmacol 1981;20(2):123–5.

38. Jamali F, Stevens DR. Naproxen excretion in milk and its uptake by the infant. Drug Intell Clin Pharm 1983;17(12):910–1.

39. Feilberg VL, Rosenborg D, Broen CC, et al. Excretion of morphine in human breast milk. Acta Anaesthesiol Scand 1989;33(5):426–8.

40. Sauberan JB, Anderson PO, Lane JR, et al. Breast milk hydrocodone and hydromorphone levels in mothers using hydrocodone for postpartum pain. Obstet Gynecol 2011;117(3):611–7.

41. Bodley V, Powers D. Long-term treatment of a breastfeeding mother with fluconazole-resolved nipple pain caused by yeast: a case study. J Hum Lact 1997;13(4):307–11.

42. Meyer D, Tobias JD. Adverse effects following the inadvertent administration of opioids to infants and children. Clin Pediatr 2005;44:499–503.

43. Koren G, Cairns J, Chitayat D, et al. Pharmacogenetics of morphine poisoning in a breastfed neonate of a codeine-prescribed mother. Lancet 2006;368(9536):704.

44. Lam J, Kelly L, Ciszkowski C, et al. Central nervous system depression of neonates breastfed by mothers receiving oxycodone for postpartum analgesia. J Pediatr 2012;160:33–7.

45. Sandstrom B, Regardh CG. Metoprolol excretion into breast milk. Br J Clin Pharmacol 1980;9(5):518–9.
46. Taylor EA, Turner P. Anti-hypertensive therapy with propranolol during pregnancy and lactation. Postgrad Med J 1981;57:427–30.
47. Lunell NO, Kulas J, Rane A. Transfer of labetalol into amniotic fluid and breast milk in lactating women. Eur J Clin Pharmacol 1985;28(5):597–9.
48. Schimmel MS, Eidelman AI, Wilschanski MA, et al. Toxic effects of atenolol consumed during breast feeding. J Pediatr 1989;114:476–8.
49. Boutroy MJ, Bianchetti G, Dubruc C, et al. To nurse when receiving acebutolol: is it dangerous for the neonate? Eur J Clin Pharmacol 1986;30(6):737–9.
50. Ehrenkranz RA, Ackerman BA, Hulse JD. Nifedipine transfer into human milk. J Pediatr 1989;114(3):478–80.
51. Anderson P, Bondesson U, Mattiasson I, et al. Verapamil and norverapamil in plasma and breast milk during breast feeding. Eur J Clin Pharmacol 1987;31:625–7.
52. Okada M, Inoue H, Nakamura Y, et al. Excretion of diltiazem in human milk. N Engl J Med 1985;312(15):992–3.
53. Devlin RG. Selective resistance to the passage of captopril into human milk. Clin Pharmacol Ther 1980;27:250.
54. Redman CW, Kelly JG, Cooper WD. The excretion of enalapril and enalaprilat in human breast milk. Eur J Clin Pharmacol 1990;38(1):99.
55. Miller ME, Cohn RD, Burghart PH. Hydrochlorothiazide disposition in a mother and her breast-fed infant. J Pediatr 1982;101(5):789–91.
56. Healy M. Suppressing lactation with oral diuretics. Lancet 1961;277(1790):1353–4.
57. Courtney TP, Shaw RW. Excretion of famotidine in breast milk. Br J Clin Pharmacol 1988;26:639.
58. Kearns GL, McConnell RF Jr, Trang JM, et al. Appearance of ranitidine in breast milk following multiple dosing. Clin Pharm 1985;4(3):322–4.
59. Marshall JK, Thompson AB, Armstrong D. Omeprazole for refractory gastroesophageal reflux disease during pregnancy and lactation. Can J Gastroenterol 1998;12(3):225–7.
60. Plante L, Ferron GM, Unruh M, et al. Excretion of pantoprazole in human breast. J Reprod Med 2004;49(10):825–7.
61. Guikontes E, Spantideas A, Diakakis J. Ondansetron and hyperemesis gravidarum. Lancet 1992;340:1223.
62. Khalil SN, Roth AG, Cohen IT, et al. A double-blind comparison of intravenous ondansetron and placebo for preventing postoperative emesis in 1 to 24 month old pediatric patients after surgery under general anesthesia. Anesth Analg 2005;101:356–61.
63. Kafetzis DA, Siafas CA, Georgakopoulos PA, et al. Passage of cephalosporins and amoxicillin into the breast milk. Acta Paediatr Scand 1981;70(3):285–8.
64. Benyamini L, Merlob P, Stahl B, et al. The safety of amoxicillin/clavulanic acid and cefuroxime during lactation. Ther Drug Monit 2005;27:499–502.
65. Morganti G, Ceccarelli G, Ciaffi G. Comparative concentrations of a tetracycline antibiotic in serum and maternal milk. Antibiotica 1968;6(3):216–23 [Multiple languages].
66. Ghaffar F, McCracken GH, Hooper DC, et al. Quinolones in pediatrics. Quinolone antimicrobial agents. Washington, DC: ASM Press; 2003. p. 343–54.
67. Giamarellou H, Kolokythas E, Petrikkos G, et al. Pharmacokinetics of three newer quinolones in pregnant and lactating women. Am J Med 1989;87(5A):49S–51S.

68. Shetty AK. Tetracyclines in pediatrics revisited. Clin Pediatr 2002;41:203–9.

69. Posner AC, Prigot A, Konicoff NG. Further observations on the use of tetracycline hydrochloride in prophylaxis and treatment of obstetric infections. In: Welch H, Marti-Ibañez H, editors. Antibiotics annual 1954-1955. New York: Medical Encyclopedia; 1955.

70. von Keutz E, Ruhl-Fehlert C, Drommer W, et al. Effects of ciprofloxacin on joint cartilage in immature dogs immediately after dosing and after a 5-month treatment-free period. Arch Toxicol 2004;78:418–24.

71. Schwebke JR. Metronidazole: utilization in the obstetric and gynecologic patient. Sex Transm Dis 1995;22(6):370–6.

72. Passmore CM, McElnay JC, Rainey EA, et al. Metronidazole excretion in human milk and its effect on the suckling neonate. Br J Clin Pharmacol 1988;26(1): 45–51.

73. Erickson SH, Oppenheim GL, Smith GH. Metronidazole in breast milk. Obstet Gynecol 1981;57(1):48–50.

74. Putter J, Satravaha P, Stockhausen H. Quantitative analysis of the main metabolites of acetylsalicylic acid. Comparative analysis in the blood and milk of lactating women (author's transl). Z Geburtshilfe Perinatol 1974;178(2):135–8 [in German].

75. Briggs GG, Ambrose PJ, Nageotte MP, et al. Excretion of metformin into breast milk and the effect on nursing infants. Obstet Gynecol 2005;105(6):1437–41.

76. Feig DS, Briggs GG, Kraemer JM, et al. Transfer of glyburide and glipizide into breast milk. Diabetes Care 2005;28(8):1851–5.

77. Product monograph: human insulin Novolin®ge. Mississauga (Ontario): Novo Nordisk Canada Inc; 2011.

78. Kennedy KI, Short RV, Tully MR. Premature introduction of progestin-only contraceptive methods during lactation. Contraception 1997;55(6):347–50.

79. Espey E, Ogburn T, Leeman L, et al. Effect of progestin compared with combined oral contraceptive pills on lactation. Obstet Gynecol 2012;119(1): 5–13.

80. Croxatto HB, Diaz S, Peralta O, et al. Fertility regulation in nursing women: IV. Long-term influence of a low-dose combined oral contraceptive initiated at day 30 postpartum upon lactation and infant growth. Contraception 1983; 27(1):13–25.

81. Queenan J. Exploring contraceptive options for breastfeeding mothers. Obstet Gynecol 2012;119(1):1–2.

82. Cox DB, Owens RA, Hartmann PE. Blood and milk prolactin and the rate of milk synthesis in women. Exp Physiol 1996;81(6):1007–20.

83. Kauppila A, Kivinen S, Ylikorkala O. A dose response relation between improved lactation and metoclopramide. Lancet 1981;1(8231):1175–7.

84. Kauppila A, Arvela P, Koivisto M, et al. Metoclopramide and breast feeding: transfer into milk and the newborn. Eur J Clin Pharmacol 1983;25:819–23.

85. da Silva OP, Knoppert DC, Angelini MM, et al. Effect of domperidone on milk production in mothers of premature newborns: a randomized, double-blind, placebo-controlled trial. CMAJ 2001;164(1):17–21.

86. Reeder C, Legrand A, O'Conner-Von S. The effect of fenugreek on milk production and prolactin levels in mothers of premature infants [abstract]. J Hum Lact 2011;27:74.

87. Rampono J, Kristensen JH, Hackett LP, et al. Citalopram and demethylcitalopram in human milk; distribution, excretion and effects in breast fed infants. Br J Clin Pharmacol 2000;50(10):263–8.

88. Schmidt K, Olesen OV, Jensen PN. Citalopram and breast-feeding: serum concentration and side effects in the infant. Biol Psychiatry 2000;47(2):164–5.

89. Frannsen EJ. Citalopram serum and milk levels in mother and infant during lactation. Ther Drug Monit 2006;28(1):2–4.

90. Taddio A, Ito S, Koren G. Excretion of fluoxetine and its metabolite, norfluoxetine, in human breast milk. J Clin Pharmacol 1996;36(1):42–7.

91. Lester BM, Cucca J, Andreozzi L, et al. Possible association between fluoxetine hydrochloride and colic in an infant. J Am Acad Child Adolesc Psychiatry 1993; 32(6):1253–5.

92. Rampono J, Hackett LP, Kristensen JH, et al. Transfer of escitalopram and its metabolite demethylescitalopram into breastmilk. Br J Clin Pharmacol 2006; 62(3):316–22.

93. Newport DJ, Ritchie JC, Knight BT, et al. Venlafaxine in human breast milk and nursing infant plasma: determination of exposure. J Clin Psychiatry 2009;70(9): 1304–10.

94. Rampono J, Teoh S, Hackett LP, et al. Estimation of desvenlafaxine transfer into milk and infant exposure during its use in lactating women withpostnatal depression. Arch Womens Ment Health 2011;14(1):49–53.

95. Lobo ED, Loghin C, Knadler MP, et al. Pharmacokinetics of duloxetine in breast milk and plasma of healthy postpartum women. Clin Pharmacokinet 2008;47(2): 103–9.

96. Stahl MM, Neiderud J, Vinge E. Thrombocytopenic purpura and anemia in a breast-fed infant whose mother was treated with valproic acid. J Pediatr 1997;130:1001–3.

97. Meador KJ, Baker GA, Browning N, et al. Effects of breastfeeding in children of women taking antiepileptic drugs. Neurology 2010;75(22):1954–60.

98. Shimoyama R, Ohkubo T, Sugawara K. Monitoring of carbamazepine and carbamazepine 10,11-epoxide in breast milk and plasma by high-performance liquid chromatography. Ann Clin Biochem 2000;37(Pt 2):210–5.

99. Moretti ME, Koren G, Verjee Z, et al. Monitoring lithium in breast milk: an individualized approach for breast-feeding mothers. Ther Drug Monit 2003;25(3): 364–6.

100. Viguera AC, Newport DJ, Ritchie J, et al. Lithium in breast milk and nursing infants: clinical implications. Am J Psychiatry 2007;164(2):342–5.

101. Ohman I, Vitols S, Tomson T. Lamotrigine in pregnancy: pharmacokinetics during delivery, in the neonate, and during lactation. Epilepsia 2000;41(6):709–13.

102. Steen B, Rane A, Lonnerholm G, et al. Phenytoin excretion in human breast milk and plasma levels in nursed infants. Ther Drug Monit 1982;4(4):331–4.

103. Matsuda S. Transfer of antibiotics into maternal milk. Biol Res Pregnancy Perinatol 1984;5(2):57–60.

104. Foulds G, Miller RD, Knirsch AK, et al. Sulbactam kinetics and excretion into breast milk in postpartum women. Clin Pharmacol Ther 1985;38(6):692–6.

105. Celiloglu M, Celiker S, Guven H, et al. Gentamicin excretion and uptake from breast milk by nursing infants. Obstet Gynecol 1994;84(2):263–5.

106. Festini F, Ciuti R, Taccetti G, et al. Breast-feeding in a woman with cystic fibrosis undergoing antibiotic intravenous treatment. J Matern Fetal Neonatal Med 2006; 19(6):375–6.

107. Uwaydah M, Bibi S, Salman S. Therapeutic efficacy of tobramycin–a clinical and laboratory evaluation. J Antimicrob Chemother 1975;1(4):429–37.

108. Yoshioka H, Cho K, Takimoto M, et al. Transfer of cefazolin into human milk. J Pediatr 1979;94(1):151–2.

109. Ilett KF, Hackett LP, Ingle B, et al. Transfer of probenecid and cephalexin into breast milk. Ann Pharmacother 2006;40(5):986–9.
110. Takase Z, Shirofuji H, Uchida M. Fundamental and clinical studies of cefuroxime in the field of obstetrics and gynecology. Chemotherapy (Tokyo) 1979;27(Suppl 6): 600–2.
111. Bourget P, Quinquis-Desmaris V, Fernandez H. Ceftriaxone distribution and protein binding between maternal blood and milk postpartum. Ann Pharmacother 1993;27(3):294–7.
112. Kafetzis DA, Lazarides CV, Siafas CA, et al. Transfer of cefotaxime in human milk and from mother to foetus. J Antimicrob Chemother 1980;6(Suppl A):135–41.
113. Blanco JD, Jorgensen JH, Castaneda YS, et al. Ceftazidime levels in human breast milk. Antimicrob Agents Chemother 1983;23(3):479–80.
114. Sauberan J, Bradley J, Blumer J, et al. Transmission of meropenem in breast milk. Pediatr Infect Dis J 2012;31:832–4.
115. Bailey DN, Weibert RT, Naylor AJ, et al. A study of salicylate and caffeine excretion in the breast milk of two nursing mothers. J Anal Toxicol 1982;6:64–8.
116. Orme ML, Lewis PJ, De Swiet M, et al. May mothers given warfarin breast-feed their infants? Br Med J 1977;1(6076):1564–5.
117. McEvoy GE, editor. Heparin Sodium. AHFS Drug Information. Bethesda (MD): American Society of Health-System Pharmacists; 2012. Available at: http://www.medicinescomplete.com.
118. Richter C, Sitzmann J, Lang P, et al. Excretion of low molecular weight heparin in human milk. Br J Clin Pharmacol 2001;52(6):708–10.
119. Product monograph: Plavix. Clopidogrel tablets. Laval (Quebec): Sanofi-Aventis Canada Inc; 2012.

Circumstances when Breastfeeding is Contraindicated

Robert M. Lawrence, MD

KEYWORDS

- Breastfeeding • Breastmilk • Human milk • Contraindications • Infectious diseases
- Environmental contaminants • Chemicals • Heavy metals

KEY POINTS

- The infectious diseases in the mother that remain contraindications to breastfeeding, at this time, are HIV-1 and HIV-2 (in industrialized settings) and human T-cell lymphotropic virus I and II. Temporary interruption (either for an initial period of treatment in the mother or for the finite period equal to the duration of illness) of breastfeeding and provision of breast milk is appropriate for a few infections with potential serious consequences.
- In some infectious situations, preventive interventions are available for the infant (immune serum globulin, vaccination, or prophylactic antimicrobial medication) while continuing to provide breast milk to the infant. Yellow fever vaccine and smallpox vaccine are the only contraindicated vaccines during breastfeeding.
- Coordinated medical care and lactation assistance are essential for successful breastfeeding in the face of maternal illness. Restrictive diets or malnutrition in the mother are not contraindications to breastfeeding.
- The substance exposure should be accurately identified and assessed for the individual mother-infant dyad, and temporary cessation as a potential intervention to decrease the infant's toxic exposure should be discussed.
- When faced with the question of a possible contraindication to breastfeeding, a balanced assessment of the potential risks versus the probable, known benefits of breastfeeding must be completed and discussed with the mother and family.

INTRODUCTION

Universal and exclusive breastfeeding for the first 6 months of every infant's life remain the recommendation and stated goal for infant feeding by numerous national and international organizations including; World Health Organization (WHO), United Nations International Children's Emergency Fund, US Department of Health and Human Services, and the American Academy of Pediatrics (AAP). Human milk has

Pediatric Infectious Diseases, Department of Pediatrics, Health Science Center, University of Florida, 1600 Southwest Archer Road, ARB1-118, Box 100296, Gainesville, FL 32610-0296, USA
E-mail address: lawrerm@peds.ufl.edu

Pediatr Clin N Am 60 (2013) 295–318
http://dx.doi.org/10.1016/j.pcl.2012.09.012
0031-3955/13/$ – see front matter © 2013 Elsevier Inc. All rights reserved.
pediatric.theclinics.com

evolved as a unique nutritional substance that is specific and ideal for the optimal growth and development of human infants.[1–3] The numerous, important benefits of exclusive breastfeeding for the mother and infant have been well documented in evidence-based medicine literature[4–6] and in this issue. Any circumstance, situation, condition, or illness that interferes with exclusive breastfeeding is a threat to the infant's growth and development and the health of the mother-infant dyad. The question of contraindications to breastfeeding, relative or absolute, is a crucial topic for pediatricians in their role as knowledgeable advocates for breastfeeding.

There are few absolute contraindications to breastfeeding or the use of human milk for infant nutrition. Among the relative contraindications there are numerous circumstances or situations that constitute theoretical or potential risks to the infant or mother-infant dyad. A balanced discussion of the potential risks versus the probable, known benefits of breastfeeding must be considered. That discussion should include the scientific, evidence-based data on the potential risks; the specific facts of the situation for the mother-infant dyad; and the cultural and personal conceptions, beliefs, and preferences of the mother and family. In certain situations, it may also be appropriate to discuss the risks of not breastfeeding for the mother and infant.[7] Additionally, a distinction should be made whether the potential risk or contraindication exists in the act of breastfeeding (eg, pulmonary tuberculosis in the mother and the potential for respiratory transmission of tuberculosis during the close contact of breastfeeding) or in the substance of the mother's breast milk (eg, medication that is potentially toxic to an infant in the mother's milk).

This article summarizes the potential contraindications to breastfeeding with a focus on infectious diseases and exposure to environmental contaminants. Potential contraindications to breastfeeding due to restrictive diets or malnutrition in the mother by Valentine and colleagues and medication and drug use by the mother are discussed by Hale and colleagues elsewhere in this issue.

CIRCUMSTANCES

Circumstances that pose potential contraindications are highly varied and include infectious diseases in the mother or infant, other medical conditions in the mother or in the infant (particularly metabolic diseases in the infant that necessitate special changes in the infant's diet), environmental contaminants in the milk due to maternal exposure, and medications or drugs in the milk due to maternal use (prescribed or not prescribed) of those substances (**Box 1**).

Infectious Diseases

Most infectious diseases occurring in the mother are not contraindications for breastfeeding (**Tables 1** and **2**). In most cases, by the time the diagnosis is made in the mother, the infant has already been exposed through contact with the mother or others in the household. There is extensive evidence that breastfeeding protects infants against many common infections, including upper respiratory or lower respiratory tract infection, otitis media, respiratory syncytial virus bronchiolitis, and gastroenteritis.[5,6,8–11] To interrupt or stop breastfeeding in this scenario would only deprive the infant of potentially beneficial antibodies (secretory IgA), and antiinflammatory or immunomodulating substances contained in human milk.[12–16]

In general, other mechanisms of transmission (blood or body fluids, contact, droplet, or airborne) are the more common risk for transmission of infection between a mother and her infant. In rare situations, temporary separation of the mother and infant (related to the risk of transmission via another mechanism) can be considered

Box 1
Selected conditions for which the question of contraindication to breastfeeding is frequently raised

Infectious diseases

    Human immunodeficiency virus

    Human T-cell lymphotropic virus I and II

    Hepatitis: A, B, C, E

    Measles

    Cytomegalovirus

    Herpes simplex virus

    Varicella-zoster virus

    Human papilloma virus

    Syphilis

    Lyme disease

    Tuberculosis

    Brucellosis

    Candida infection

    West Nile virus

    Influenza

    Localized infection of the breast: mastitis, breast abscess

    Staphylococcus aureus

    Streptococcus (Group A or B)

    Vaccinations in the lactating mother

Medical conditions in the infant

    Galactosemia

    Phenylketonuria

    Inborn errors of metabolism

    Lactose intolerance

    Milk protein allergy

    Hyperbilirubinemia (breastfeeding jaundice, breast milk jaundice)

Medical conditions in the mother

    Wilson disease

    Galactosemia

    Phenylketonuria

    Cystic fibrosis

    Cancer

    Rheumatologic disorders and/or inflammatory bowel disease

    Obesity and/or gastric bypass surgery

    Polycystic ovarian disorder

    Renal failure and/or dialysis

Diabetes

Hyperlipidemia

Restrictive diet or malnutrition in the mother (see discussion elsewhere in this issue on nutrition management by Valentine and colleagues)

Caloric restriction

Protein deficiency

Vitamin A, C, D, or B6 deficiency

Nutrients: Calcium, iron, zinc

Exposure to environmental contaminants

Herbicides

Insecticides

Heavy metals

Radionuclides

Medications and drug use (see discussion elsewhere in this issue for a complete list and discussion by Hale and colleagues)

along with maintaining the milk supply and providing the infant with expressed breast milk (eg, active pulmonary tuberculosis, pertussis). There are a few rare and serious infections in the mother in which breast milk should temporarily not be provided to the infant until the mother is clinically well (eg, Ebola and Marburg hemorrhagic fevers). In other serious invasive infections (bacteremia, meningitis, osteomyelitis, septic arthritis) due to specific organisms (*Brucellosis*, Group B *Streptococcus, Staphylococcus aureus, Haemophilus influenza b, Streptococcus pneumonia* or *Neisseria meningitidis*), temporary suspension of breastfeeding from an infected mother should occur until an initial period (usually 24–96 hours) of treatment of the mother has occurred and there is evidence of some clinical improvement. Mastitis and breast abscesses are not considered invasive infections (see later discussion). In other rare situations in which specific infections involve the mother's nipple or breast (eg, herpes simplex virus, tuberculosis), if the milk cannot be expressed and/or collected without contamination it should not be given to the infant until the mother is treated and the lesions resolved.[17] The infectious agents are not in the breast milk unless contaminated at the time of expression. In some situations, prophylactic or empiric therapy for the infant against the identified organism can be considered and, once instituted, breastfeeding can continue (eg, azithromycin for pertussis, varicella immune globulin or acyclovir for varicella, immune serum globulin and vaccine for hepatitis A, rabies immune globulin and rabies vaccine for maternal rabies, isoniazid for pulmonary tuberculosis).[18–22] The only real infectious contraindications to breastfeeding are human T-cell lymphotropic viruses (HTLV) I and II, and HIV-1 and HIV-2, in resource-rich regions.[6,23] The WHO continues to recommend exclusive breastfeeding for at least 6 months for HIV-positive mothers in resource-poor regions, and combining complementary feeds and continued breastfeeding through the first 12 months of life, for improved overall survival, child growth and development, and greater HIV-free survival. In situations when the mother is too ill to breastfeed or severely immune suppressed, she should be encouraged to consider alternative feeding when that choice of feeding is affordable, feasible, accessible, sustainable and safe (AFASS criteria).[23–27] Breastfeeding in resource-poor settings offers a significant mortality and morbidity benefit regardless of whether or not the infant becomes HIV infected

Table 1
Summary of selected bacterial infections and concern as a contraindication to breastfeeding

Problem or Infection	Mode of Transmission	Breastfeeding	Use of Expressed Breast Milk	Preventive Interventions	Special Conditions
Staphylococcus	Contact	TI 24–48 h of Rx	OK after 24–48 h of Rx	Prophylactic antibiotics	Severe MI, toxin-mediated disease
Streptococcus Group B	Contact	TI 24–48 h of Rx	OK after 24–48 h of Rx	Prophylactic antibiotics	Severe, invasive MI, recurrent infections
Brucellosis	Milk, contact	TI 48–96 h of Rx	OK after 48–96 h of Rx	None	Severe MI
Listeria	Contact, perinatal	OK	OK	None	Severe MI
Meningococcus	Respiratory droplets	TI 24 h of Rx	OK	Prophylactic antibiotics	Severe MI
Pertussis	Respiratory droplet	TI 5 d of Rx	OK	Prophylactic antibiotics, vaccine	—
Latent TB infection	None	OK	OK	None	Maternal Rx with INH, B6
Active Pulmonary TB	Respiratory, Airborne	TI for 7–14 d, or until infant on INH	OK	INH for the infant, subsequent testing and f/u	Insure adherence to therapy by mother
TB Mastitis	Contact	TI for Rx	TI until lesions resolved, Cx negative	INH for the infant	Insure adherence, f/u
Syphilis	Sexual, secretions, contact with skin lesions	TI for 24 h of Rx	OK after 24 h of Rx If a nipple or breast lesion, no BM until healed	Empiric or prophylactic Rx for the infant	Isolation and Rx for the infant if congenital infection and/or rhagades, f/u
Lyme disease, *Borrelia burdorferi*	Tick borne, rarely other modes	TI for 24–48 h of initial Rx of mother	OK after initial Rx of mother	None	Informed discussion

Abbreviations: B6, vitamin B6; BM, breast milk; Cx, culture; f/u, follow-up, including testing of the infant; INH, isoniazid; MI, maternal illness; Rx, therapy; TB, tuberculosis; TI, temporary interruption.

Table 2
Summary of selected viral infections and concern as a contraindication to breastfeeding

Problem or Infection	Mode of Transmission	Breastfeeding	Use of Expressed Breast Milk	Preventive Interventions	Special Conditions
Acute hemorrhagic fevers (Ebola virus, Lassa fever)	Contact, body fluids, blood	No for DI	No for DI	None	Separation and isolation
Cytomegalovirus	Body fluids	OK, caution in premature infants	OK, caution in premature infants Freeze-thaw or pasteurize milk	None	Extremely premature or VLBW infants
HAV	Fecal-oral, food, water	OK after intervention	OK after intervention	SIG or HAV vaccination	—
HBV	Blood, body fluids, vertical	OK after intervention	OK after intervention	HBIG, and HBV vaccination	Standard protocol for HBV surface Ag + mothers
Hepatitis C	Blood, IVDU	OK	OK	None	Informed discussion
HSV	Perinatal, contact	OK, except if a lesion involves the nipple or breast	No, if a lesion involves the nipple or areola and contamination of expressed BM is unavoidable	Systemic and topical Rx for mother, cover any lesions	Can consider prophylactic Rx for the infant
HHV 6 and 7	Oral secretions	OK	OK	None	—
Parvovirus	Oral secretions vertical	OK	OK	None	—

HTLV I and II	Blood, sexual contact, BM	No	No	None	Avoid BF when alternate infant feeding is AFASS
HIV-1	Blood, sexual, perinatal, vertical, BM	Yes in resource-poor settings No in resource-rich settings	Yes in resource-poor settings No in resource-rich settings	Exclusive BF, antiretroviral Rx or prophylaxis for the mother and/or the infant	When avoiding BF alternate infant feeding should be AFASS
HIV-2	Blood, sexual, perinatal, vertical, BM	Yes in resource-poor settings No in resource-rich settings	Yes in resource-poor settings No in resource-rich settings	None	When avoiding BF alternate infant feeding should be AFASS
Smallpox	Contact, airborne	No	No	None	Avoid contact with lesions
Vaccinia virus (smallpox vaccine)	Contact, airborne	OK if local lesion can be covered	No, if a lesion involves the nipple or areola and contamination of expressed BM is unavoidable	—	Do not vaccinate pregnant women
West Nile virus	Mosquito, blood	Yes	Yes	—	Severe maternal illness can interfere with BF
VZV	Contact, Airborne	No, until lesions are crusting and dried	Yes, if no lesions on the breast	VariZIG, acyclovir	5 d before delivery up to 2 d after[a]

Abbreviations: AFASS, acceptable, feasible, affordable, safe, sustainable; Ag +, antigen positive; BF, breastfeeding; BM, breast milk; DI, duration of illness; HAV, Hepatitis A virus; HBIG, Hepatitis B immune globulin; HBV, Hepatitis B virus; HHV, human herpesvirus; HIV, human immunodeficiency virus; HTLV, human T-cell lymphotrophic virus; HSV, herpes simplex virus; IVDU, intravenous drug use; Rx, therapy; SIG, immune serum globulin; VLBW, very low birth weight; VZV, varicella zoster virus.

a American Academy of Pediatrics. Varicella-Zoster Infections. In: Pickering LK, Baker CJ, Kimberlin DW, et al, editors. Red Book: 2012 Report of the Committee on infectious diseases. Elk Grove Village (IL): American Academy of Pediatrics; 2012. p. 774–89.

because of the significant risk in many settings for other infections and malnutrition in the absence of breastfeeding. Exclusive breastfeeding reduces the risk of transmission of HIV from the mother to the infant compared with mixed feeding. Breastfeeding does not adversely affect the HIV-infected mother's health.[23] Now, there are possible situations in which ongoing breastfeeding by an HIV-1–infected mother while the mother, infant, or both receive effective antiretroviral medication regimens throughout the breastfeeding period can improve HIV-free survival of the infant.[23,28,29] There are multiple prospective studies demonstrating the proof of this concept. The true efficacy of such an approach and an optimal regimen for prevention in various situations and/or locations has not been studied in well-controlled prospective trials. The WHO does state that continued breastfeeding with antiretroviral therapy for the mother or prophylaxis for the mother or infant is a strategy that, in certain situations, can offer the child the greatest chance of HIV-free survival.[23] The American Academy of Pediatrics has not changed the recommendations for the United States; breastfeeding by an HIV-infected mother is proscribed.[6] In Great Britain, the British HIV Association has commented that, in very rare instances, breastfeeding by an HIV-positive mother can be considered with effective antiretroviral treatment of the mother, infant, or both.[30] There are limited data concerning the risk of transmission of HIV-2 via breastfeeding. Breastfeeding by mothers with confirmed HIV-2 infection should currently follow the guidelines for HIV-1 in the mother's locale.

HTLV-1 and HTLV-2, which cause leukemia or lymphoma and chronic neurologic disorders, are associated with significant transmission through breastfeeding because both are present in human milk, associated with a longer duration of breastfeeding, and demonstrate an increased risk of transmission in breastfed infants in comparison with formula-fed infants. There are no immunologic or pharmacologic interventions currently available to prevent HTLV I and II infections; however, a shorter duration of breastfeeding, freezing and thawing breast milk, and complete avoidance of breast milk have shown decreased transmission to the infant.[31–33] For each of these retroviruses (HIV-1, HIV-2, and HTLV I and II), avoidance of breastfeeding is one form of prevention that still requires that the use of a formula or alternative feeding meets AFASS criteria, whether the circumstances are in a resource-rich or resource-poor country.

Transmission of *Brucella* from human to human is exceedingly rare and there are only a handful of cases that describe breastfeeding or breast milk as a possible source of infection for the infant. *Brucella* is readily identified in animal milks but has been cultured from human milk in only one reported case. Other, more likely, routes of transmission include direct contact with infected animals or their unpasteurized milk or milk products. Other uncommon routes of infection include intrauterine infection, exposure during delivery, blood transfusion, bone marrow transplantation, and sexual contact.[34] Documented *Brucella* infection in a mother is a situation in which temporary suspension of breastfeeding should occur. Breast milk should not be given to the infant until at least 72 to 96 hours of maternal treatment of *Brucella* with evidence of clinical improvement. Then the use of breast milk can be resumed or breastfeeding continued if the mother is able.[35,36]

Although invasive *Candida* infection occurs in premature, low-birth weight or very-low birth weight infants, mild mucocutaneous infection is the most common form of this infection in infants. Several aspects of mammary candidosis or candidiasis remain areas in need of further study including; how to make the clinical diagnosis, the significance of associated pain, and the presence or absence of *Candida albicans* isolated from human milk of symptomatic and asymptomatic women. *Candida* does survive to a large extent in frozen-thawed breast milk. The direct contact during breastfeeding of the infant-mother dyad is the probable source of ongoing recolonization and reinfection. Simultaneous treatment of the dyad should occur when one or both of the pair are symptomatic. Treatment of mucocutaneous candidiasis and mammary candidiasis can begin with topical agents, including nystatin, clotrimazole, miconazole, econazole, terconazole, ciclopirox, or gentian violet solution. Various other topical preparations (mupirocin, grapefruit seed extract, or mixtures of mupirocin, betamethasone, and miconazole) have been recommended for the mother's breast without available clinical trials for efficacy and toxicity. Systemic therapy is sometimes necessary, and oral fluconazole is the most commonly used preparation because of its favorable side-effect profile. Other antifungal agents can be considered if systemic or invasive disease is present in the infant or mother because of other predisposing factors. Risk factors predisposing for candidal infections in the mother or infant should be addressed (eg, eliminating antibiotic use as soon as possible). Breastfeeding can continue without cessation in the full-term infant with the professional assistance of someone knowledgeable in the management of breastfeeding.

Local infections of the breast, mastitis or breast abscess, are not contraindications to continued breastfeeding. Antimicrobial therapy should be chosen with consideration of the most common organisms (penicillin-resistant *Staphylococcus aureus*, *Streptococcus*, *Escherichia coli*) and agents that are compatible with breastfeeding.[37] In most instances the infecting organism has not been identified unless a culture has been done. Possible factors predisposing to mastitis or milk stasis should be addressed and effective milk-removal strategies encouraged along with more frequent breastfeeding. Pumping and discarding the milk for a short period while optimizing continued effective milk removal has been recommended for invasive Group B *Streptococcus* infection in the mother or infant.[38] In most scenarios, appropriate empiric therapy has already been initiated for 1 to 2 days before culture results are available and no temporary interruption of breastfeeding or breast milk is indicated. As long as drainage from the abscess does not directly contact the infant's mouth, continued breastfeeding from the affected breast is appropriate.

It is infrequently useful to culture breast milk to guide decision-making about ongoing therapy and breastfeeding. If there is an initial failure of empiric therapy (after 48–96 hours of therapy) for mastitis, frequent recurrences of mastitis despite apparently appropriate therapy, or pain out of proportion to the clinical findings, then culturing the breast milk (collected as a "midstream collection" after gently cleaning the nipple and areola) may provide culture and sensitivity information to alter subsequent antimicrobial therapy. Material obtained from a discrete abscess that has been drained should always be cultured. Culturing breast milk may also be appropriate in outbreak or epidemiologic investigations.

Immunization of the mothers with common live virus vaccines (eg, varicella vaccine; measles, mumps, and rubella vaccine) is not a contraindication to initiating or continuing breastfeeding. Yellow fever vaccine and smallpox vaccine should not be given to breastfeeding mothers, although it is acceptable (if truly necessary) to give Japanese encephalitis vaccine, typhoid live vaccine, and rabies vaccine. The use of the inactivated influenza vaccine should be encouraged for breastfeeding mothers. Refer to the Centers for Disease Control and Prevention Web site for additional information.[39]

Medical Conditions in the Infant

Galactosemia is a rare disorder, identified by neonatal screening in most states, which is caused by deficiency of galactose 1-phosphate uridyltransferase (GALT) enzyme (**Table 3**). There are several genetic variants of the disease due to mutations in the GALT gene. "Classic" galactosemia is the most severe, necessitating strict

Table 3
Medical conditions in the infant and concerns regarding breastfeeding or human milk

Condition	BF or BM	Supplement with Animal Milk or Special Formula	Comments
Alpha-1 antitrypsin deficiency	OK	Not necessary	Potential benefit from BM
Adrenal hyperplasia	OK	Not necessary	—
Amino acid inborn errors of metabolism (methionine, leucine, isoleucine, tyrosine)	OK in combination with a special formula or feeding	Formula or feeding without the amino acid for needed protein and calories	Monitoring of infant is important: calories, nutrients, growth and amino acid levels
Cow's milk protein allergy	OK in most instances	Uncommonly need a formula without cow's milk protein	Elimination diet for the mother
Cystic fibrosis	OK	Usually not necessary, can use a hydrolyzed formula	Can give infant pancreatic enzymes
Galactosemia, classic	No	No lactose-containing foods	Close monitoring
Galactosemia, variants	OK, combined with some lactose-free formula	Supplement with lactose-free formula for needed extra calories	Close monitoring is crucial, gal-1-p levels, medical specialists involved
Hypothyroidism	OK	Not necessary	—
Hyperbilirubinemia, BF or BM jaundice	OK	BF jaundice—optimize BF, BM jaundice—rarely requires temporary interruption of BF	See text and references
Lactose intolerance	OK	BF—benefit in temporary lactase deficiency with gastroenteritis in infant	Rarely—truly a problem vs changes to lactose-free formula due to worry or fear
Ornithine transcarbamylase deficiency	OK with supplementation	Supplementation with a nonprotein source of calories	Close monitoring of ammonia levels and growth
Phenylketonuria	OK with supplementation	Use BM in combination with a phenylalanine-free formula to provide adequate calories and nutrients	Close monitoring, measure phenylalanine levels

Abbreviations: BF, breastfeeding; BM, breast milk; vs, versus; gal-1-p, galactose-1-phosphate.

diets without any lactose, whereas other variants (with the Duarte allele, D1, or D2) have milder disease with reduced enzyme activity and can be managed with a less restrictive diet. It may be appropriate in the first 14 days of life to avoid any lactose-containing milk or formula (pumping and saving breast milk for possible later use) until the exact genetic diagnosis can be made. When possible, in situations with only reduced GALT enzyme activity, a modified diet can balance the use of breast milk and a non–lactose containing formula can maintain blood galactose-1-phosphate (gal-1-p) levels less than 3 to 4 mg/100 mL. These infants should be managed by a geneticist and a genetic nutritionist, along with someone knowledgeable in breastfeeding.

Phenylketonuria is another genetic error of metabolism necessitating a modified diet with limited amounts of phenylalanine for optimal growth and development of the infant. Human milk contains small amounts of phenylalanine and tyrosine. The use of a phenylalanine-free formula can be combined with breast milk in a regimen to provide adequate nutrients and calories as well as essential manageable amounts of phenylalanine. Detailed approaches to management of breastfeeding in the infant with phenylketonuria have been described by Clark[40] and Ernest and colleagues.[41] Mothers who have phenylketonuria can breastfeed their infants and provide caloric and nutrient-appropriate milk for the infant.

Other inborn errors of metabolism involving amino acids can be managed with breastfeeding and careful monitoring of the blood and urine levels of the specific amino acid accumulating based on the specific enzyme defect (eg, methionine, leucine, isoleucine, and tyrosine). A regimen combining breast milk and another milk or formula without the specific amino acid can be developed in conjunction with a geneticist and/or endocrinologist. Careful monitoring of growth, diet, caloric and nutrient intake, and amino acid levels is essential. Ornithine transcarbamylase deficiency, one of several urea cycle disorders, results in severe illness due to the accumulation of ammonia. Infants can be breastfed combined with a nonprotein caloric supplement. Alpha1-antitrypsin deficiency has more than 24 genetic variants and children with this deficiency are at increased risk for progressive liver disease, sometimes presenting in infancy. Breastfeeding a child with alpha1-antitrypsin deficiency can be beneficial and potentially reduce the risk of subsequent liver disease.[42] Cystic fibrosis is another condition often identified in infancy for which breastfeeding is appropriate. The addition of pancreatic enzymes or hydrolyzed formula to the infant's diet may be appropriate for certain infants to optimize growth and development.

Neither hypothyroidism nor adrenal hyperplasia is a contraindication to breastfeeding. Congenital hypothyroidism can be diagnosed by neonatal screening. Breast milk does contain T4 and T3 and may delay the diagnosis or mask the presentation of hypothyroidism.[43,44] Neonatal lupus, another rare condition manifesting in infancy, is not a contraindication to breastfeeding.[45,46]

Jaundice and hyperbilirubinemia are not contraindications to breastfeeding (see elsewhere in this issue for additional discussion by Chantry and colleagues). The management of hyperbilirubinemia is completely reviewed in the AAP guidelines.[47,48] Specific guidelines for the management of jaundice in the breastfeeding infant are detailed in the Academy of Breastfeeding Medicine Clinical Protocol #22 on hyperbilirubinemia in infants equal to or greater than 35 weeks gestational age.[49] Optimization of breastfeeding technique, maintenance of the maternal milk supply and support are recommended during the management of hyperbilirubinemia in any infant. Uncommonly, supplementation with a hydrolyzed protein formula may be initiated to decrease intestinal absorption of bilirubin and, rarely, temporary interruption of breastfeeding for 24 to 48 hours is appropriate as treatment options in cases with very high bilirubin levels.[49]

Cow's milk protein allergy can occur when a breastfeeding infant is transitioned from breast milk to formula or whole cow's milk or other animal milk-based products. Human milk contains some foreign proteins in small amounts, so some children may react while exclusively breastfeeding and cow's milk protein allergy should be considered when the infant has symptoms suggestive of cow's milk protein allergy. Reinstitution or continuation of breastfeeding in the former situation is appropriate and, in the latter situation, the strict elimination of cow's milk protein from the diet of the mother can be attempted with expected disappearance of symptoms in the infant. If the infant's symptoms do resolve, cow's milk protein can be slowly replaced in the mother's diet, to a degree still tolerated by the breastfeeding infant. It has also been recommended, in severe cases of allergic proctocolitis, that the mother be given pancreatic enzymes that, theoretically, break down potential protein allergens in the mother's intestine.[50] Occasionally, supplementation with a formula that contains no cow's milk protein is necessary. Calcium intake or supplements are essential for the mother on any cow's milk protein elimination diet.[51,52] Lactose intolerance is not a contraindication to breastfeeding.

Lactose intolerance is a clinical syndrome characterized by abdominal pain, diarrhea, nausea, flatulence, and/or bloating after ingestion of lactose containing foods.[53] It is very rare in infants except as a transient, secondary lactase deficiency due to intestinal mucosal injury as might occur with acute gastroenteritis or persistent diarrhea. Congenital lactase deficiency is the extremely rare condition of complete lactase deficiency. Developmental lactase deficiency is the relative lactase deficiency that occurs in premature infants, usually less than 34-weeks gestation. As children get older, often at 3 to 5 years of age, they can develop intolerance of lactose. Symptoms that are consistent with lactose intolerance do need evaluation in infants, especially if the infant is failing to thrive. This does not require an immediate switch from breast milk to a lactose free formula.

Medical Conditions in the Mother

There are no medical conditions (the condition itself) in the mother that are absolute contraindications to breastfeeding (**Table 4**). The most common issues related to a mother's medical condition that can be relative contraindications, or simply interferences, to breastfeeding include: (1) the severity of maternal illness, (2) exposure to radionuclides for diagnostic purposes (eg, fibrinogen leg scan using iodine-125 for detecting deep vein thrombosis requires discarding the mother's milk for approximately 2 weeks until the radioactive material is out of the milk), or (3) medications used to treat the condition that are not compatible with breastfeeding (eg, tamoxifen as an antiestrogen, anticancer medication) or not amenable to continued breastfeeding with intermittent discarding of breast milk containing the proscribed agent (eg, antineoplastic agent such as vincristine that would require discarding mother's milk for 35 days). Some maternal conditions or illness may make the mother too sick to breastfeed (eg, adult respiratory distress syndrome requiring intubation, renal failure with or without dialysis, systemic lupus erythematosus with central nervous system vasculitis, or encephalitis). Mothers on dialysis produce caloric and nutrient appropriate milk for the infant without an accumulation of urea nitrogen or creatinine in their breast milk. Other conditions may hinder or interfere with the initiation (eg, cesarean section delivery or toxemia) or maintenance of adequate milk production (eg, polycystic ovary syndrome) for the nutritional needs of the growing infant. A review and meta-analysis of breastfeeding after cesarean section reported that early

Table 4
Selected medical conditions in the mother that can affect breastfeeding but are not contraindications

Condition	Additional Benefit of BF for the Mother or Infant	Can Interfere with BF	Diagnostic Testing a Concern	Medications a Concern	Comments
Cesarean Delivery	Yes—oxytocin and uterine involution	Yes	No	Yes	—
Toxemia	Yes, oxytocin, prolactin	Yes—severe maternal illness	No	Yes—sedation, anti-hypertensives	—
Retention of placenta, lactation failure	Yes	Yes	No	No	BF improves after surgical removal
Venous thrombosis, pulmonary embolus	—	Yes—severe maternal illness	No, angiography, MRI are OK	No, heparin, low-molecular weight heparin, warfarin	Important to diagnose and treat
Mastitis, abscess	Yes, effective removal of milk	Temporarily	No	No, alternatives are commonly available	Treat engorgement, pain and infection
Sheehan syndrome and hypopituitarism	—	Yes	No	Yes, bromocriptine	Nasal oxytocin spray plus lactation supplement
Diabetes mellitus	Yes, weight loss, decreased insulin requirement	Yes, prematurity, respiratory distress, hypoglycemia, poor feeding, hyperbilirubinemia in the infant	No	No	Adjust diet, monitor insulin and glucose, early education plus support
Thyroid disease	—	Yes	Careful test selection	Careful choices of medications	Coordinated care for successful BF
Polycystic Ovarian Syndrome	—	Yes, insufficient milk supply	No	No	Coordinated care for successful BF
CF	Yes	Yes, if severely underweight or sick	No	No	Plan with CF physicians during pregnancy

(continued on next page)

Table 4
(continued)

Condition	Additional Benefit of BF for the Mother or Infant	Can Interfere with BF	Diagnostic Testing a Concern	Medications a Concern	Comments
Celiac disease	Yes	No	No	No	Mother needs additional vitamins and nutrients for herself
Galactosemia	Yes	No	No	No	Calcium and Vitamin D for the mother
Phenylketonuria	Yes	No	No	No	Infant may need a source of phenylalanine
Connective tissue disorders	—	Yes, Sjögren syndrome, Raynaud phenomenon of the nipple	No	Yes—dose, timing, drug interactions	Coordinated care for successful BF
Cardiovascular disease	—	Severe MI	No	Yes—choice of medications	—
Solid organ transplant	—	Severe MI	No	Yes	Coordinated care for successful BF
Glomerular disease and hypertension	—	Severe MI	No	Yes	Coordinated care for successful BF
Osteoporosis	—	No	Bone density scan OK	No	Maternal therapy appropriate, Vitamins D for infant (400 IU)
Inflammatory bowel disease	—	No	No	No	Maternal nutrition is important
Epilepsy	—	Plus uncontrolled seizures	No	Sometimes	Monitor medication levels in mother
Breast Cancer	—	Yes, surgery, radiation	No	Yes	Depending on stage of treatment, BF can be done

Fibrocystic breast disease	—	Yes	No	No	—
Gigantomastia	—	Yes, medication or surgery	No	Yes, bromocriptine	Surgery—reduction mammoplasty
Augmentation Mammoplasty	—	Yes, if minimal functional breast tissue	No	No	—
Reduction mammoplasty	—	Yes—if interruption of nerves or ductal structures	No	No	Options of different procedures, consider BF preoperatively
Multiple sclerosis	Yes, decreased risk of postpartum relapses	Yes, severity of illness	No	No	—
Postpartum Depression	—	Yes, early termination of BF	No	Yes, medication choices	Early diagnosis crucial, combined therapy

Abbreviations: BF, breastfeeding; CF, cystic fibrosis; MI, maternal illness; MRI, magnetic resonance imaging.

breastfeeding (initiation or breastfeeding at discharge) was significantly lower after cesarean section compared with vaginal delivery. In a separate analysis of mothers who initiated breastfeeding, cesarean delivery had no significant effect on breastfeeding at 6 months of age.[54]

Restrictive Diets in the Mother

Exclusive human milk is the preferred food source for human infants for the first 6 months of age. Breastfeeding is recommended in usual circumstances, even when the maternal diet may be poor or restricted. In 1991, the Subcommittee on Nutrition During Lactation of the Committee on Nutritional Status During Pregnancy and Lactation of the Food and Nutrition Board of the Institute of Medicine at the National Academy of Science noted in their report that there is a large body of evidence demonstrating that women are able to "produce milk of sufficient quantity and quality to support the growth and promote the health of infants—even when the mother's supply of nutrients is limited."[55] A poor or restrictive maternal diet is not a contraindication to breastfeeding. Nevertheless, women on such diets should be counseled concerning possible nutritional deficiencies caused by such diets and the potential effect on their milk.[56] Nutritional needs during lactation and restrictive diets are discussed in more detail elsewhere in this issue by Valentine and colleagues.

Exposure to Environmental Contaminants

The possibility of environmental contamination of human milk by chemicals exists; however, most individuals are not at significantly increased risk of exposure (**Table 5**). Specific exposures, in the workplace (to chemicals or heavy metals), in the food chain in a geographic area (eg, polybrominated biphenyls in bovine milk and meat products in Michigan in the 1970s or high levels of mercury in the fish food supply in Japan),[57] or during a specific period of time (eg, the herbicide Agent Orange exposure during the Vietnam War) are rare events. When the mother is exposed, the greatest risk to the infant is during pregnancy as a fetus, compared with the relatively smaller exposure during breastfeeding.

Pesticide and herbicide use in the United States has decreased dramatically since the 1970s, but the most common ongoing source of exposure is through working with or eating fish caught in sport fishing in contaminated waters. Pesticide and herbicide exposure continues to be a significant problem in many other parts of the world. Nevertheless, the WHO has stated that, despite the possible contamination of breast milk with dioxins and other herbicides and pesticides, the benefits of breastfeeding outweigh the potential risk to the infant and has recommended breastfeeding except in specific situations of high-level acute exposures.[58] This recommendation is supported by the recommendations of a technical workshop on Human Milk Surveillance and Biomonitoring for Environmental Chemicals in the United States and recommendations from experts.[59,60]

Many herbicides and pesticides are deposited in the fat stores in the body. The concern with breast milk is that they will enter the fat component of the milk. Chlorinated hydrocarbons (polychlorinated biphenyls, including DDT and its metabolites, dieldrin and aldrin) are the most familiar to the public. Although these and related products have been identified in breast milk, in most cases these levels are lower than what is found in cow's milk.[61,62] See **Table 5** for consideration of selected compounds.

Specific heavy metals that have been identified in human milk include lead, arsenic, mercury, and cadmium. Whenever a significant maternal exposure occurs, leading to a documented, elevated level of the compound in the mother, the breastfed infant and/or the human milk should be tested. In the case of lead, a level of 40 mg/dL or less

Table 5
Environmental contaminants and breast milk

Class	Agent	Sources	BF and BM are OK	Comments
Herbicides	Dioxin	Contaminated water, food supply	Yes	WHO statement says OK
	Furans	Contaminated water	Yes	—
Pesticides	DDT, DDE	Contaminated water, animals, food supply	Yes	Lower levels in human milk than in cow's milk
	PCBs, PBBs	Contaminated water, animals, food supply, waste disposal, "spills"	Yes	Very low levels in milk
	Cyclodiene pesticides	—	Yes	Rare exposures
Heavy Metals	Arsenic	Water, water supply	Yes	Little arsenic in breast milk
	Cadmium	Contaminated shellfish, industrial exposures, smokers	Yes	—
	Lead	Lead-based paints, lead pipes, water supply, industrial pollutants	Yes, when mother's blood level is <40 mg/dL (little or no lead in BM)	Pregnancy is the greater risk, check family members, increase calcium and iron in diet
	Mercury	Seafood, "spills," herbs and tonics	Yes	See text

Abbreviations: BM, breast milk; DDE, dichlorodiphenyldichloroethane; DDT, dichlorodiphenyltrichloroethane; PBBs, polybrominated biphenyls; PCBs, polychlorinated biphenyls.

measured in the mother's blood is reported to be less than the level of transfer into the breast milk; therefore, testing of the breast milk is unnecessary.[63] Lead remains a significant concern throughout the world. Common sources are old paint, contaminated ground water, gasoline, lead batteries, and even herbs and herbal teas (exported from China). In addition to testing for lead, once found, identifying the source and performing adequate lead abatement is the next step. Mothers and infants should receive extra iron and calcium in their diets to diminish absorption from the intestine and mobilization from bone. Arsenic is commonly found contaminating bodies of water and water supplies from industrial sources. In several arsenic-contaminated areas, high levels of arsenic were detected in some of the women but low levels were detected in the breastfeeding babies, suggesting little arsenic is excreted in breast milk and that breastfeeding is appropriate.[64] Mercury is being detected in food around the world, especially in fish, herbs, and tonics. In the Faroe and Seychelles Islands, there are two studies reporting on the good growth and health of breastfed infants chronically exposed to high levels of methylmercury in breast milk.[65,66] Breastfeeding is acceptable in the face of methylmercury exposure, although acute industrial or environmental exposures should be investigated carefully and decision-making should be analyzed relative to the individual's and the mother-infant dyad's health situation. Cadmium exposure usually occurs from industrial waste or eating large amounts of contaminated shellfish and is often worse in smokers (who seem to accumulate cadmium). The greatest risk of exposure is to the fetus during pregnancy. Breastfeeding is not contraindicated; however, significant or unusual exposures should be investigated and assessed.[67]

Volatile chemicals are most commonly found in paint shops, repair shops, garages, and industrial chemical workplaces. Protective gear, as recommended by the Occupational Safety and Health Administration and the Environmental Protection Agency, is crucial to minimizing the exposure to mothers and their infants. "Protective reassignment" of pregnant or breastfeeding employees is another appropriate option. Of the thousands of chemicals that humans can be exposed to, Fisher and colleagues[68] reported on 19 chemicals that they analyzed via a physiologically based pharmacokinetic model. The three chemicals they reported as the highest risk exposure for infants were bromochloromethane, perchloroethylene and 1,4-dioxane. There is a low relative risk to breastfed infants for 153 of 5736 substances (2.2%), which show evidence of transfer into human milk, as listed in the Toxicological Index of Quebec.[69] Selected databases that can be useful in assessing a specific chemical exposure in the mother include: Toxicological Index maintained by the Division of Occupational Health and Safety of the Nova Scotia Department of Labor and Workforce Development, found at www.gov.ns.ca/lwd/healthandsafety and LactMed in TOXNET, the Toxicology Data Network of the National institutes of Health, and Health and Human Services found at http://toxnet.nlm.nih.gov. Overall, there are inadequate data concerning exposure to volatile chemicals through breast milk.[68,70] The benefits of long-term breastfeeding probably outweigh the risks related to an acute short-term exposure; especially if the mother temporarily suspends breastfeeding immediately after the exposure and expresses and discards the milk (or saves it for subsequent testing of the milk for the identified chemicals). The period of temporary cessation of the use of human milk depends on the chemical involved and the type and period of exposure. Temporary cessation of breastfeeding and discarding the milk in situations of longer term exposures to lipophilic chemicals based on the concept that the concentration of the chemical in the milk will decrease over time has been called into question.[71] Each individual exposure situation should be assessed with the assistance of experts in chemistry, toxicology, maternal and infant health, and breastfeeding.

Phthalates, or "plasticizers," to soften plastic products are ubiquitous in our environment. They are commonly found in polyvinyl chloride, various other polymers, wiring insulation, automotive parts, personal care products, toys, and pharmaceuticals. Phthalate intake for formula-fed and exclusively breastfed infants, estimated from median values measured in breast milk and formula, are approximately equal and correlate with approximately 2% to 7% of the recommended tolerable daily intake. Potential exposure to phthalates and their metabolites through breast milk is not a contraindication to breastfeeding.[72]

Radionuclides are another class of potentially toxic substances that are most commonly encountered through contact with the health care system as part of a diagnostic evaluation or therapeutic intervention. These are described elsewhere in this issue by Valentine and colleagues. The American College of Radiology summarizes their review of the use of contrast media in breastfeeding mothers by stating that less than 1% of an administered maternal dose of contrast agent is excreted into the breast milk and less than 1% of the contrast media in breast milk ingested is absorbed from the gastrointestinal tract of the infant. They also note that, if the mother remains concerned about the potential exposure to the infant, temporary abstention from breastfeeding, actively expressing and discarding breast milk from both breasts for 24 hours after the procedure, and feeding the infant saved breast milk expressed before the radiologic study is appropriate.[73] Radionuclides associated with nuclear accidents, specifically strontium 90, are measured at lower levels in breast milk than in cow's milk, formula (produced in the area of the exposure), the water supply, and other portions of the food supply.[74] Breastfeeding is not contraindicated after exposure from nuclear accidents.

Medication and Drug Use

These are discussed elsewhere in this issue by Hale and colleagues and are not considered here.

SUMMARY

Concerns and questions about various health-related conditions or exposures and the potential risks to the breastfed infant will continue to be discussed and reevaluated. The infectious diseases in the mother that remain contraindications to breastfeeding at this time, are HIV-1, HIV-2 (in industrialized settings), and HTLV I and II. Temporary interruption (either for an initial period of treatment in the mother or for the finite period equal to the duration of illness) of breastfeeding and provision of breast milk is appropriate for a few infections with potential serious consequences. In some infectious situations, preventive interventions are available for the infant (immune serum globulin, vaccination, or prophylactic antimicrobial medication) while continuing to provide breast milk to the infant. Yellow fever vaccine and smallpox vaccine are the only contraindicated vaccines during breastfeeding. Classic galactosemia is the only medical condition in an infant that is a true contraindication to breastfeeding. For others conditions, breastfeeding remains an important component of infant nutrition. There are no medical conditions in the mother that, by themselves, are contraindications to breastfeeding; however, diagnostic procedures, treatment, or severe medical illness in the mother can interfere with breastfeeding. Coordinated medical care and lactation assistance are essential for successful breastfeeding in the face of maternal illness. Restrictive diets or malnutrition in the mother are not contraindications to breastfeeding. They are important opportunities to provide understandable nutritional counseling and guidelines to breastfeeding mothers. In the uncommon instance of a significant environmental toxic exposure within the United States, breastfeeding is not contraindicated. The substance exposure should be accurately identified and assessed for the individual mother-infant dyad, and temporary cessation as a potential intervention to decrease the infant's toxic exposure should be discussed. When faced with the question of a possible contraindication to breastfeeding, a balanced assessment of the potential risks versus the probable, known benefits of breastfeeding must be completed and discussed with the mother and family.

REFERENCES

1. WHO Multicentre Growth Reference Study Group. WHO child growth standards: length/height-for-age, weight-for-age, weight-for-length, weight-for-height and body mass index-for-age: technical report. Geneva (Switzerland): World Health Organization; 2006. p. 1–312. Available at: http://www.who.int/childgrowth/standards/technical_report/en/. Accessed August 1, 2012.
2. Butte NF, Lopez-Alarcon MG, Garza C. Nutrient adequacy of exclusive breastfeeding for the term infant during the first six months of life. Geneva (Switzerland): World Health Organization; 2002. Available at: http://whqlibdoc.who.int/publications/9241562110.pdf. Accessed August 29, 2012.
3. Goldman AS. Evolution of immune functions of the mammary gland and protection of the infant. Breastfeed Med 2012;7:132–42.
4. Ip S, Chung M, Raman G, et al. Breastfeeding and maternal and infant health outcomes in developed countries. Evid Rep Technol Assess (Full Rep) 2007; 153:1–186.
5. Ip S, Chung M, Raman G, et al. A summary of the Agency for Healthcare Research and Quality's evidence report on breastfeeding in developed countries. Breastfeed Med 2009;4(Suppl 1):S17–30.
6. AAP Section on Breastfeeding. Breastfeeding and the use of human milk. Pediatrics 2012;129:e827–41. Available at: http://pediatrics.aappublications.org/content/129/3/e827.full.html. Accessed August 20, 2012.
7. Steube A. The risks of not breastfeeding for mothers and infants. Rev Obstet Gynecol 2009;2:222–31.
8. Chantry CJ, Howard CR, Auinger P. Full breastfeeding duration and associated decrease in respiratory tract infection in US children. Pediatrics 2006;117: 425–32.
9. Dujits L, Jaddoe VW, Hoffman A, et al. Prolonged and exclusive breastfeeding reduces the risk of infectious diseases in infancy. Pediatrics 2010;126:e18–25. Available at: http://pediatrics.aappublications.org/content/126/1/e18.full.html. Accessed August 29, 2012.
10. Nishimura T, Suzue J, Kaji H. Breastfeeding reduces the severity of respiratory syncytial virus infection among young infants: a multi-center prospective study. Pediatr Int 2009;51:812–6.
11. Quigley MA, Kelly YJ, Sacker A. Breastfeeding and hospitalization for diarrheal and respiratory infection in the United Kingdom Millennium Cohort Study. Pediatrics 2007;119(4):e837–42. Available at: http://pediatrics.aappublications.org/content/119/4/e837.full. Accessed October 22, 2012.
12. Goldman AS. The immune system of human milk: antimicrobial, anti-inflammatory and immunomodulating properties. Pediatr Infect Dis J 1993;12:664–71.
13. Goldman AS. Modulation of the gastrointestinal tract of infants by human milk. Interfaces and interactions. An evolutionary perspective. J Nutr 2000;130(Suppl 2S): 426S–31S.

14. Goldman AS. Evolution of the immune functions of the mammary gland and protection of the infant. Pediatr Infect Dis J 2012;7:132–42.
15. Hanson LA, Silfverdal SA, Korotkova M, et al. Immune system modulation by human milk. Adv Exp Med Biol 2002;503:99–106.
16. Wheeler TT, Hodgkinson AJ, Prosser CG, et al. Immune components of colostrums and milk: a historical perspective. J Mammary Gland Biol Neoplasia 2007;12:237–47.
17. Lawrence RM. Transmission of infectious diseases through breast milk and breastfeeding. In: Lawrence RA, Lawrence RM, editors. Breastfeeding: a guide for the medical profession. 7th edition. Maryland Heights (MO): Elsevier Mosby; 2011. p. 406–73.
18. AAP Red Book Committee. Hepatitis A. In: Pickering LK, Baker CJ, Kimberlin DW, et al, editors. Red Book: 2012 Report of the Committee on the infectious diseases. 29th edition. Elk Grove Village (IL): American Academy of Pediatrics; 2012. p. 361–5.
19. AAP Red Book Committee. Pertussis. In: Pickering LK, Baker CJ, Kimberlin DW, et al, editors. Red Book: 2012 Report of the Committee on the infectious diseases. 29th edition. Elk Grove Village (IL): American Academy of Pediatrics; 2012. p. 553–66.
20. AAP Red Book Committee. Rabies. In: Pickering LK, Baker CJ, Kimberlin DW, et al, editors. Red Book: 2012 Report of the Committee on the infectious diseases. 29th edition. Elk Grove Village (IL): American Academy of Pediatrics; 2012. p. 600–7.
21. AAP Red Book Committee. Varicella. In: Pickering LK, Baker CJ, Kimberlin DW, et al, editors. Red Book: 2012 Report of the Committee on the infectious diseases. 29th edition. Elk Grove Village (IL): American Academy of Pediatrics; 2012. p. 774–89.
22. AAP Red Book Committee. Tuberculosis. In: Pickering LK, Baker CJ, Kimberlin DW, et al, editors. Red Book: 2012 Report of the Committee on the infectious diseases. 29th edition. Elk Grove Village (IL): American Academy of Pediatrics; 2012. p. 736–59.
23. World Health Organization. Guidelines on HIV and infant feeding. In: Maternal, newborn, child and adolescent health. 2010 Available at: http://www.who.int/maternal_child_adolescent/documents/9789241599535/en/. Accessed August 26, 2012.
24. Horvath T, Madi BC, Iuppa IM, et al. Interventions for preventing late postnatal mother-to-child transmission of HIV. Cochrane Database Syst Rev 2009;(1):CD006734. http://dx.doi.org/10.1002/14651858.CD006734.pub2.
25. Kindra G, Coutsoudis A, Esposito F, et al. Breastfeeding in HIV exposed infants significantly improves child health: a prospective study. Matern Child Health J 2012;16:632–40.
26. Becquet R, Bland R, Leroy V, et al. Duration, pattern of breastfeeding and postnatal transmission of HIV: pooled analysis of individual data from West and South African Cohorts. PLoS One 2009;4:e7397–415.
27. Coutsoudis A. Breastfeeding and HIV. Best Pract Res Clin Obstet Gynaecol 2005; 19:185–96.
28. Mofenson LM. Protecting the next generation—eliminating perinatal HIV-1 infection. N Engl J Med 2010;362:2316–8.
29. Morrison P, Israel-Ballard K, Greiner T. Informed choice in infant feeding decisions can be supported for HIV-infected women even in industrialized countries. AIDS 2011;25:1807–11.
30. Taylor GP, Anderson J, Clayden P, et al. British HIV Association and Children's HIV Association position statement on infant feeding in the UK 2011. HIV Med 2011; 12:389–93.

31. Hino S, Katamine S, Miyata H, et al. Primary prevention of HTLV-1 in Japan. Leukemia 1997;11(Suppl 3):57–9.
32. Ando Y, Kakimoto K, Tanigawa T, et al. Effect of freeze-thawing breast milk on vertical HTLV-I transmission from seropositive mothers to children. Jpn J Cancer Res 1989;80:405–7.
33. Ando Y, Saito K, Nakano S, et al. Bottle-feeding can prevent transmission of HTLV-I from mothers to their babies. J Infect 1989;19:25–9.
34. Palanduz A, Palanduz S, Guler K, et al. Brucellosis in a mother and her young infant: probable transmission by breast milk. Int J Infect Dis 2000;4:55–6.
35. Arroyo Carrera I, Lopez Rodriguez MJ, Sapina AM, et al. Probable transmission of brucellosis by breast milk. J Trop Pediatr 2006;52:380–1.
36. Tikare NV, Mantur BG, Bidari LH. Brucellar meningitis in an infant—evidence for human breast milk transmission. J Trop Pediatr 2008;54:272–4.
37. Academy of Breastfeeding Medicine Protocol Committee. ABM clinical protocol #4: mastitis. Breastfeed Med 2008;3:177–80.
38. Byrne PA, Miller C, Justus K. Neonatal group B streptococcal infection related to breast milk. Breastfeed Med 2006;1:263–70.
39. CDCP. Vaccinations. In: Breastfeeding: recommendations for vaccinations. 2012. Available at: http://www.cdc.gov/breastfeeding/recommendations/vaccinations.htm. Accessed August 27, 2012.
40. Clark BJ. After a positive Guthrie—what next? Dietary management for the child with phenylketonuria. Eur J Clin Nutr 1992;46(Suppl 1):S33–9.
41. Ernest AE, McCabe ER, Neifert MR, et al. Guide to breastfeeding the infant with PKU. DHHS Publication No. HAS 79-5110. Washington, DC: US Governement Printing Office; 1979.
42. Udall JN, Dixon M, Newman AP, et al. Liver disease in α1-antitrypsin deficiency. A retrospective analysis of the influence of early breast- vs bottle-feeding. JAMA 1985;253:2679–82.
43. Sack J, Anado O, Lunenfeld B. Thyroxine concentration in human milk. J Clin Endocrinol Metab 1977;45:171–3.
44. Varma SK, Collins M, Row A, et al. Thyroxine, tri-iodothyronine and reverse tri-iodothyronine concentrations in human milk. J Pediatr 1978;93:803–6.
45. Izmirly PM, Llanos C, Lee LA, et al. Cutaneous manifestations of neonatal lupus and risk of subsequent congenital heart block. Arthritis Rheum 2010;62:1153–7.
46. US DHHS Office on Women's Health. Lupus fact sheet. In: A–Z health topics. Available at: http://www.womenshealth.gov/publications/our-publications/fact-sheet/lupus.cfm. Accessed August 21, 2012.
47. American Academy Pediatrics Subcommittee of Hyperbilirubinemia. Management of hyperbilirubinemia in the newborn infant 35 or more weeks of gestation. Pediatrics 2004;114:297–316.
48. Maisels MJ, Bhutani VK, Bogen D, et al. Hyperbilirubinemia in the newborn infant >/= 35 weeks' gestation: an update with clarifications. Pediatrics 2009;124:1193–8.
49. Academy of Breastfeeding Medicine Protocol Committee. ABM clinical protocol #22: guidelines for management of jaundice in the breastfeeding infant equal to or greater than 35 weeks' gestation. Breastfeed Med 2010;5:87–93.
50. Academy of Breastfeeding Medicine Protocol Committee. ABM clinical protocol #24: allergic proctocolitis in the exclusively breastfed infant. Breastfeed Med 2011;6:35–40.
51. De Greef E, Hauser B, Devreker T, et al. Diagnosis and management of cow's milk protein allergy in infants. World J Pediatr 2012;8:19–24.

52. Dupont C, Chouraqui JP, de Boissieu D, et al. Dietary treatment of cow's milk protein allergy in childhood: a commentary by the Committee on Nutrition of the French Society of Paediatrics. Br J Nutr 2012;107:325–38.
53. Heyman MB, Committee on Nutrition. Lactose intolerance in infants, children, and adolescents. Pediatrics 2006;118:1279–86.
54. Prior E, Santhakumaran S, Gale C, et al. Breastfeeding after Cesarean delivery: a systematic review and meta-analysis of world literature. Am J Clin Nutr 2012; 95:1113–35.
55. Subcommittee on Nutrition During Lactation, Committee on Nutritional Status During Preganancy, Lactation of the Food and Nutrition Board of the Institute of Medicine, National Academy of Sciences. Summary, conclusions and recommendations. In: Nutrition during lactation. Washington, DC: National Academy Press; 1991. p. 1–19.
56. Thomas MR, Kawamoto J. Dietary evaluation of lactating women with or without vitamin and mineral supplementation. J Am Diet Assoc 1979;74:669–72.
57. Poland RL, Cohen SN. The contamination of the food chain in Michigan with PPB: the breastfeeding question. In: Liss AR, editor. Drugs and chemical risks to the fetus and newborn. New York: Alan R. Liss; 1980. p. 129–37.
58. World Health Organization. Consultation on assessment of the health risks of dioxins: re-evaluation of the Tolerable Daily Intake (TDI): executive summary. Food Addit Contam 2000;17:223–40.
59. Berlin CM, LaKind JS, Fenton SE, et al. Conclusions and recommendations off the expert panel: technical workshop on human milk surveillance and biomonitoring for environmental chemicals in the United States. J Toxicol Environ Health 2005; 68:1825–31.
60. LaKind JS, Berlin CM, Mattison DR. The heart of the matter on breastmilk and environmental chemicals: essential points for healthcare providers and new parents. Breastfeed Med 2008;3:251–9.
61. Lakind JS, Berlin CM. Technical workshop on human milk surveillance and research on environmental chemicals in the United States: an overview. J Toxicol Environ Health 2002;65:1829–37.
62. Rogan WJ, Gladen B. Monitoring breast milk contamination to detect hazards from waste disposal. Environ Health Perspect 1983;48:87–91.
63. Namihira D, Saldivar L, Pustilnik N, et al. Lead in human blood and milk from nursing women living near a smelter in Mexico City. J Toxicol Environ Health 1993;38:225–32.
64. Fangstrom B, Moore S, Nermell B, et al. Breastfeeding protects from arsenic exposure in Bangladeshi infants. Environ Health Perspect 2008;116:963–9.
65. Grandjean P, Wiehe P, White RF. Milestone development in infants exposed to methyl mercury from human milk. Neurotoxicology 1995;16:27–33.
66. Marsh DO, Clarkson TW, Meyers GJ, et al. Seychelles study of fetal methylmercury exposure and child development. Neurotoxicology 1995;16:583–96.
67. Rogan WI, Ragan NB. Chemical contaminants, pharmacokinetics and the lactating mother. Environ Health Perspect 1994;102(Suppl 11):89–95.
68. Fisher J, Mahle D, Bankston L, et al. Lactation transfer of volatile chemicals in breast milk. Am Ind Hyg Assoc J 1997;58:425–31.
69. Giroux D, Lapointe G, Baril M. Toxicological index and the presence in the workplace of chemical hazards for workers who breast-feed infants. Am Ind Hyg Assoc J 1992;53:471–4.
70. Lakind JS, Wilkins AA, Berlin CM. Environmental chemicals in human milk: a review of levels, infant exposures and health, and guidance for future research. Toxicol Appl Pharmacol 2004;198:184–208.

71. Lakind JS, Berlin CM, Sjodin A, et al. Do human milk concentrations of persistent organic chemicals really decline during lactation? Chemical concentrations during lactation and milk/serum partitioning. Environ Health Perspect 2009;117: 1625–31.
72. Fromme H, Gruber L, Seckin E, et al. Phthalates and their metabolites in breast milk—results from the Bavarian Monitoring of Breast Milk (BAMBI). Environ Int 2011;37:715–22.
73. American College of Radiology (ACR). Manuel on Contrast Media v8. In: Quality and safety of the ACR 2012. Available at: http://www.acr.org/Quality-Safety/Resources/Contrast-Manual. Accessed on August 27, 2012.
74. Gori G, Cama G, Guerresi E, et al. Radioactivity in breast milk and placenta after Chernobyl accident. Am J Obstet Gynecol 1988;158:1243–4.

Index

Note: Page numbers of article titles are in **boldface** type.

A

Academy of Breastfeeding Medicine, 6–7, 15, 20, **75–113**, 235
Acetaminophen, in breast milk, 282
Adiponectin, in breast milk, 57, 59
Adolescent mothers, breastfeeding support for, 179
Adrenal hyperplasia, breastfeeding in, 304–305
Advanced practice nurses, breastfeeding promotion by, 175
Alcohol, in breast milk, 279–280
Allergic proctocolitis, breastfeeding protocols for, 86, 108
Alpha-1 antitrypsin deficiency, breastfeeding in, 304–305
Amenorrhea, lactational, 43
American Academy of Pediatrics, breastfeeding support by, 1–2, 6–7, 115–116
Amniotic fluid, swallowing of, 190
Amoxicillin, in breast milk, 285
Ampicillin, in breast milk, 285
Analgesics and anesthetics, in breast milk, 82, 101, 282
Angiotensin receptor blockers, in breast milk, 283
Angiotensin-converting enzyme inhibitors, in breast milk, 282–283
Ankyloglossia, breastfeeding protocols for, 81, 99
Antibiotics, in breast milk, 284–285
Antibodies, in breast milk, 34–35, 60–61
Anticoagulants, in breast milk, 285–286
Antidepressants, in breast milk, 84, 103–104, 200, 277–278
Antiemetics, in breast milk, 284
Antiepileptic drugs, in breast milk, 279
Antihistamines, in breast milk, 278
Antihypertensives, in breast milk, 282–283
Antiplatelet agents, in breast milk, 285–286
Antipsychotics, in breast milk, 278–279
Anxiolytics, in breast milk, 278–279
Arsenic exposure, breastfeeding in, 310–312
Aspirin, in breast milk, 285–286
Asthma, in breastfed versus formula-fed infants, 37
Atopic allergies, in breastfed versus formula-fed infants, 37
Attitudes, toward breastfeeding, 33

B

Baby-Friendly Hospital Initiative, 33–34, 119–120, 154–160, 172–174, 180
Banks, milk. *See* Donor milk and donor milk banks.
Benzodiazepines, in breast milk, 278
Beta blockers, in breast milk, 282–283
Bile salt-stimulating lipase, in breast milk, 60–61

Pediatr Clin N Am 60 (2013) 319–334
http://dx.doi.org/10.1016/S0031-3955(12)00198-8
0031-3955/13/$ – see front matter © 2013 Elsevier Inc. All rights reserved.

pediatric.theclinics.com